Handbook of Pediatric Cardiovascular Drugs

Handbook of
Pediatric
Cardiovascular Drugs

Ricardo Munoz,

Carol G. Schmitt,

Stephen J. Roth, and

Eduardo da Cruz
(Eds.)

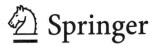 Springer

Ricardo Munoz, MD, FAAP, FCCM
Chief
Cardiac Intensive Care Division
Director
Cardiac Recovery Program
Associate Professor
Critical Care Medicine, Pediatrics
    and Surgery
Children's Hospital of Pittsburgh
    of UPMC
Pittsburgh, PA
USA

Stephen J. Roth, MD, MPH
James Baxter and Yvonne Craig Wood
    Director, Cardiovascular ICU
Lucile Packard Children's Hospital
    at Stanford
Associate Professor of Pediatrics
    (Cardiology)
Stanford University School of Medicine
Palo Alto, CA
USA

Carol G. Schmitt, PharmD
Clinical Pharmacy Specialist
Pediatric Critical Care
Clinical Instructor
School of Pharmacy
University of Pittsburgh
Children's Hospital of Pittsburgh of UPMC
Pittsburgh, PA
USA

Eduardo da Cruz, MD
Director of the Cardiac Intensive Care Unit
Associate Professor of Pediatrics
    (Pediatric Cardiology & Intensive Care)
The Heart Institute
Department of Pediatrics
The Children's Hospital of Denver
University of Colorado at Denver & Health
    Sciences Center
Denver, CO
USA (since the 1st of April 2007)
Senior Consultant & Lecturer
Pediatric Cardiology Unit
Service of Pediatric and Neonatal Intensive
    Care
Department of Pediatrics
Children's University Hospital of Geneva
Geneva, Switzerland (until 31st of
    March 2007)

British Library Cataloguing in Publication Data
Handbook of pediatric cardiovascular drugs
    1. Cardiovascular agents   2. Cardiovascular system - Diseases - Chemotherapy
    3. Pediatric cardiology
    I.   Munoz, Ricardo
    618.9'21061

ISBN: 978-1-84628-952-1   e-ISBN: 978-1-84628-953-9

Library of Congress Control Number: 2007928820

9 8 7 6 5 4 3 2 1

Springer Science + Business Media

springer.com

Foreword

The treatment of pediatric patients with congenital or acquired cardiac disease remains an important challenge for physicians in charge of these often precarious patients. It is well known that most of the drugs used in this field are either unlicensed or off-label. We have to face a very heterogeneous group of patients not only in pathologies but also in size, weight, and metabolism, particularly when we face problems in premature or newborns. Not only have very few studies offered evidenced-based data for our pediatric patients, but even simple pharmacokinetics data are lacking. This is, to a great extent, caused by the difficulties of conducting research in pediatrics, particularly large-scale double-blinded randomized and controlled studies. This may change in the close future as authorities throughout the world have clearly stated that they will support this type of study. However, for the time being, we must rely on the available pharmacological knowledge, on the rare clinical trials and case series, and, most of all, on the international cumulative clinical experience.

This comprehensive handbook on pediatric cardiovascular drugs offers a wide source of useful information for specialists in different fields, such as pediatricians, pediatric cardiologists, intensivists, neonatologists, anesthesiologists, cardiac surgeons, nurses, and others involved in the management of cardiovascular disorders. It presents the updated knowledge and experience regarding the use of the currently available therapies for pediatric patients with primary or secondary cardiac and circulatory disorders. All authors are recognized as worldwide experts in their field. This book will be an important tool for professionals in charge of these patients, instrumental in choosing the most appropriate drugs and the most appropriate dosages with minimal side effects. It may also lead to underlining the need of formal pharmacokinetics and adequate studies for our very special patients.

Maurice Beghetti, MD
Associate Professor
Pediatric Cardiology Unit
Department of Pediatrics
Children's University Hospital of Geneva
Switzerland

Preface

Our main purpose in editing this book is to provide the health care practitioner with general clinical practical guidelines regarding the use of pediatric cardiovascular drugs. We also intend to provide an overview of basic pediatric cardiovascular principles. We realize the need for a pocket reference handbook that is tailored to meet the daily challenges of practitioners that care for pediatric cardiac patients.

This book is not intended to provide an extensive review of all cardiovascular medications, but hopefully, this reference will compile the necessary information required to assist the practitioner involved in the care of pediatric patients with heart disease in their day-to-day practice.

We expect this manual to be helpful for physicans, fellows, residents, pharmacists, and nurses in the multiple disciplines of anesthesia, critical care, cardiology, and cardiac intensive care.

Notice

The authors, editors, and publisher have exerted every effort to ensure that the information and dosages set forth in this handbook are accurate and in accordance with current recommendations at the time of publication. However, in view of ongoing research, evolving information relating to drug therapy and drug reactions, changes in drug labeling, as well as clinical experience, the reader is advised to consult the most current product information or other standard references for more detailed information, including changes in indication, dosage, interactions, and any added warnings or precautions prior to drug use. The authors, editors, and publisher cannot be responsible for the continued currency of the information in the book or for any omissions, errors, or the application of this information, or for any consequences from application of the information in this book and make no warranty, expressed or implied, with respect to the currency, completeness, or accuracy of the contents. Therefore, the author(s) or editors shall have no liability to any person or entity with regard to claims, losses, or damage caused, or alleged to be caused, directly or indirectly, by the use of information contained in this handbook. The application of the information in a clinical situation is the professional responsibility of the practitioner.

Ricardo Munoz, MD, FAAP, FCCM
Carol G. Schmitt, PharmD
Stephen J. Roth, MD, MPH
Eduardo da Cruz, MD

Contents

Contributors

Donald Berry, BSPharm
Pharmacy Department
Children's Hospital of Pittsburgh
Pittsburgh, PA, USA

Constantinos Chrysostomou, MD
Department of Pediatrics and Critical
    Care
Children's Hospital of Pittsburgh
University of Pittsburgh
    Medical Center
Pittsburgh, PA, USA

Eduardo da Cruz, MD
Director of the Cardiac Intensive
    Care Unit
Associate Professor of Pediatrics
    (Pediatric Cardiology & Intensive
    Care)
The Heart Institute
Department of Pediatrics
The Children's Hospital of Denver
University of Colorado at Denver &
    Health Sciences Center
Denver, CO
USA (since the 1st of April 2007)
Senior Consultant & Lecturer
Pediatric Cardiology Unit
Service of Pediatric and Neonatal
    Intensive Care
Department of Pediatrics
Children's University Hospital of
    Geneva
Geneva, Switzerland (until 31st of
    March 2007)

Peter J. Davis, MD
Anesthesiology and Critical Care
    Medicine

University of Pittsburgh School
    of Medicine
Children's Hospital of Pittsburgh
Pittsburgh, PA, USA

Sarah D. de Ferranti, MD, MPH
Department of Cardiology
Children's Hospital Boston
Boston, MA, USA

Anne M. Dubin, MD
Division of Pediatric Cardiology
Stanford University
Palo Alto, CA, USA

Brian Feingold, MD
Division of Pediatric Cardiology
Children's Hospital of Pittsburgh
Pittsburgh, PA, USA

Denise L. Howrie, PharmD
Pharmacy and Pediatrics
University of Pittsburgh School of
    Pharmacy and Medicine
Pittsburgh, PA, USA

Jonathan Kaufman, MD
The Heart Institute
Children's Hospital of Denver
Denver, CO, USA

Traci M. Kazmerski, BS
University of Notre Dame
University of Pittsburgh School
    of Medicine
Cardiac Intensive Care Unit
Children's Hospital of Pittsburgh
Pittsburgh, PA, USA

Indira A. Khimji, PharmD
Pharmacy Department
Children's Hospital of Pittsburgh
Pittsburgh, PA, USA

Victor O. Morell, MD
Department of Pediatric
    Cardiothoracic Surgery
Children's Hospital of Pittsburgh
Pittsburgh, PA, USA

Mary P. Mullen, MD, PhD
Department of Cardiac
    Intensive Care
Children's Hospital Boston
Boston, MA, USA

Ricardo Munoz, MD, FAAP, FCCM
Cardiac Intensive Care Division
Cardiac Recovery Program
Critical Care Medicine,
    Pediatrics and Surgery
Children's Hospital of Pittsburgh
Pittsburgh, PA, USA

Phuong-Tan Nguyen, PharmD
General Pediatrics
School of Pharmacy
University of Pittsburgh
Children's Hospital of Pittsburgh
Pittsburgh, PA, USA

Robert L. Poole, PharmD
Pharmacy Department
Lucile Packard Children's
    Hospital at Stanford
Palo Alto, CA, USA

Peter C. Rimensberger, MD
Pediatric and Neonatal ICU
Department of Pediatrics
University Hospital
    of Geneva
Geneva, Switzerland

Stephen J. Roth, MD, MPH
James Baxter and Yvonne Craig Wood
    Director, Cardiovascular ICU
Lucile Packard Children's Hospital
    at Stanford
Associate Professor of Pediatrics
    (Cardiology)
Stanford University School of
    Medicine
Palo Alto, CA, USA

Jessica Erin Sandy, PharmD
Neonatal Intensive Care
School of Pharmacy
University of Pittsburgh
Children's Hospital of Pittsburgh
Pittsburgh, PA, USA

Carol G. Schmitt, PharmD
Pediatric Critical Care
School of Pharmacy
University of Pittsburgh
Children's Hospital of Pittsburgh
Pittsburgh, PA, USA

Pravin Taneja, MD
University of Pittsburgh School of
    Medicine
Children's Hospital of Pittsburgh
Pittsburgh, PA, USA

Cécile Tissot, *MD*
Pediatric Cardiology Unit
University Hospital of Geneva
Geneva, Switzerland
The Heart Institute
Children's Hospital of Denver
Denver, CO, USA

Peter D. Wearden, MD, PhD
Department of Cardiothoracic
    Surgery
Children's Hospital of Pittsburgh
University of Pittsburgh Medical
    Center
Pittsburgh, PA, USA

Steven A. Webber, MBChB, MRCP
Department of Pediatrics
University of Pittsburgh School of
    Medicine
Division of Cardiology
Children's Hospital of Pittsburgh
Pittsburgh, PA, USA

David L. Wessel, MD
Department of Pediatrics
    (Anasthesia)

Harvard Medical School
Cardiology and Anesthesia
Cardiac Intensive Care
Children's Hospital Boston
Boston, MA, USA

Charles I. Yang, MD
University of Pittsburgh School
    of Medicine
Pittsburgh, PA, USA

1. Cardiac Physiology Review

Brian Feingold and Ricardo Munoz

A basic understanding of cardiovascular physiology is fundamental to the comprehension of the conditions and pharmacological mechanisms described throughout this Handbook. With that goal in mind, this chapter provides an overview of cardiovascular physiology and highlights the unique aspects of the neonatal and pediatric heart. Although not intended to be an exhaustive review, this chapter should serve to familiarize the reader with concepts to be discussed in greater detail in later chapters. For those seeking further knowledge, a list of more comprehensive sources is provided at the conclusion of this chapter.

Basic Cardiac Structure and Function

The human heart is, in essence, two pumps connected in series, delivering blood to the pulmonary and systemic circulations. It is comprised of two atria, which receive venous blood; two ventricles, which pump blood; valves, which prevent the backflow of blood; and a conduction system, which transmits the electrical impulses that drive cardiac activity. The electrical signal is propagated and converted to mechanical activity through a series of biochemical interactions, which involve stereotyped ion fluxes (mainly Na^+, Ca^{++}, and K^+) through voltage-gated ion "pores" and downstream protein interactions. Although inherited or acquired defects in these components may result in cardiac disease, these same mechanisms form the basis of pharmacological therapies.

Electrophysiology

Rhythmic and coordinated contraction of the heart is accomplished by the propagation of an electrical impulse (action potential) in a precise manner (Figure 1-1). Each action potential is normally initiated by the sinoatrial (SA) node, a specialized group of myocardial cells in the high right atrium. These cells exhibit automaticity, meaning they spontaneously become electrically active (depolarize). The impulse then spreads to adjacent atrial myocytes via cell-to-cell connections termed gap junctions. Ultimately, the wave of depolarization reaches a second group of specialized cells at the bottom of the right atrium, the atrioventricular (AV) node. Because the atria and ventricles are electrically isolated from one another by a circumferential band of fibrous tissue at the level of the tricuspid and mitral valves, the only path for impulse propagation is via the AV node. After a brief (approximately 0.1 s), intrinsic delay at the AV

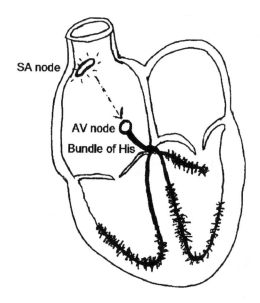

Figure 1-1. Diagrammatic representation of structures involved in normal cardiac conduction.

node, the action potential is propagated quickly down the bundle of His and Purkinje fibers within the ventricular myocardium. This rapidly conducting network acts as "wiring" to convey the impulse to the apex of the heart, allowing for a coordinated, mechanically efficient contraction of the ventricles.

Action and Resting Potentials

At rest, cardiac myocytes maintain a net negative electrical gradient with respect to the extracellular environment (resting potential). The gradient results from the activities of ion channels and transporters within the cell membrane and is essential to the ability of the myocyte (and heart) to propagate electrical impulses. With sufficient stimulus, alterations in the myocyte's permeability to Na^+ result in a net positive electrical gradient with respect to the extracellular environment (depolarization). Further, changes in the myocyte's ion permeability to K^+, Cl^-, and Ca^{++} result in the eventual restoration of the negative intracellular environment. When plotted against time, the changes in electrical potential are conventionally described as having five distinct phases (Figure 1-2), which correspond to the stereotyped alterations in membrane permeability of the cardiac myocyte. Antiarrhythmic medications exert their influence by altering membrane permeability, affecting the characteristics of the action potential. For example, Class Ia agents (procainamide, disopyramide, and quinidine) affect Na^+ influx, resulting in a decreased rate of Phase 0 depolarization and mild prolongation of repolarization.[1]

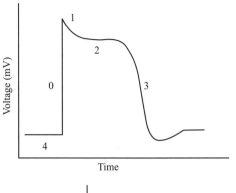

Figure 1-2. The action potential of a Purkinje fiber. Phase 4 is the resting state before electrical stimulation. Phase 0 is the rapid depolarization as a result of Na^+ influx. Phase 1 is the initial stage of repolarization caused by closure of Na^+ channels and efflux of Cl^-. Phase 2, or the plateau phase, is mediated primarily by Ca^{++} influx. Phase 3 is the rapid repolarization and is facilitated primarily by K^+ efflux.

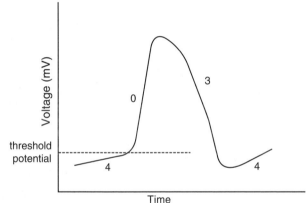

Figure 1-3. Diagrammatic representation of the action potential of SA or AV nodal cells. Phase 4 is characterized by the positive slope, indicating gradual depolarization toward threshold, at which point the Phase 0 upstroke is observed.

Automaticity

Automaticity refers to the intrinsic ability of a cardiomyocyte or cluster of cardiomyocytes to spontaneously depolarize and, thus, initiate propagation of an action potential. Such cells are termed "pacemaker cells" and include those of the SA and AV nodes. Cells of the His-Purkinje system and the ventricular myocardium may also spontaneously depolarize under circumstances of particularly slow cardiac rhythms (e.g., sinus node arrest, complete heart block). Because of the more rapid depolarization of the heart's usual pacemakers, the automaticity of these cells is often not manifested. Furthermore, after cardiac injury, cells that typically do not possess automaticity may acquire altered membrane conductance with resultant current leakage and spontaneous depolarization. Figure 1-3 depicts the action potential for cells of the SA and AV nodes. Notice the positively sloped Phase 4, progressing toward the threshold potential, at which point, Phase 0 occurs. The slope of the Phase 4 depolarization is a key determinant in the rate of initiation of an action potential and, thus, overall heart rate. Modulation of automaticity occurs via the autonomic nervous system and may, thus, be affected by pharmacological agents acting centrally (dexmedetomidine, clonidine) or those affecting action potential initiation and propagation at the level of the myocytes (digoxin, β-blockers). In clinical practice, there is often an overlap of direct and autonomic effects with many pharmacological agents.

Electromechanical Coupling

On a macroscopic level, propagation of the action potential from the high right atrium to the AV node, His-Purkinje system, and, finally, the ventricular myocardium allows for ordered, coordinated myocardial contraction and relaxation. On a cellular level, this is accomplished by coupling the changes in electrical environment to changes in mechanical activity (myocardial contraction and relaxation) via fluctuations of cytosolic Ca^{++} concentration. As a consequence of depolarization, cytosolic Ca^{++} concentration markedly increases via influx across the cell membrane as well as release of intracellular calcium stores within the sarcoplasmic reticulum. Ca^{++} directly enables the interaction of the contractile elements actin and myosin, the result of which is myofiber shortening. Just as the process of myocyte contraction is reliant on Ca^{++}, myocardial relaxation is an *active* process, requiring the expenditure of energy in the form of adenosine triphosphate (ATP) to remove Ca^{++} from the cytosol quickly and inhibit continued contraction.[2] For further detail regarding the downstream interactions between contractile elements and the process of electromechanical coupling, the reader is referred to selections referenced at the conclusion of this chapter.

Dysrhythmias

Although an extensive review of all dysrhythmias is outside the scope of this chapter, a brief overview of the mechanisms of the basic categories of dysrhythmias is provided. On the simplest level, heart rhythm abnormalities can be divided into those that are "too slow" (bradyarrhythmias) and those that are "too fast" (tachyarrhythmias). Bradyarrhythmias primarily result from delay or block in conduction of the impulse from the high right atrium to the AV node and His-Purkinje system. Most involve disease of the AV nodal tissue (first degree and second degree type I [Wenckebach] heart block) or of the His-Purkinje system (second degree type II [Mobitz] and third degree [complete] heart block). Bradyarrhythmias may also result from disease of the sinus node (ineffective automaticity), such that no appropriate pacemaker is available to establish a physiological heart rate. Tachyarrhythmias are more varied in terms of etiologies and can originate from the atria, ventricles, or AV node. However, the mechanism that underlies each can often be categorized as automatic or reentrant. An automatic tachycardia results from a cell or cluster of cells acquiring abnormal automaticity, such that this region of the heart spontaneously depolarizes more rapidly than the sinus node, establishing the heart rate at greater than physiological rates. Examples of automatic tachycardias include ectopic atrial tachycardia, multifocal atrial tachycardia, and junctional ectopic tachycardia. Automatic tachycardias tend to exhibit "warm-up" and/or "cool-down" phases at onset and termination, and, despite the overall rapid rate, there is subtle variability in heart rate over time. In contrast, reentrant tachycardias result from nonphysiological electrical pathways that allow conduction of an impulse back to a region of the heart that has repolarized after the earlier conduction of the *same* impulse. Such "short circuits" essentially allow the same impulse to recycle itself and lead to successive depolarizations. Reentrant tachyarrhythmias characteristically have an abrupt onset and termination and a nonvarying rate during the tachycardia. The reentrant circuit may exist exclusively within the atria (atrial flutter), ventricles (ventricular tachycardia), or AV node (AV node reentrant tachycardia), or may be comprised of tissue that connects the atria, AV node, and/or ventricles (accessory pathway tachycardia).

Cardiovascular Physiology

Care of the patient with hemodynamic derangements remains rooted in basic physiological concepts—preload, contractility, and afterload—first described in the late 19th century. These factors directly impact stroke volume, which, along with heart rate, are the key determinants of cardiac output (Figure 1-4).

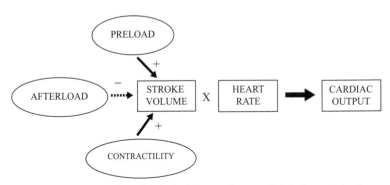

Figure 1-4. Preload, contractility, and afterload each impact cardiac output via their effects on stroke volume.

Preload

Preload refers to the ventricle's intrinsic ability, within a physiological range, to alter the force of contraction based on the degree of ventricular filling just before contraction (end-diastolic volume/fiber length). The greater the end-diastolic volume, and, thus, ventricular myofiber stretch, the greater the force of contraction. Conceptually, preload is most often equated with the intravascular volume status of a patient. Under conditions of relatively low-volume status (e.g., dehydration), the force of myocardial contraction, and, thus, cardiac output, is diminished. Volume status is most often gauged clinically by measuring the central venous pressure (CVP), which is usually equivalent to right ventricular end-diastolic pressure. Assuming normal ventricular compliance (pressure-volume relationship) and absence of significant tricuspid (or mitral) stenosis, CVP is a clinically useful surrogate for preload. Caution must be used when interpreting the CVP in light of the clinical scenario (i.e., a "normal" CVP may in fact be too low if there is a poorly compliant ventricle, as occurs with diastolic dysfunction or constrictive pericarditis).

Contractility

As already noted, within physiological range, the greater the myofiber stretch (preload), the greater the force of contraction. However, contractility (or inotropic state) specifically refers to the magnitude of response to a given preload and can be thought of as the "multiplication factor" for any given preload (Figure 1-5). Contractility is an intrinsic property of the muscle fiber that is relatively independent of changes in preload or afterload. In other words, for any given preload, the force of contraction will be greater under conditions of increased inotropy (e.g., dobutamine infusion) and less under conditions of depressed inotropy (e.g., systolic dysfunction). In the setting of low cardiac output (e.g., dilated cardiomyopathy), improvement is sought by administration of medication (e.g., dobutamine, low-dose epinephrine, milrinone, or digoxin) to augment contractility. Each of these therapies has multiple effects, aside from enhanced inotropy, which may limit their therapeutic efficacy (e.g., increased myocardial oxygen consumption, excessive tachycardia, or arrhythmias).

Afterload

Afterload is defined as the ventricular wall stress during contraction and is often conceptualized as the load against which the ventricle contracts. In clinical practice, afterload is usually identified with systemic vascular resistance (SVR), which is primarily determined by the arteriolar resistance. However,

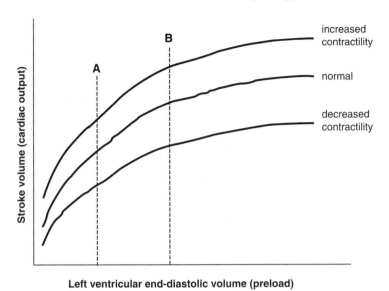

Left ventricular end-diastolic volume (preload)

Figure 1-5. Frank-Starling curve illustrating the relationship between various preloads inotropic states and cardiac output. At preload **A**, cardiac output is less than that at preload **B**. However, for a given preload **A** or **B**, cardiac output is, in part, determined by the inotropic state (contractility).

from LaPlace's principle, wall stress is directly proportional not only to the ventricular pressure, but also to ventricular chamber diameter, while it is inversely proportional to ventricular wall thickness. Thus, for the left ventricle (LV), the major components of afterload are peripheral vascular resistance, arterial wall stiffness, mass of the column of blood in the aorta, blood viscosity, and LV wall thickness and diameter. Similarly, for the right ventricle (RV), afterload is primarily influenced by pulmonary artery impedance, pulmonary vascular resistance (PVR), mass of the column of blood in the pulmonary circulation, viscosity of the blood, and RV chamber characteristics. Examples of clinical scenarios in which the LV faces increased afterload include aortic stenosis (increased resistance), coarctation of the aorta and systemic hypertension (increased resistance and wall stiffness), and dilated cardiomyopathy (increased chamber diameter). For any given preload, greater afterload results in more limited myofiber shortening during contraction and decreased stroke volume as compared with contraction in the face of lesser afterload (see next section and baseline stroke volume [SV_B] versus decreased afterload stroke volume [SV_{DA}] of Figure 1-6b). In other words, afterload determines the size of the ventricular cavity at the end of contraction, independent of the ventricular volume before contraction (preload).

Pressure-Volume Loops

Visual representations of these physiological concepts can be helpful to best appreciate their individual characteristics and their impact on one another *in vivo*. One particularly useful way to appreciate the contributions of and interactions between preload, contractility, and afterload is by examination of pressure-volume loops. As shown in Figure 1-6a, ventricular diastolic performance (compliance) and changes in preload are illustrated by the curve at the bottom of the graph (end-diastolic pressure volume relationship), ventricular volume throughout the cardiac cycle is illustrated by the rectangle, and contractility is illustrated by the diagonal line (end-systolic pressure volume relationship). With the onset of systole (Point A), there is an increase in pressure (isovolumic contraction) until ventricular pressure exceeds aortic pressure, at which point, the aortic valve opens and blood is ejected from the ventricle (Point B). As the ventricle continues to empty, there is the onset of relaxation of the ventricle, with an eventual drop in pressure below that of the aorta (Point C). At this point, ventricular pressure falls but the volume remains unchanged (isovolumic relaxation) until the pressure drops below that of the left atrium and the mitral valve opens (Point D). The ventricular volume then increases during diastole, until the cycle repeats itself with the next contraction. The area within the rectangle represents stroke work, and the distance along the x axis between the vertical lines is the stroke volume. As illustrated in Figure 1-6b, increased preload results in a greater stroke volume as compared with baseline, but the end-systolic volume in both instances is limited by the afterload (and contractility). With decreased afterload (dash-dot line), a lesser end-systolic volume and a greater stroke volume are achieved. Conversely, increased afterload results in greater end-systolic volumes (i.e., decreased myofiber shortening) and diminished stroke volume. As shown in Figure 1-6c, alterations in contractility (inotropic state) also affect changes in stroke volume. Finally, differences in ventricular compliance (slope and shape of curve at bottom of graphs) result in differences in end-diastolic volume (myofiber stretch) for a given preload (Figure 1-6d), and, thus, also impact stroke volume.

Clinical Measures of Cardiac Function and Contractility

Bedside assessment and care of patients is driven, in part, by the technology available for clinical assessment. For example, although the use of impedance catheters to ascertain pressure-volume loops might best inform clinicians regarding the changing cardiovascular status of their patients (and the response to therapies), this technology is impractical in most cases because it requires an invasive procedure for placement and impractical levels of continuous monitoring. Thus, most clinicians rely on surrogate measures and their clinical experience to manage patients. Just as CVP is commonly used to estimate preload and systemic blood pressure is commonly used to estimate afterload, echocardiographic assessments of ventricular systolic function are often relied

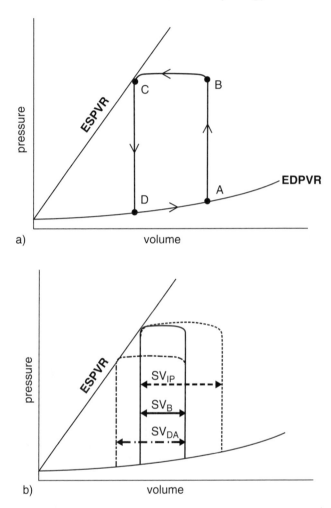

Figure 1-6. a) Stylized pressure-volume loop. Followed in the counterclockwise direction are end-diastolic volume and onset of systole (**A**), isovolumic contraction (**A** to **B**), aortic valve opening (**B**), ventricular ejection (**B** to **C**), aortic valve closure (**C**) and isovolumic relaxation (**C** to **D**), mitral valve opening (**D**), and diastolic filling of the ventricle (**D** to **A**). The volume difference between lines **AB** and **CD** is the stroke volume. ESPVR, end-systolic pressure-volume relationship; EDPVR, end-diastolic pressure-volume relationship. **b)** Increased preload results in a greater stroke volume (SV_{IP}) as compared with baseline (SV_B), but the end-systolic volume in both instances is limited by the afterload (height of the pressure-volume curve) and contractility (slope of the ESPVR line). In the setting of decreased afterload, stroke volume (SV_{DA}) is increased by achieving a lower end-systolic volume.

(Continued)

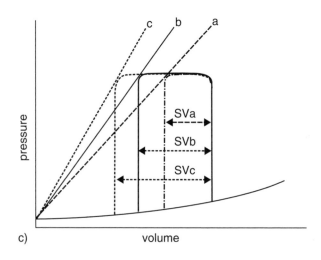

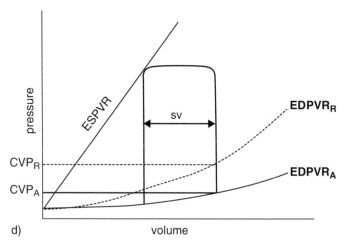

Figure 1-6. (Continued)   **c)** For a given preload and afterload, stroke volume (SV) varies based on contractility. ESPVR lines **A**, **B**, and **C** represent progressively increased inotropic states. **d)** The impact of changes in ventricular compliance are depicted by the two EDPVR curves. In the setting of decreased compliance (EDPVR$_B$), a greater CVP$_B$ is required to achieve the same ventricular end-diastolic volume and stroke volume (SV). (Figures adapted from Chang and Towbin, eds. Heart Failure in children and young adults, From Molecular Mechanisms to Medical and Surgical Strategies, page 253, Copyright © Elsevier 2006.)

on to assess contractility. Specific estimators of contractility include shortening fraction (SF), ejection fraction (EF), and mean velocity of circumferential fiber shortening (Vcf_c). Both SF and EF are similar in their approach, in that they measure the extent of shortening of LV chamber size to assess function. For EF, the end-systolic and end-diastolic parameters are estimated LV volumes (LV end-systolic volume [LVESV] and LV end-diastolic volume [LVEDV]), whereas for SF, the parameters are linear measurements of LV cavity length or dimension (LV end-systolic dimension [LVESD] or LV end-diastolic dimension [LVEDD]). The formulas for each are given below:

$$EF = (LVEDV - LVESV) / LVEDV \times 100$$
$$SF = (LVEDD - LVESD) / LVEDD \times 100$$

For EF, the volumes are estimated from echocardiography, whereas, for SF, the dimensions are measured using M-mode echocardiography. Although both are relatively easy to ascertain and provide some quantification of LV systolic function, these measures are dependent on preload and afterload, which vary over time and are unlikely to be the same at serial evaluations. Another measure of ventricular function, mean Vcf_c, makes use of the rate of LV ejection to assess systolic function and has the advantage of being independent of preload and heart rate, but still does not account for afterload.

Wall stress, the tension per unit cross-sectional area of myocardium, is thought to be the best estimator of ventricular afterload because it accounts for LV wall thickness (mass). Comparison of the mean Vcf_c to LV wall stress enables assessment of contractility free from the biases of alterations in preload, heart rate, and afterload. Unfortunately, none of these measures account for ventricular diastolic function, an often under appreciated but increasingly recognized contributor to symptomatic heart failure. Indices of diastolic function are available, but discussion of them is outside the scope of this chapter.

Unique Features of the Pediatric Heart

From structural, physiological, and anatomic perspectives, neonatal and pediatric hearts differ from the adult heart. Studies in experimental animals have shown that both systolic and diastolic cardiac function in the neonate are reduced as compared with adults. From a structural perspective, this results, in large part, from differences in calcium handling by the cardiomyocyte. Because the immature cardiomyocyte has less sarcoplasmic reticulum, intracellular calcium stores are limited.[3] The diminished numbers and activities of sarcoplasmic reticulum membrane transport proteins further differentiates the calcium flux of the immature heart from that of the adult heart. As a result of these differences in calcium handling, the immature cardiomyocyte has a greater reliance on extracellular calcium to enable myofibril contraction and relaxation.[4] Also contributing to the unique physiological profile of neonatal and infant hearts are fewer numbers of contractile elements per myocyte and a greater relative proportion of noncardiomyocytes to cardiomyocytes as compared with the mature heart. The former likely impacts the ability to generate systolic tension, whereas the latter is thought to contribute to the relative noncompliance of neonatal and infant hearts.

Many of these structural differences impact the clinical characteristics of neonatal and infant hearts. For example, neonatal and infant hearts are exquisitely sensitive to serum calcium concentration, such that, after cardiac surgery, calcium infusions are often used for inotropic support. In addition, limited ventricular compliance results in the inability to augment stroke volume as a means of increasing cardiac output. Thus, neonates, infants, and (to a lesser extent) young children rely much more on increases in heart rate as the primary mechanism to augment cardiac output. Clinically, this explains the relatively fast heart rates of infants and young children, and their inability to tolerate heart rates that are normally for adults.

When evaluating a neonate, infant, or young child, it is mandatory that a thorough assessment of the underlying cardiac anatomy be conducted, because significant structural lesions can go undetected before clinical presentation. Some of these lesions result in heart failure from low cardiac output (e.g., left heart obstruction from coarctation of the aorta, hypoplastic left heart syndrome, or critical aortic stenosis), whereas others result in heart failure from pulmonary overcirculation (e.g., large left-to-right shunts from a ventricular septal defects, or a patent ductus arteriosus).

Shunt Lesions and Calculations

Common to the practice of pediatric cardiology is the care of patients with structural lesions that cause shunting of blood. An explanation of the terms and calculations used to describe shunted blood flow follows. A key principle to keep in mind when considering congenital heart disease and quantification of shunts is that marked changes in systemic vascular resistance (SVR) and pulmonary vascular resistance (SPVR) occur around the time of birth and continue for some time thereafter. These changes impact the direction and magnitude of shunt flow, and multiple therapeutic maneuvers (e.g., pharmacotherapy, mechanical ventilation, and inhaled gases) are often used to affect the degree and minimize the impact of shunting during the management of patients. It is also essential to appreciate the relationship that exists between cardiac output, vascular resistance, and blood pressure. This relationship is conceptualized as Ohm's Law (voltage = current × resistance), with the substitution of pressure (P) for voltage and cardiac output (Q) for current, to yield the equation $\Delta P = Q \times R$.

As was noted at the onset of this chapter, the heart is, in essence, two pumps that are connected in series. The right heart pumps to the pulmonary circulation and the left heart to the systemic circulation. In the absence of a shunt, right heart cardiac output (Qp) is equal to left heart cardiac output (Qs), i.e., Qp/Qs equals 1. In the setting of a net left-to-right shunt, Qp/Qs is greater than 1, and in the setting of a net right-to-left shunt, Qp/Qs is less than 1. A simple rule of thumb (analogous to electrical current) is that "blood flows down the path of least resistance." Thus, the relative resistances of the pulmonary and systemic circulations are a primary determinant of the net direction and magnitude of a shunt (although this holds true for shunts at the ventricular [ventricular septal defects] and vascular levels [aortopulmonary window, patent ductus arteriosus, and surgically created arterial shunts], the direction and magnitude of shunts at the atrial level are determined instead by the relative compliance of the left and right ventricles). In clinical practice, both flow and pressure are relatively easily measured, whereas resistance is usually calculated. Rearranging the equation noted above, PVR equals ΔP divided by Qp, where ΔP is the transpulmonary gradient (mean pulmonary artery pressure minus mean pulmonary vein [or left atrial] pressure). Likewise, SVR equals ΔP divided by Qs, where ΔP equals the transsystemic gradient (the mean arterial pressure minus CVP).

In day-to-day practice, knowledge of the normal physiological changes in PVR and SVR from fetus to neonate to adulthood enables clinicians to make reasonably valid assumptions regarding a particular patient's condition and to direct appropriate therapies. However, there are instances in which the clinical picture is not entirely clear and quantification of the magnitude, or even net direction, of a shunt is necessary. Clinically, much of the information necessary to quantify a shunt or calculate resistance can be achieved at cardiac catheterization, with the measurement of oxygen saturations and pressures in the various cardiac chambers and major blood vessels. Furthermore, quantification of Qp may be achieved at the bedside in the intensive care unit or at the time of catheterization with the use of a thermodilution catheter (aka, Swann-Ganz catheter) or measurement of oxygen consumption (VO_2) and application of the Fick principle. Although detailed descriptions of each of these techniques is outside the scope of this Handbook, a thermodilution catheter enables measurement of Qp and the pressures necessary to calculate PVR, whereas measurement of VO_2 and appropriate oxygen saturations enables calculation of Qp and Qs. The reader is directed to "Hemodynamic Calculations" for examples in Tables 1-1 to 1-4, and a list of commonly used formulas, and to the end of this chapter for suggested reference texts.

Hemodynamic Calculations

Table 1-1. Large, unrestrictive ventricular septal defect in an 8-week-old infant [a]

	Pressure (mmHg)	Oxygen saturation
Superior vena cava	8	68%
Right ventricle	85/55	88%
Pulmonary artery	70 (mean)	88%
PCWP	15	98%
Aorta	85/55	98%

[a]PCWP, pulmonary capillary wedge pressure. Hemoglobin (Hgb), 13.0 g/dL; VO_2, 55.8 mL/min; body surface area (BSA), 0.25 m^2.

(continued)

Table 1-1. (Continued)

Using Fick Equation:

$Qp = VO_2 / [Hgb (g/dL) \times 13.6 \times (PV_{sat} - PA_{sat})] = 55.8 / [13 \times 13.6 \times (0.98 - 0.88)] = 3.2$ L/min

$Qs = VO_2 / [Hgb (g/dL) \times 13.6 \times (Ao_{sat} - MV_{sat})] = 55.8 / [13 \times 13.6 \times (0.98 - 0.68)] = 1.1$ L/min

Thus, Qp:Qs = 3.2/1.1 ~ 3:1. Alternately, because all other terms cancel out, if only saturations are known, can use $(Ao_{sat} - MV_{sat}) / (PV_{sat} - PA_{sat}) = (0.98 - 0.68) / (0.98 - 0.88) = 3:1$.

$Qp_i = Qp / BSA = 12.6$ L/min/m^2

$PVR = TPG / Qp_i = (70 - 15 \text{ mmHg}) / 12.6$ L/min/m^2 = 3.97 indexed Wood units

PV_{sat}, pulmonary vein saturation; PA_{sat}, pulmonary artery saturation; Ao_{sat}, aortic saturation; MV_{sat}, mixed venous saturation; Q_{pi}, Qp indexed to body surface area; Q_{si}, Qs indexed to body surface area.

Table 1-2. Large, unrestrictive ventricular septal defect in a 5-year-old child[a]

	Pressure (mmHg)	Oxygen saturation
Superior vena cava	8	68%
Right ventricle	85/55	73%
Pulmonary artery	70 (mean)	73%
PCWP	15	98%
Aorta	85/55	98%

[a]Hgb, 13.0 g/dL; VO$_2$, 55.8 mL/min; BSA, 0.7 m^2.

$Qp_i = 5.0$ L/min/m^2

Qp:Qs = (0.98 − 0.68) / (0.98 − 0.73) = 1.2:1

Thus, $Qs_i = 5.0$ L/min/m^2 / 1.2 = 4.2 L/min/m^2

$PVR = TPG / Qp_i = (70 - 15 \text{ mmHg}) / 5.0$ L/min/m^2 = 11.0 indexed Wood units

Table 1-3. Large atrial septal defect[a]

	Pressure (mmHg)	Oxygen saturation
Superior vena cava	10	72%
Right atrium	10	79%
Right ventricle	32/14	83%
Pulmonary artery	20 (mean)	83%
PCWP	11	99%
Aorta	85/55	99%

[a]Hgb, 12.6 g/dL; VO$_2$, 86 mL/min; BSA, 0.7 m^2.

$Qp_i = 4.48$ L/min/m^2

$Qs_i = 2.65$ L/min/m^2

Qp:Qs = 4.48 / 2.65 = 1.69:1

$PVR = TPG / Qp_i = (20 - 11 \text{ mmHg}) / 2.65$ L/min/m^2 = 3.4 indexed Wood units

Table 1-4. Tetralogy of Fallot[a]

	Pressure (mmHg)	Oxygen saturation
Right atrium	10	63%
Right ventricle	85/55	63%
Pulmonary artery	16 (mean)	63%
PCWP	11	
Aorta	85/55	87%

[a]$Hgb = 14.2 \, g/dL, VO_2 = 62 \, mL/min, BSA = 0.3 \, m^2$
$Qp_i = 2.97 \, L/min/m^2$
$Qs_i = 4.43 \, L/min/m^2$
$Qp{:}Qs = 2.97 \, / \, 4.43 = 0.67{:}1$
$PVR = TPG \, / \, Qp_i = (16 - 11 \, mmHg) \, / \, 2.97 \, L/min/m^2 = 1.68$ indexed Wood units

Suggested Reading

Colan SD. Assessment of ventricular and myocardial performance. In: Keane FJ, Lock JE, Flyer CD, editors. Nadas' Pediatric Cardiology. Philadelphia: Saunders Elsevier, 2006:251–273.

Fogoros RN. Practical Cardiac Diagnosis: Electrophysiologic Testing, 3rd ed. Oxford: Blackwell Publishing, 1999:1–33.

Lilly LS, editor. Pathophysiology of Heart Disease. Philadelphia: Lea & Febiger, 1993.

Mahony L. Development of myocardial structure and function. In: Allen HD, Gutgesell HP, Clark EB, Driscoll DJ, editors. Moss and Adams' Heart Disease in Infants, Children, and Adolescents, 6th ed. Philadelphia: Lippincott Williams & Wilkins, 2001:24–40.

Vargo TA. Cardiac catheterization: hemodynamic measurements. In: Garson A, Bricker JT, Fisher DJ, Neish SR, editors. The Science and Practice of Pediatric Cardiology, 2nd ed. Baltimore: Williams & Wilkins, 1998:961–993.

References

1. DiMarco JP, Gersh BJ, Opie LH. Antiarrhythmic drugs and strategies. In: Opie LH, Gersh BJ, editors. Drugs for the Heart, 6th ed. Philadelphia: Elsevier Saunders, 2005:218–219.

2. Schwartz SM. Cellular and molecular aspects of myocardial dysfunction. In: Shaddy RE, Wernovsky G, editors. Pediatric Heart Failure. Boca Raton: Taylor & Francis Group, 2005:71–73.

3. Fisher DJ. Basic science of cardiovascular development. In: Garson A, Bricker JT, Fisher DJ, Neish SR, editors. The Science and Practice of Pediatric Cardiology. Baltimore: Williams and Wilkins, 1998:201–209.

4. Ralphe JC. Pathophysiology of chronic myocardial dysfunction. In: Slonim AD, Pollack MM, editors. Pediatric Critical Care Medicine. Philadelphia: Lippincott Williams & Wilkins, 2005:230–234.

Formulas

Qp:Qs = (aortic − mixed venous saturation) / (pulmonary venous − pulmonary arterial saturation)

Qp = VO_2 / [13.6 × Hgb (g/dL) × (pulmonary venous − pulmonary arterial saturation)]

Qs = CO = VO_2 / [13.6 × Hgb (g/dL) × (aortic − mixed venous saturation)]

PVR = transpulmonary gradient (TPG) / Qp

TPG = mean pulmonary artery pressure − pulmonary capillary wedge (or left atrial) pressure

SVR = (mean arterial pressure − central venous pressure) / Qs

2. Clinical Pharmacokinetics: Applications in Pediatric Practice

Denise L. Howrie and Carol G. Schmitt

The statement "Children are not little adults" is a foundation of pediatric drug therapy referring to well-documented differences in pharmacokinetics and pharmacodynamics existing between children and adults.[1-6] It is, therefore, important to understand the influence of age on drug disposition, especially in neonates and infants, and resulting effects on drug activity. This chapter provides brief discussions of principles of pediatric pharmacokinetics and knowledge of the effects of disease states on disposition of cardiovascular drugs affecting safe and effective drug therapy.

Pediatric Pharmacokinetics

Drug Absorption

Oral Administration

The rate of drug absorption is generally slowed in infancy when compared with older children and adults.[1,3] Efficiency of absorption of drugs after oral administration may be variable, especially during infancy in the presence of prolonged gastrointestinal emptying time (6–8 h), unpredictable gastric peristalsis, and delayed time to peak concentrations.[1,3] Gastric pH values of 1 to 3 are achieved within 24 hours after birth,[1] gastric pH values become acid neutral by 1 week of age, and slowly decline over 2 to 3 years to adult values.[4] These changes may result in greater absorption of basic drugs, such as amoxicillin, erythromycin, and penicillin G, while reducing absorption of weak acidic drugs, including phenobarbital, in infants.[1,3,4]

Reduced bile acid pool and low lipase production decrease absorption of fat-soluble vitamins.[1] Irregular peristalsis may affect small intestinal drug absorption in childhood. Improvement in antral contractions occurs through the first week of life and intestinal motility through early infancy.[3] Other developmental differences include reduced glutathione-*S*-transferase, altered microflora, and changes in splanchnic blood flow.[3] Diarrhea, as well as variation in intestinal transit, may accelerate transit, with reduced and variable absorption from sustained-release products.[1,4]

Other Routes of Administration

Percutaneous absorption of drugs, including adrenal corticosteroids and alcohols, may be increased in infancy because of greater relative body surface area, enhanced hydration of epidermis, and decreased thickness of the epidermis and stratum corneum.[1,3,4] The ratio of total body surface area to body mass is greater in infants and children when compared with adults.[3,4]

Absorption from intramuscular injection sites may be less predictable in neonates because of variation in peripheral perfusion[1,3,4] and limited muscle mass. However, intramuscular absorption in neonates may be more efficient because of higher density of skeletal muscle capillaries.[3]

Rectal administration of drugs, such as diazepam or midazolam, may result in higher serum concentrations as compared with oral administration, although this is not an age-dependent observation for these drugs.[1] Immaturity of hepatic metabolism may increase rectal drug bioavailability in neonates, although enhanced expulsion of rectal products could also reduce drug bioavailability.[3]

Bioavailability

The amount of a drug dose that reaches the systemic circulation is the "bioavailability" of the drug. It is affected by drug absorption, metabolism in the intestinal wall (referred to as presystemic metabolism), and hepatic metabolism (referred to as "first-pass effects"). Low bioavailability values reflect either poor absorption or high rates of metabolism.

Drug Distribution

Drug transport through body compartments occurs under the influence of factors including protein binding, body fluids, membrane transport, and blood and tissue hemodynamics. Drugs generally distribute rapidly through blood to more highly perfused organs, such as the liver and kidneys, then more slowly to other compartments. Drug movement occurs into and out of multiple compartments over time to maintain equilibrium, with disease states, drug lipid solubility, characteristics of body tissues, regional pH differences, and protein binding as determinants.

Volume of Distribution

The volume of distribution (Vd) of a drug indicates the extent of drug distribution into body fluids and tissues and relates the amount of drug in the body to measured plasma concentration (Css) and is defined as:

$$Vd\ (L/Kg) = \frac{Amount\ of\ drug\ (mg)}{Css\ (mg/L)}$$

In clinical practice, this value permits rapid calculation of "Loading Doses" to rapidly achieve therapeutic serum concentrations for drugs such as phenytoin and lidocaine by use of measured mean Vd values for the defined patient population. For example, if the average population Vd for a particular drug is 1 L/kg and the desired plasma concentration is 15 mg/L, the required average loading dose would be 15 mg/kg. Drugs with extensive extraplasma distribution seem to have large Vd values.

Total Body Water and Extracellular Fluid Volume

Expanded total body water values relative to body weight are observed in newborns, infants, and children when compared with adults: 80% total body weight in premature infants and 70 to 75% in newborns as compared with 50 to 60% in adults.[1,4] Neonates and young infants also have a greater extracellular fluid compartment relative to body weight when compared with adults.[1,3,4] For water-soluble drugs demonstrating distribution through total body water, including aminoglycosides, penicillins, and cephalosporins, larger doses (expressed as milligram per kilogram doses) will be required in infants to achieve comparable serum concentrations to those achieved in adults.

Total Body Fat

Preterm infants have significantly lower body fat (1%) when compared with full-term infants (15%) and adults (20%). Lipid-soluble drugs, such as benzodiazepines, would, therefore, demonstrate lower Vd estimates in premature infants, leading to augmented clinical effects.[1]

Protein-Binding Effects

Drugs in plasma bind to proteins, including albumin, α-1-acid-glycoprotein (α-1-AG), and lipoproteins. Albumin is the major serum protein that binds anionic drugs at two binding sites. Site I has binding sites for drugs such as warfarin, sulfonamides, phenytoin, and valproate; whereas Site II is the binding site for penicillins and benzodiazepines. In the presence of lower concentrations of albumin in the first year of life (75–80% of adult values[5]), the presence of fetal albumin with reduced affinity for many drugs; endogenous competitive substances, such as bilirubin and free fatty acids; and higher free-drug concentrations for drugs such as phenytoin, salicylates, and valproic acid may result in augmented response.[3,4] The potential competition of drugs that are highly bound to albumin with endogenous substrates such as bilirubin that are also bound to albumin dictates cautious use of drugs such as ceftriaxone and sulfonamides in infants with or at risk of hyperbilirubinemia.[4]

Although emphasis is placed on albumin and drug binding, the role α-1-AG cannot be overlooked because this protein binds important cationic and neutral drugs. Changes in α-1-AG in an acute phase reaction caused by inflammation, as seen after myocardial infarction, may result in lower free concentrations of drugs, including lidocaine, propranolol, and quinidine. Additionally, concentrations of this protein are 50% of adult levels during infancy and increase slowly during the first year of life.[4,5]

Drug Elimination

Drug elimination from the body generally occurs via the liver or other sites of metabolism and/or the kidney through excretion of active drug or biotransformed metabolites. Total body elimination is the sum of all metabolism and excretion.

Metabolism

Drug metabolism occurs through biotransformation through Phase I reactions (oxidation, reduction, sulfoxidation, and hydrolysis)[4] by conversion of a functional group such as hydroxyl, amine, or sulfhydryl.[7] Oxidation proceeds via mixed-function oxidase systems including cytochrome P(CYP) 450 reductase enzymes through hydroxylation, dealkylation, and deamination. Both Phase I and II reactions mature over time.[4] Phase I reactions generally mature by 1 year of age.[1] Phase II reactions, also called synthetic or conjugation reactions, combine these byproducts with substances such as glucuronide, sulfate, or glycine. After Phase II reactions, the more polar metabolites are more readily excreted via the urine.[7] Phase II processes mature at a slower rate, for example, glucuronidation activity by 3 to 4 years of age.[1]

Hepatic Extraction of Drugs

Efficiency of drug removal by the liver (hepatic extraction ratio) is affected by hepatic blood flow, protein binding, and intrinsic metabolic activity. Hepatic clearance of a drug (CLh) describes the volume of blood from which the drug is completely removed per unit time, which is a function of hepatic blood flow and extraction ratio of drug, as follows:

$$CLh = Q \times \frac{C_i - C_o}{C_i}$$

where Q is hepatic blood flow, C_i is concentration of drug entering the liver, and C_o is concentration of drug leaving the liver. High clearance drugs include metoprolol, propranolol, lidocaine, nitroglycerin, and verapamil. For these drugs, clearance is greatly dependent on hepatic blood flow, necessitating dosage adjustment when diseases affect hepatic blood flow.[8]

Cytochrome P-450 Isoenzymes

Drug metabolism to pharmacologically inactive or less active compounds may occur in many tissues, although the greatest sites of drug metabolism are the liver and gastrointestinal tract through activity of specific drug-metabolizing enzymes, referred to as cytochrome P(CYP) 450 enzymes. These enzymes, present in highest concentrations in the liver, small intestine, kidney, lung, and brain, are responsible for drug metabolism, with more than 30 types of human enzymes identified to date. CYP enzymes are classified in families and sub-families based on amino acid sequences.

Intense interest is focused on these pathways, because observed genetic polymorphism affects drug metabolism and, therefore, effects. More than 90% of common medications are metabolized by seven isoenzymes: 3A4, 3A5, 1A2, 2C9, 2C19, 2D6, and 2E1.[1,7] Knowledge of patterns of drug metabolism through CYP-450 isoenzymes permits assessment of potential drug-drug interactions for prescribed medications.

Multiple factors affect individual CYP activity, including genetics and ethnicity, environmental factors such as nicotine and ethanol, and diseases.[7] For example, in cirrhosis, reduced CYP activity occurs through loss of func-tional tissue. CYP activity is reduced in inflammation and infection, increasing potential toxicity risk. CYP activity can also be affected through substances that inhibit activity either via simple competitive inhibition or as an irreversi-ble inhibition effect. Examples of irreversible inhibitors include clarithromycin and erythromycin, isoniazid, carbamazepine, irinotecan, verapamil, midazolam, fluoxetine, and grapefruit products including bergamottin.[7]

The CYP3A4 isoenzyme pathway is responsible for metabolism of the greatest number of drugs commonly used in clinical care, with sites of metab-olism in hepatocytes and intestinal mucosa as well as the duodenum and esophagus.[6] Approximately 40% of CYP3A4 activity is in the small intestine,[6] producing the "first pass" phenomenon of drug metabolism before systemic exposure and determining bioavailability of drugs, including opioids, calcium channel blockers, and β-blockers.

Common examples of drug substrates for the CYP3A4 family include cisapride, prednisone, cyclosporine, tacrolimus, quinidine, amiodarone, calcium channel blockers, many benzodiazepines, common "statins," lidocaine, car-bamazepine, and dextromethorphan.[9] Potent inhibitors of 3A4 activity include macrolide antibiotics, such as erythromycin, azole antifungals, and psychotropic agents such as sertraline, fluoxetine, and nefazodone. Isoenzyme activity may be affected by potent inducing compounds, including phenytoin, phenobarbital, and carbamazepine, as well as rifampin. Dramatic variations in CYP3A4 activity are documented, with 4-to 13-fold differences in clearance rates.[6]

The CYP2D6 isoenzyme pathway, affecting approximately 25% of drugs, demonstrates important variability based on genetic polymorphisms, with dextromethorphan as a marker of drug-metabolizing capacity. As many as 3 to 10% of the white and 0 to 2% of Asian and African American populations may demonstrate slowed rates of drug metabolism ("poor metabolizers") for substrates including opioids, tricyclic antidepressants, flecainide, fluoxetine, β-blockers, and mexilitine.[9] Inhibiting drugs include cardiovascular agents, such as amiodarone and quinidine; cimetidine; and psychotropic agents, such as fluoxetine, paroxetine, and sertraline. Again, enzyme induction is seen with concurrent use of phenytoin, phenobarbital, and carbamazepine.

The CYP2C isoenzyme pathway also demonstrates significant genetic variability caused by polymorphisms, potentially affecting approximately 15% of clinically useful drugs. Approximately 3 to 5% of whites, 18 to 23% of Asians, and 5% of African Americans demonstrate reduced CYP2C19 activity, increasing the risk of delayed drug metabolism and toxicity.[9] Substrates for this isoenzyme system include omeprazole, S-warfarin, propranolol, topiramate, and diazepam. Examples of drugs that may inhibit this system include fluconazole and potentially other azole antifungals, omeprazole, sertraline, fluoxetine, and isoniazid. Inducing substances include phenytoin, phenobarbital, and carbamazepine, as well as rifampin.

A fourth isoenzyme pathway responsible for metabolism of approximately 5% of drugs is the CYP1A2 system, with important substrates, including theophylline, R-warfarin, and caffeine, and notable inhibitors, including azole antifungals; macrolides, including erythromycin; fluvoxamine; paroxetine; and isoniazid.

Development of Metabolic Functionality with Age

Maturation of CYP-450 microsomal activity occurs at different ages and rates.[4–6] CYP activity is present at 30 to 60% of adult values in infancy[4,6] and each CYP-450 enzyme undergoes a unique maturation process. For example, CYP3A7 demonstrates greater expression in fetal liver and regresses to 10% after age 3 months and undetectable levels in adults.[3,4,6] CYP3A4 is reported to be expressed at 50% of adult values between the ages 6 to 12 months of age, with low activity in utero but rapid development within a week of life.[3,4,6] These lower levels of CYP3A4 in infancy may cause an inability to clear cisapride and, therefore, increase drug toxicity risk.[4]

CYP2C, involved in metabolism of warfarin, phenytoin, and diazepam, demonstrates 33% of eventual activity in the first month of life.[4] Interestingly, elevated CYP2C content has been reported in Sudden Infant Death Syndrome, with a possible role of pulmonary smooth relaxation by endogenous substances metabolized through this system.[4]

CYP1A2, involved in metabolism of acetaminophen, warfarin, caffeine, and theophylline, is low in neonates,[1] develops in 1 to 3 months,[3] and achieves 50% adult activity by age 1 year.[4] N-demethylation patterns of caffeine metabolism vary by age, with N3-demethylation more prominent in infants.[4] CYP2D isoenzymes involved in metabolism of β-blockers, codeine, captopril, and ondansetron increase in activity over several years of age, achieving 66% of adult values by that age.[4] Deficiency in infancy may contribute to adverse effects in infants of selective serotonin reuptake inhibitor (SSRI)-treated mothers.[1] CYP2E1 isoenzymes develop to 40% of adult values by age 1 year, with eventual adult values at 1 to 10 years.[4]

Age-dependent increases in drug clearance in children younger than 10 years of age are reported for many drugs when compared with clearance values in adults. The mechanism(s) for these observed differences have not been described.[3]

Phase II reaction functions also mature over time,[3] as exemplified by slowed development of acetyltransferase that limits accurate assessment of acetylation status until after several years of age.[4] Slowed glucuronidation activity may contribute to the observed toxicity of chloramphenicol in infants and may also determine detoxification of morphine in infancy[3] and in bilirubin metabolism.[4]

Development of glucuronidation activity to adult values has been reported to occur over widely variable time periods, from 3 months to older than 3 years of age.[4] Sulfate conjugation can be an alternative pathway of metabolism for morphine and acetaminophen during infancy.[4]

Drug-Drug Interactions

Drug interactions result from physical or chemical effects, pharmacokinetic competition, or as pharmacodynamic effects at receptor sites. These are considered adverse drug effects that are usually predictable and, ideally, avoidable. Although more than 100,000 drug interactions have been documented, only a subset of these are clinically significant because of potential for harm.[7] Glintborg et al. detected 476 potential drug interactions in 63% of a cohort of 200 elderly patients, although only 4.4% were classified as relative contraindications for use and none resulted in adverse events documented in patient records. Patients receiving multiple medications were at greatest risk for drug-drug interactions.[10] In approximately 46 million individuals, as reported by Malone et al., 2.5 million persons have been exposed to a drug-drug combination judged to be clinically important, with more women than men and more older individuals than younger individuals exposed. The highest prevalence of drug-drug interaction involved a nonsteroidal anti-inflammatory drug-warfarin exposure.[11] Data in pediatric populations are generally lacking, although Novak et al. reported a 3% incidence of serious drug-drug interactions in pediatric patients receiving chronic antiepilepsy drugs.[12]

Implications of CYP-450 Drug-Drug Interactions of Cardiovascular Drugs

The CYP-450 system may have significant effects on cardiovascular drug therapy. β-adrenergic-blocking agents, such as propranolol, metoprolol, carvedilol, and timolol undergo metabolism via the CYP2D6 pathway and would be affected by "inducers," such as rifampin, and "inhibitors," including quinidine, amiodarone, and cimetidine. Carvedilol is a racemic mixture of both R- and S-enantiomers, with metabolism by CYP2C9, CYP1A2, and CYP3A4, as well as CYP2D6; this complex pattern of metabolism may mitigate effects of inhibitor drugs on carvedilol.[13]

Although angiotensin-converting enzyme (ACE) inhibitor prodrugs may undergo metabolism via CYP-450 enzyme systems, no significant CYP-450-mediated drug-drug interactions have been documented. However, inhibitor compounds, such as fluconazole, and inducers, such as rifampin, may affect plasma concentrations of losartan, which undergoes transformation via CYP2C9 to an active metabolite.[13]

Calcium channel-blocking drugs are substrates for CYP3A4 and are, therefore, subject to significant drug-drug interactions. Decreased effectiveness of verapamil and nifedipine has been noted with rifampin, whereas increased bioavailability and potential toxicity may be seen when CYP3A4 inhibitors like azole antifungals or quinidine are used with members of this drug class. Conversely, drugs in this class such as diltiazem and verapamil may exert clinically significant inhibitory effects on cyclosporine metabolism through CYP3A4 and have been proposed as means to reduce cyclosporine dose requirements for potential cost savings. Diltiazem also may reduce metabolism of triazolam, midazolam, and methylprednisolone.[13]

Antiarrhythmic agents are also subject to important drug-drug interactions involving CYP-450 enzyme pathways, and agents in this class may act as substrates, inducers, or inhibitors of various isoenzymes. Quinidine, for example, undergoes metabolism through CYP3A4 pathways and may achieve higher serum levels in the presence of inhibitors, including azole antifungals and cimetidine, and lower levels with classic inducers, such as phenytoin and phenobarbital. In addition, quinidine may reduce codeine effectiveness by inhibiting CYP2D6 conversion to morphine. Disopyramide may be affected by cytochrome inducers such as rifampin and by inhibitors, including macrolides and human immunodeficiency virus (HIV) protease inhibitors.[9]

In addition to documented interactions with propranolol caused by hepatic blood flow, lidocaine is also affected by CYP-450 inducers such as rifampin and inhibitors such as HIV protease inhibitors, necessitating close monitoring of serum concentrations. Mexiletine, subject to rifampin-induced CYP2D6 metabolism, may also increase theophylline concentrations related to its inhibitory effects on CYP1A2. Flecainide toxicity may result from concurrent use of SSRIs that affect CYP2D6 pathways as well as amiodarone.[9]

Amiodarone demonstrates complex potential drug-drug interactions related to CYP-450 effects as well as other mechanisms. Amiodarone-related inhibition of CYP2C9 may result in toxicity during concurrent phenytoin, theophylline, or cyclosporine therapy, whereas phenytoin may decrease amiodarone concentrations and increase metabolite concentrations.[9]

Furanocoumarin(s), including bergamottin contained in grapefruit, may cause irreversible inhibition of intestinal CYP3A4 within 24 hours of ingestion of 200 to 300 ml juice; ingestion of fresh grapefruit may decrease CYP3A4 activity by 47% within several hours of ingestion.[14,15] Although initial recommendations included timing of medications several hours after ingestion of grapefruit products, inhibitory effects may continue for up to 72 hours. Variability in CYP3A4 between individual patients leads to variability in effect and lack of predictability because of this interaction. Pharmacokinetics of parenterally administered drugs, however, are unaffected.[14,15] High-dose consumption may also affect hepatic CYP3A4 enzymes.[14] Overall, grapefruit effects would be expected to increase oral bioavailability (and, therefore, effects) of drugs metabolized via CYP3A4 through decreased presystemic clearance.

Diverse cardiovascular agents have been documented as affected by grapefruit juice constituents. The HMG-CoA inhibitors, atorvastatin, simvastatin, and lovastatin have the greatest potential for enhanced bioavailability because of significant CYP3A4 intestinal metabolism, whereas pravastatin or fluvastatin do not rely on this pathway for metabolism. Dihydropyridines, such as felodipine, nicardipine, and nifedipine, are examples of calcium channel blockers that may demonstrate enhanced systemic bioavailability (1.5- to 4-fold), producing augmented effects on blood pressure, especially significant in the elderly. The angiotensin II type 1 inhibitor, losartan, is metabolized via CYP3A4 and CYP2C9 to its active metabolite; grapefruit juice may reduce conversion and, therefore, its therapeutic effects. Other agents that may be significantly affected include amiodarone, quinidine, sildenafil, and propafenone.[14,15]

Excretion

Drugs can be excreted through urine, bile, sweat, air, or other fluids. However, the most important routes are the bile and the kidney. The kidney is the major organ responsible for elimination of parent drug and/or metabolite, with renal excretion the product of glomerular filtration, tubular secretion, and tubular reabsorption. Factors affecting glomerular filtration include molecular size, protein binding, and number of functional nephrons. Tubular secretion of weak organic acids or bases occurs via active transport subject to competition with other substances. Tubular reabsorption of drugs occurs via active or passive transport in the distal tubule, and may be dependent on urine pH, urine flow rates, and drug properties, including ionization.

In pediatrics, glomerular filtration function is dramatically reduced in newborns,[5] with greater immaturity in premature infants when compared with full-term infants; increases in glomerular filtration rate (GFR) occur in the first weeks of life, reaching 50 to 60% of adult function by the third week of life,[1,3] and adult values by 8 to 12 months of age.[3] Premature infants show slower improvements of GFR when compared with full-term infants,[1] with continued reduced drug clearance despite chronological age. By 3 to 6 years of life, GFR values (expressed per kilogram) exceed adult values.[1] Therefore, drugs dependent on glomerular filtration will show reduced drug clearance through early infancy, more evident in premature infants, and likely require dosage reduction. However, during early childhood, higher daily doses are likely when corrected for weight and in comparison with adult doses because of increased GFR.

Tubular secretion rates are also reduced in neonates[1,3] and mature during the first year of life, reaching adult values by age 7 months[4] and maturing much later than glomerular filtration function.

The development of renal excretion pathways must be appreciated for appropriate prescribing of many drugs in infancy, especially when drugs with narrow therapeutic indices are administered, such as vancomycin and aminoglycosides. The use of therapeutic drug monitoring by measuring serum concentrations is helpful in guiding drug dosing to individualize therapy in infants and children.

Alterations in Pharmacokinetics in Disease States

Liver Disease

Pharmacokinetic changes and the need for dosing adjustments of cardiovascular drugs in the presence of liver disease have been extensively discussed.[8,16] Liver disease may produce significant changes in plasma protein binding, hepatic blood flow, and oxidative metabolism via CYP-450 isoenzymes. The need for dosing adjustment in the presence of liver diseases is most clearly evident when cirrhosis is present because of factors including variable CYP-450 activity and altered blood flow to functional hepatocytes.[8] CYP-450 activity may be decreased overall, but selectivity of enzyme systems may be present, with CYP1A2 susceptible to degree of liver damage as well as variable activity of CYP3A4. Other liver diseases, including chronic active hepatitis, do not uniformly affect hepatic drug elimination.[8] Unfortunately, in both liver disease and congestive heart failure (CHF), liver function test values are not indicative of altered drug metabolism and, thus, do not aid dosing adjustments.

Cardiovascular Agents in Liver Disease

The angiotensin II receptor antagonists may show significant alterations in pharmacokinetics and effects in the presence of liver disease. Losartan and its active metabolites achieve higher serum concentrations with lower plasma clearance rates (approximately 50%) and higher bioavailability in the presence of alcoholic cirrhosis. Valsartan also demonstrates significantly increased plasma concentrations with potentiation of effects in the presence of liver dysfunction with a two-fold increase in the area under the curve (AUC).[8]

ACE inhibitors, as prodrugs, may be affected in liver disease, with reduced conversion to active forms in the presence of liver cirrhosis. Lisinopril, as a non-prodrug form, may be preferred in this setting.[8,16]

Antiarrhythmic agents may also show significant alteration in pharmacokinetics in the presence of liver dysfunction, with serum concentrations useful for assessing patient-specific dosage adjustment. Dosage reduction may be required for quinidine in the presence of heart failure or cirrhosis. Serum level monitoring of procainamide is recommended because of variability in reported pharmacokinetic parameters by various investigators. Liver dysfunction may necessitate dosage alterations of lidocaine, mexiletine, disopyramide, tocainide, and flecainide. Dramatic dose reduction of propafenone by 50 to 80% is recommended in cirrhosis because of increased bioavailability, prolonged half-life, and increased plasma levels.[8]

Propranolol, a high-extraction drug, demonstrates significant alterations in pharmacokinetics in states of altered liver blood flow, as well as impaired activity of microsomal enzymes and inhibition of its own metabolism resulting from altered hepatic flow. Cirrhosis is associated with prolonged drug clearance rates. Additionally, propranolol has also been reported to reduce lidocaine clearance by 40 to 50%.[8]

Carvedilol demonstrates increased bioavailability, reduced drug clearance rates and increased Vd (280%) in the presence of cirrhosis, with initial dose reductions and careful monitoring recommended.[8]

Calcium channel blockers generally require dosage adjustments and close monitoring in the presence of cirrhotic liver disease because of multiple factors, including increased bioavailability, altered protein binding, prolonged drug half-lives, and decreased drug clearances. Verapamil, amlodipine, felodipine, isradipine, nimodipine, and nicardipine are examples of drugs in this class affected by liver disease.[16]

Renal Disease

The kidney is of great importance in excretion of drugs, both parent drug or metabolites, which may also possess significant pharmacological activity. Drug elimination may be dramatically altered in the presence of severe renal dysfunction and during supportive renal replacement therapies.

Although dosing guidelines may have been developed from studies in adults, pediatric-specific dosing adjustment data are generally unavailable. In these situations, dosage adjustments must be extrapolated from adult pharmacokinetic studies and patient-specific estimates of creatinine clearance using age-appropriate formulas. However, age-related differences in GFR, Vd estimates, and plasma protein concentrations, and drug affinity in infants and children limit our ability to rely on data from adult populations.[17,18]

Other changes in pharmacokinetic parameters exist that determine dosing regimens in the setting of renal dysfunction. Drug absorption may be reduced via oral administration routes through changes in gastric pH, use of phosphate binders and other antacids, and enhanced bioavailability because of reduced presystemic clearance in the intestine through decreased CYP-450 activity and altered P-glycoprotein drug transport.[19]

Drug distribution may be altered through decreased plasma protein-binding capacity caused by reduced plasma albumin concentrations, reduced albumin affinity, or the presence of compounds competing for drug binding sites, as well as elevations in α-1-AG. Changes in Vd may also be present because of fluctuations in body water, muscle mass, and adipose tissue.[19]

Although often overlooked in renal dysfunction, changes in drug metabolism in chronic renal disease exert important effects on drug clearance. Phase I hydrolysis and reduction reactions are decreased, as well as reduced activity of CYP2C9, CYP3A4, and CYP2D6. Phase II reactions through acetylation, sulfation, and methylation are also slowed. Renal metabolism can be significant, because renal tissue contains 15% of the metabolic activity of the liver and is involved in metabolism of acetaminophen, imipenem, insulin, isoproterenol, morphine, vasopressin, and other drugs.[19]

Renal dysfunction obviously reduces clearance of drugs that rely on glomerular filtration, tubular secretion, or both processes, and produces prolonged elimination rates. Also important is the role of delayed renal clearance of drug metabolites with pharmacological activity, such as allopurinol, cefotaxime, meperidine, midazolam, morphine, and propranolol.[19]

Drug Elimination During Dialysis Procedures

Drug removal during dialysis is influenced by many factors, including molecular weight, protein binding, Vd, water solubility, as well as technical influences of equipment (filter properties) and technique (blood flow, dialysate flow, and ultrafiltration rates). In patients receiving therapy with intermittent hemodialysis, estimation of residual renal function is important to avoid underestimation of dosing requirements. Pediatric-specific dosing guidelines should be used as a basis for estimating supplemental doses for drugs removed via hemodialysis.[17]

In continuous renal replacement therapies (CRRT) in children, dosage determination is best based on estimation of total drug clearance reflecting residual renal function, nonrenal clearance, and clearance via the CRRT circuit. Veltri et al. used pharmacokinetic data from previous investigators and/or extrapolated data to develop extensive guidelines for dosing of commonly used medications for pediatric patients with renal dysfunction or when undergoing intermittent hemodialysis or other CRRT therapies.[17]

Cardiovascular Drugs in Renal Disease

Numerous drugs demonstrate significant alterations in pharmacokinetics and/or pharmacodynamics in the setting of renal dysfunction. ACE inhibitors undergo significant renal clearance, with dosage adjustments required. However, fosinopril is an exception. Careful monitoring of serum electrolytes, especially potassium, and renal function is required. β-blockers, such as atenolol, nadolol, sotalol, and acebutolol, may also require dosage adjustment. Other antihypertensive agents and/or active metabolites, such as methyldopa, reserpine, and prazosin, may also accumulate in renal disease.[19]

Other cardiovascular drugs also require dosage adjustment. Digoxin demonstrates altered Vd (approximately 50% of normal) and both the loading dose and maintenance dose should be reduced with decreased renal clearance. Procainamide and its active metabolite n-acetyl-procainamide will accumulate to toxic concentrations in the presence of renal disease, necessitating dosage adjustment and close monitoring of serum concentrations of both antiarrhythmic agents.[19]

Congestive Heart Failure

In CHF, hypoperfusion of the liver and passive congestion of liver sinusoids can affect drug metabolism. Total hepatic blood flow is reduced proportional to cardiac output, with significant effects on high-extraction drugs, such as lidocaine. Additionally, depression of CYP-450 activity also has been reported in the presence of CHF, with improvement after effective treatment. As in liver disease, liver function test values are not indicative of altered drug metabolism and, thus, do not aid in dosing adjustments.[8]

Cardiovascular Drugs in CHF

Sokol et al. have also summarized the effects of CHF on important cardiovascular drug classes, although only limited data are available. ACE inhibitors, such as ramipril, may show higher peak concentrations and prolonged half-lives in the presence of severe CHF, although no significant changes are reported with lisinopril, captopril, or fosinopril.[8]

Antiarrhythmic agents may be affected in the presence of CHF. Close monitoring of serum levels of quinidine is recommended, because lower doses may be required because of reduced plasma clearance and higher serum concentrations. Variability in pharmacokinetics may occur also with procainamide, and close monitoring of serum procainamide and n-acetyl-procainamide concentrations and QTc is also recommended.[8]

As previously described, CHF may greatly affect lidocaine pharmacokinetics, with reduction in drug clearance correlated with cardiac output. Dosage reduction by 40 to 50% has been advocated, with close monitoring of serum levels. Reduction in loading doses associated with decreased Vd is also recommended. Doses of mexiletine, tocainide, flecainide, and amiodarone may also require adjustment in CHF.[8]

Critical Care Settings

Absorption

Redistribution of blood flow to central organs in shock states may reduce oral, sublingual, intramuscular, or subcutaneous absorption profiles of drugs. Additionally, use of vasoactive drug infusions may also affect drug absorption profiles indirectly through perfusion changes. Use of enteral feedings may result in altered absorption of drugs, as demonstrated for phenytoin, quinolones, and fluconazole.[20]

Distribution

Theoretically, changes in pH may alter drug ionization and affect tissue penetration. Changes in body fluid concentrations and shifts can more dramatically affect those drugs that demonstrate distribution through total body water, such as aminoglycosides, with expanded Vd values in fluid overload or "third spacing" of fluids (e.g., ascites or effusions) and contracted Vd with fluid depletion (e.g., with diuretics).[20] Increased cardiac output may also result in increased clearance of drugs. Plasma protein-binding changes, including decreased production of albumin and increased production of α-1-AG, may affect "free" (unbound) drug concentrations with increased free concentrations of acidic drugs, such as phenytoin, and reduced free concentrations of basic drugs, such as meperidine and lidocaine. Other drugs affected by protein-binding changes include fentanyl, nicardipine, verapamil, milrinone, and propofol.

Metabolism

Sepsis, hemorrhage, mechanical ventilation, and acute heart failure may affect drug metabolism through effects on hepatic blood flow and impact high-extraction drugs, including midazolam and morphine. Additionally, drugs such as vasopressin and α-agonists may detrimentally affect hepatic blood flow during critical care support. Phase I reactions via CYP-450 enzymes in drug metabolism may also be reduced in the presence of inflammatory mediators in acute stress.[20]

Excretion

The frequency of renal dysfunction in the critical care setting results in significant pharmacokinetic changes and dosage adjustments. Delayed renal clearance with resulting risk of toxicity necessitates careful assessment of renal function and resulting dosage adjustments using the many sources of dosing guidelines available from manufacturers, scientific literature, and drug dosing tables, as discussed above.

Pharmacogenomics

Pharmacogenomics is the study of inherited variation in drug disposition and response, and focuses on genetic polymorphisms. This new field in pharmaceutical science holds the promise of improved drug design and selection based on unique individual genetic patterns of drug disposition, improved drug dosing, and avoidance of unnecessary drug toxicity. Examples of applications of pharmacogenomics as described by Hines and McCarver include polymorphism of CYP2D6 and response to β-blockers, codeine and antidepressants, thiopurine methyltransferase and use of chemotherapeutic agents for pediatric leukemias, and response to corticosteroids and other drugs in pediatric asthma. Many issues remain in this field, including the ethics of genetic screening, validity of phenotype screening and associations, ethnicity, conduct of clinical trials, reasonable cost, patient autonomy, and practicality in clinical practice.[21]

Conclusion

Pharmacokinetic variations in drug handling between adults and infants and children are important determinants of effective and safe drug dosing and use. Knowledge of age-related differences in drug absorption, distribution, metabolism, and excretion may assist in anticipating potential differences to improve drug use and monitoring. It is particularly important to review the role of the CYP-450 enzyme system in metabolism for many common drugs used in pediatric therapy to anticipate possible changes in drug clearance caused by drug-disease or drug-drug interactions. There is, unfortunately, limited published experience describing pharmacokinetics of major cardiovascular drugs or the influence of liver or renal dysfunction or CHF in children, necessitating continued study and vigilance in drug use. However, knowledge of alterations of pharmacokinetics of major cardiovascular drug classes in adults in the setting of hepatic and renal disease and in the presence of CHF may assist rationale drug use in pediatrics. Finally, the field of pharmacogenomics holds promise as a science to enhance drug selection and safety in pediatric practice.

References

1. Tetelbaum M, Finkelstein Y, Nava-Ocampo AA, Koren G. Understanding drugs in children: pharmacokinetic maturation. Pediatr Rev 2005;26:321–327.
2. Pal VB, Nahata MC. Drug Dosing in Pediatric Patients. In: Murphy JE, ed. Clinical Pharmacokinetics, 2nd ed. Bethesda, MD: American Society of Health-System Pharmacists, Inc, pp. 439–465, 2001.
3. Kearns GL, Abdel-Rahman SM, Alander SW, Blowey DL, Leeder JS, Kauffman RE. Developmental pharmacology—drug disposition, action, and therapy in infants and children. N Engl J Med 2003;349:1157–1167.
4. Benedetti MS, Blates EL. Drug metabolism and disposition in children. Fund Clin Pharmacol 2003;17:281–299.
5. Alcorn J, McNamara PJ. Ontogeny of hepatic and renal systemic clearance pathways in infants. Clin Pharmacokinet 2002;41:1077–1094.
6. deWildt SN, Kearns GL, Leeder JS, van den Anker JN. Cytochrome P450 3A: ontogeny and drug disposition. Clin Pharmacokinet 1999;37:485–505.
7. Mann HJ. Drug-associated disease: cytochrome P450 interactions. Crit Care Clin 2006;22:329–345.
8. Sokol SI, Cheng A, Frishman WH, Kaza CS. Cardiovascular drug therapy in patients with hepatic diseases and patients with congestive heart failure. J Clin Pharmacol 2000;40:11–30.
9. Trujillo TC, Nolan PE. Antiarrhythmic agents. Drug Safety 2000;23:509–532.
10. Glintborg B, Andersen SE, Dalhoff K. Drug-drug interactions among recently hospitalized patients—frequent but most clinically insignificant. Eur J Clin Pharmacol 2005;61:675–681.
11. Malone DC, Hutchins DS, Haupert H, Hansten P, et al. Assessment of potential drug-drug interactions with a prescription claims database. Am J Health-Syst Pharm 2005;62:1983–1991.
12. Novak PH, Ekins-Daukes S, Simpson CR, Milne RM, Helms P, McLay JS. Acute drug prescribing to children on chronic antiepilepsy therapy and the potential for adverse drug interactions in primary care. Brit J Clin Pharmacol 2005;59:712–717.
13. Flockhart DA, Tanus-Santos JE. Implications of cytochrome P450 interactions when prescribing medication for hypertension. Arch Intern Med 2002;162:405–412.
14. Bailey DG, Dresser GK. Interactions between grapefruit juice and cardiovascular drugs. Am J Cardiovasc Drugs 2004;4:281–297.
15. Stump AL, Mayo T, Blum A. Management of grapefruit-drug interactions. Amer Family Physicians 2006;74:605–608.

16. Rodighiero V. Effects of liver disease on pharmacokinetics. Clin Pharmacokinet 1999;37:399–431.

17. Veltri MA, Neu AM, Fivush BA, Parekh RS, Furth SL. Drug dosing during intermittent hemodialysis and continuous renal replacement therapy. Pediatr Drugs 2004;6:45–65.

18. Joy MS, Matzke GR, Armstrong DK, Marx MA, Zarowitz BJ. A primer on continuous renal replacement therapy for critically ill patients. Ann Pharmacother 1998;32:362–375.

19. Gabardi S, Abramson S. Drug dosing in chronic kidney disease. Med Clin N Am 2005;89:649–687.

20. Boucher BA, Wood GC, Swanson JM. Pharmacokinetic changes in critical illness. Crit Care Clin 2006;22:255–271.

21. Hines RN, McCarver DG. Pharmacogenomics and the future of drug therapy. Pediatr Clin N Am 2006;53:591–619.

3. Inotropic and Vasoactive Drugs

Eduardo da Cruz and Peter C. Rimensberger

Pediatric patients with congenital cardiac defects or with acquired cardiac diseases may develop cardiovascular dysfunction[1–4]. In the context of cardiac surgery, the low cardiac output syndrome (LCOS) probably is the most important cause of morbidity and mortality in the immediate postoperative phase, particularly in newborns and infants[5,6]. Cardiovascular performance may also be affected in many other physiopathological circumstances, such as sepsis, endocrine, and metabolic or respiratory disorders. Regardless of the etiology of cardiovascular dysfunction in the pediatric population, medical treatment must be based on a comprehensive hemodynamic and pathophysiological appraisal[7].

The main physiological factors to be assessed by noninvasive and invasive clinical methods are *heart rate, contractility, preload,* and *afterload*. It is also crucial to keep in perspective the importance of the evaluation of and the balance between *systemic* and *pulmonary vascular resistances*, the appraisal of both *right- and left-sided cardiac function*, and the importance of *diastolic* disturbances.

Inotropic and vasoactive drugs are cornerstone therapies used to support the heart and the circulatory system in circumstances of documented or potential cardiovascular failure. Pharmacological management of cardiocirculatory dysfunction is complex and targets two main receptor sites, first, myocardial receptors and, second, systemic and pulmonary vascular receptors. Inotropic drugs (mainly catecholamines and phosphodiesterase inhibitors) play a vital role in myocardial and vascular performance[8–11]. Different issues have to be considered to choose the proper inotropes that could be used alone or in combination with systemic or pulmonary vasodilators (see Chapters 4 and 10). Among the selection criteria, there are a wide array of aspects, including the pathophysiology of the cardiac or circulatory dysfunction and the adverse effects (Figures 3-1 to 3-5) and drug interactions that might be deleterious or even fatal. Hence, it is essential to distinguish between the drug properties that support the heart and those that affect the peripheral circulation. The use of these drugs may be limited by significant increases in myocardial oxygen consumption, proarrhythmogenic effects, or neurohormonal activation. Moreover, it is crucial to know that down-regulation of β-adrenergic receptors may arise with prolonged use of catecholamines. Obviously, basic principles of common sense are required to choose rational combinations and obtain maximal effects with the lowest effective doses.

Vasoconstrictors are drugs that target the peripheral systemic and/or pulmonary circulation with more or less specific effects. Some of these drugs have an inotropic action; others act specifically on peripheral receptors. In the cardiovascular intensive care scenario, these drugs are mainly used for situations

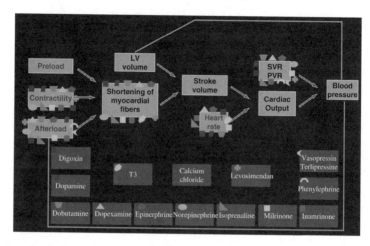

Figure 3-1. Inotropic and vasoconstrictive drugs.

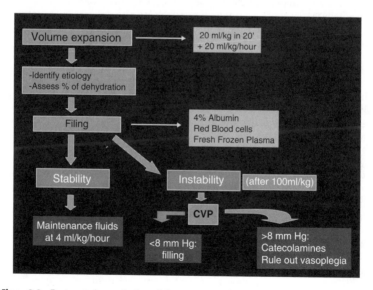

Figure 3-2. Treatment of acute circulatory failure: Hypovolemic shock.

of severe vasoplegia (low systemic vascular resistance) or else to antagonize a deleterious and marked vasodilator effect of other drugs[12, 13].

A combination of inotropic and vasoconstrictor drugs is often required in such circumstances (Figures 3-1 to 3-5).

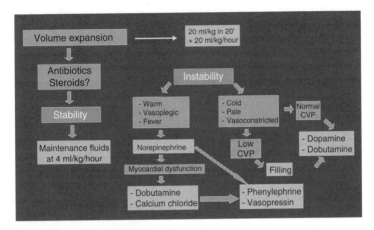

Figure 3-3. Treatment of acute circulatory failure (2).

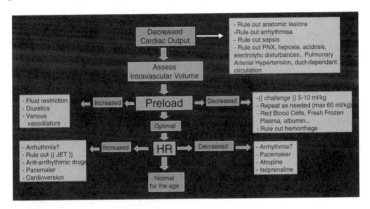

Figure 3-4. Treatment of acute circulatory failure: Cardiogenic shock (1).

Inotropic Agents

Digoxin

Indication

Digoxin is a cardiac glycoside used in the therapy of congestive cardiac failure and as an antiarrhythmic agent that decreases ventricular rate in selected tachyarrhythmias. Although still widely used, few clinical trials have provided evidence for a consistent clinical efficacy in the pediatric population. Taking into account the potential for toxicity and the lack of evidence-based data

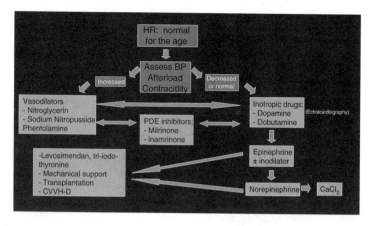

Figure 3-5. Treatment of acute circulatory failure: Cardiogenic shock (2).

supporting its use, digoxin is not currently a first choice for therapy of heart failure in children[14-19]. Paradoxically, digoxin is the most widely prescribed antiarrhythmic and inotropic agent.

Mechanisms of Action

Digoxin has a miscellaneous action. There are both direct (caused by binding to the Na^+-K^+ adenosine triphosphatase [ATPase] transport complex) and indirect (autonomic effects mediated by the parasympathetic nervous system) properties. First, by inhibition of the sodium and potassium ion movement across the myocardial membrane, digoxin increases the influx of calcium ions into the cytoplasm. In addition, it potentiates myocardial activity and contractile force by an inotropic effect. Second, digoxin inhibits ATPase and decreases conduction through the sinus and the atrioventricular (AV) nodes. Third, digoxin increases parasympathetic cardiac and arterial baroreceptor activity, which decreases central sympathetic outflow and exerts a favorable neurohormonal effect. However, evidence of increased contractility does not consistently correlate with clinical improvement.

Dosing

The following doses are recommended for patients with normal renal function. The loading dose is calculated and then half is administered initially, followed by one-quarter of the dose every 8 hours for two doses. The daily maintenance dose may be administered once or twice a day in patients younger than 10 years. The maintenance dose may be administered once a day in patients older than 10 years of age[16]. Parenteral administration is preferred in the intensive care setting

Table 3-1. Inotropic and vasoactive drugs

| | Oral/enteral | | I.V. | |
Age group	Loading dose	Maintenance dose	Loading dose	Maintenance dose
Neonates				
Preterm	20 µg/kg	5–8 µg/kg/day	15 µg/kg	3–4 µg/kg/day
Term	30 µg/kg	6–10 µg/kg/day	20 µg/kg	5–8 µg/kg/day
Infants/children				
1 mo to 2 yr	40–60 µg/kg	10–12 µg/kg/day	30–40 µg/kg	7.5–12 µg/kg/day
2–5 yr	30–40 µg/kg	7.5–10 µg/kg/day	20–30 µg/kg	6–9 µg/kg/day
5–10 yr	20–30 µg/kg	5–10 µg/kg/day	15–30 µg/kg	4–8 µg/kg/day
>10 yr	10–15 µg/kg	2.5–5 µg/kg/day	6–12 µg/kg	2–3 µg/kg/day
Adults	0.75–1.5 mg	0.125–0.5 mg/day	0.5–1 mg	0.1–0.4 mg/day

because oral absorption may be erratic because of congestive heart failure and because of the systematic use of antacids (Table 3-1).

Patients with renal failure require close monitoring of serum digoxin concentration. The loading dose should be reduced by 50% and the maintenance dose adapted to creatinine clearance (Cl_{cr}). If the Cl_{cr} is between 10 and 50 mL/min, administer 25 to 50% of the daily dose at normal intervals or administer the normal dose every 36 hours; if Cl_{cr} is below 10 mL/min, administer 10 to 25% of normal daily dose at normal intervals or administer the normal dose every 48 hours.

Pharmacokinetics

Onset of action:
  Oral: 0.5 to 2 hours
  Intravenous (I.V.): 5 to 30 minutes
Distribution phase: 6 to 8 hours
Maximum effect: oral, 2 to 8 hours; I.V., 1 to 4 hours
Protein binding: 20 to 30%
Metabolism: most of the drug is eliminated unchanged by the kidney
Half-life:
  Preterm neonates: 60 to 170 hours
  Full-term neonates: 35 to 45 hours
  Toddlers: 18 to 25 hours
  Children: 35 hours
  Adults: 38 to 48 hours
Elimination: 50 to 90% by renal excretion. *Note:* cannot be removed by dialysis

Digoxin Concentration Profile after an Oral Dose

Digoxin elimination is predominantly renal in nature (the fraction excreted unchanged in the urine is 50–90%) and is dependent on glomerular filtration and p-glycoprotein-mediated active tubular secretion. A long half-life of more than 30 hours (in normal renal function) results in steady-state concentrations taking at least 5 days to be achieved (it takes four half-lives to achieve greater than 90% of steady-state concentrations). In the elderly and in patients with renal impairment, elimination is diminished and the half-life prolonged. In these cases, the steady-state concentration may take several weeks to achieve. Measurement of concentrations before steady state is reached results in a falsely low estimate of the steady-state concentration, and inappropriate dose increases may result[20, 21].

Drug Interactions

Diuretics (furosemide, spironolactone, amiloride, triamterene), antiarrhythmics (verapamil, quinidine, amiodarone), calcium antagonists (verapamil, nifedipine, diltiazem), cholestyramine, neomycin, ketoconazole, itraconazole, cyclosporine, indomethacin, 3-hydroxy-3-methylglutaryl (HMG) CoA reductase inhibitors (atorvastatin), macrolide antibiotics (erythromycin, clarithromycin, roxithromycin), and benzodiazepines (alprazolam) may all increase the concentration or effects of digoxin.

Rifampicin and liquid antacids may decrease the concentration or effects of digoxin.

Adverse Effects

Cardiovascular: any new rhythm (especially those with induction of ectopic pacemakers and impaired conduction), sinus bradycardia, AV block, sinus block, atrial ectopic beats, bigeminy and trigeminy, atrial tachycardia with AV block, and ventricular arrhythmias. *Digoxin is contraindicated in patients with subaortic obstruction or hypertrophic cardiomyopathy, and in patients with severe electrolyte or acid-base disturbances (hypokalemia, or alkalosis) or metabolic disorders (hypothyroidism)*

Gastrointestinal: nausea, vomiting, diarrhea, abdominal pain, lack of appetite or intolerance to feeding

Metabolic: hyperkalemia in cases of toxicity

Central nervous system: fatigue, somnolence, drowsiness, vertigo, disorientation, asthenia

Neuromuscular and skeletal: neuralgia, myalgia

Ophthalmological: blurred vision, photophobia, diplopia, flashing lights, aberrations of color vision

Other: gynecomastia

Contraindications

Digoxin is contraindicated in patients with subaortic obstruction or hypertrophic cardiomyopathy, and in patients with severe electrolyte or acid-base disturbances (hypokalemia, alkalosis) or metabolic disorders (hypothyroidism). Acute rheumatic fever with pancarditis is a relative contraindication.

Poisoning Information

Digoxin therapeutic levels should be monitored in the following circumstances: suspicion of toxicity, therapeutic failure, lack of compliance with the prescribed dosing regimen, renal dysfunction, and concomitant administration of drugs that might modify digoxin concentrations[22]. *Levels should be drawn 6 hours after a dose or just before a dose*

Clinical signs or symptoms of poisoning: lack of appetite, nausea, vomiting, diarrhea, visual disturbances, arrhythmias

Electrocardiogram (EKG) signs of toxicity: premature ventricular contractions, ventricular bigeminy, AV block, supraventricular tachycardia, junctional tachycardia, ventricular arrhythmias

Laboratory: serum potassium, calcium, and magnesium levels and renal function should be closely monitored. Toxicity is usually associated with digoxin serum concentrations levels greater than 2 ng/mL (normal therapeutic range, 0.8–2 ng/mL).

Treatment: suspicion of poisoning justifies immediate hospital admission for specific antidote therapy with *digoxin immune Fab* in selected patients; in cases of life-threatening arrhythmias (ventricular dysrhythmia or supraventricular bradyarrhythmia unresponsive to atropine), hyperkalemia, hypotension, or acute ingestion of toxic doses of the drug. *Dose of digoxin immune Fab: serum digoxin (nmol/mL) × kilograms × 0.3, or milligrams ingested × 55 (if ingestion <greater than> 0.3 mg/kg).* Close monitoring of potassium levels (risk of hypokalemia) and of hemodynamic parameters is recommended. Digoxin serum levels might acutely rise, but the drug will be almost entirely bound to Fab fragments and, thus, unable to react with receptors. Therefore, this might be misleading laboratory information. Digoxin and Fab complexes will be slowly eliminated over approximately 1 week. *Other measures include:*

1. Administer Ipecac and charcoal, even several hours after ingestion of oral digoxin
2. If digoxin Fab are not immediately available and in cases of dysrhythmia:
   a. Ventricular tachyarrhythmia: consider using phenytoin, lidocaine, or bretylium
   b. Ventricular and supraventricular tachydysrhythmia: use propranolol
   c. Sinus bradycardia or AV block: use atropine or phenytoin
   d. Consider transvenous pacing and cardioversion, if necessary

Compatible Diluents

Oral digoxin should ideally be administered 1 hour before or 2 hours after meals to avoid erratic absorption secondary to diets rich in fiber or pectin content. Attention must paid to other drugs that might affect digoxin absorption.

I.V. digoxin may be administered undiluted or diluted in normal saline or in dextrose solutions over 10 minutes. More rapid I.V. administration can be hemodynamically deleterious.

Dobutamine

Indication

Dobutamine is an adrenergic agonist agent (sympathomimetic) with a potent β1 and mild β2 and α1 effect. Thus, it increases myocardial contractility, cardiac output and stroke volume (to a lesser extent than dopamine), and blood pressure by its strong inotropic and mild systemic and pulmonary vasodilator action[23–27]. When used after adequate fluid replacement, dobutamine increases urine output.

Mechanisms of Action

Dobutamine stimulates β1-adrenergic receptors, causing increased contractility and heart rate. It has minimal β2 or α effects. Its action is mediated by a direct β-adrenergic mechanism without associated norepinephrine release. Dobutamine also lowers central venous pressure and wedge pressure, but it has no selective effect on pulmonary vascular resistance[28,29]. It may also exert a beneficial effect on diastolic function. Dobutamine increases splanchnic blood flow in sepsis, particularly when combined with norepinephrine[30,31].

Dosing

Dobutamine is to be used as a continuous infusion and should be titrated within the therapeutic range and to the minimal effective dose until the desired response is achieved. It should be administered under comprehensive hemodynamic monitoring. Dobutamine should be avoided in hypovolemic patients.

Neonates: 2 to 15 µg/kg/min; Dobutamine is used in many neonatal intensive care units (NICUs) at higher doses than those used in infants and children[32–34]

Infants/children: 2 to 15 µg/kg/min; may be increased to a maximum of 30 µg/kg/min in some circumstances

Adults: 2 to 15 µg/kg/min; may be increased to a maximum of 30 µg/kg/min in some circumstances

Pharmacokinetics

Onset of action: 1 to 10 minutes
Maximum effect: 10 to 20 minutes
Metabolism: in tissues and the liver to inactive metabolites (by catechol-ortho-methyltransferase) followed by glucuronidation
Half-life: 2 minutes
Elimination: by the kidneys and in the bile

Drug Interactions

β-adrenergic blocking agents and general anesthetic drugs may interact with dobutamine.

Adverse Effects

Cardiovascular: sinus tachycardia, ectopic beats, palpitations, hypertension, chest pain, atrial and ventricular arrhythmias. *Particular attention should be paid to patients with hypertrophic subaortic stenosis*

Gastrointestinal: nausea, vomiting

Respiratory: dyspnea

Neuromuscular: paresthesia, cramps

Central nervous system: headache

Cutaneous/peripheral: dermal necrosis (extravasation), inflammatory disorders, phlebitis

Poisoning Information

Adverse effects caused by excessive doses or altered pharmacokinetics of dobutamine may be observed. In these circumstances, it is recommended to temporarily decrease or even withdraw the drug and treat symptomatically (significant individual variability). In the case of extravasation, local administration of either phentolamine or papaverine should be considered.

Compatible Diluents

Dobutamine is a stable product in various solutions, except for alkaline solutions, for 24 hours. It is recommended to dilute dobutamine with normal saline or dextrose, with a maximal concentration of 5 mg/mL. However, concentrations of up to 6 mg/mL have been used through a central line. Dobutamine must be administered into a central vein, except in urgent scenarios (and using lower concentrations), with an infusion device allowing proper and reliable titration. Dobutamine may be administered with other vasoactive drugs, muscle relaxants, lidocaine, potassium chloride, and aminoglycosides. Administration is to be avoided in the same I.V. catheter as some antibiotics (cefazolin or penicillin), sodium bicarbonate, heparin, ethacrynic acid, or furosemide. Pink discoloration of the product does not contraindicate its administration.

Dopamine

Indication

Dopamine is an adrenergic agonist agent (sympathomimetic) with moderate $\alpha 1$-, $\alpha 2$- and $\beta 1$-receptor stimulator effects and a mild $\beta 2$ effect. It also acts directly on dopaminergic (DA_1 and DA_2) receptors. Therefore, dopamine increases cardiac contractility and output and improves blood pressure[27–29,33]. When used after adequate fluid replacement, dopamine increases urine output. Its effects are dose dependant. In some postoperative cardiac pathologies, such as Fallot's tetralogy or in patients undergoing a Stage 1 Norwood procedure, high doses of dopamine may exert negative effects[35]. There is no evidence-based data supporting the use of dopamine as a renal protector, particularly after cardiac surgery[36,37].

Mechanisms of Action

Dopamine or 3-hydroxy tyramine, a precursor of norepinephrine, stimulates adrenergic and dopaminergic receptors and releases norepinephrine in the heart. Its effects are dose dependent: at *low doses*, dopamine exerts essentially a dopaminergic (DA_1 and DA_2) effect, which stimulates and produces renal, cerebral, coronary, pulmonary, and mesenteric vasodilation; at *intermediate doses*, dopamine stimulates both dopaminergic and β1-adrenergic receptors and produces cardiac stimulation, increasing heart rate and cardiac output; at *high doses*, dopamine stimulates primarily α-adrenergic receptors, inducing systemic and pulmonary vasoconstriction, and increased heart rate and blood pressure. Dopamine also increases mesenteric blood flow, although this may be associated with negative hepatic energy balance at high doses[30, 31].

Dosing

Dopamine is to be used as a continuous infusion and should be titrated within the therapeutic range and to the minimal effective dose until the desired response is achieved. Premature babies of younger than 30 weeks gestation may require higher doses to achieve the desired effect. Dopamine should be administered under comprehensive hemodynamic monitoring. Dopamine should be avoided in hypovolemic patients.

The hemodynamic effects are dose-dependent:

1 to 5 μg/kg/min (low dosage): increased renal and mesenteric blood flow, increased urine output
5 to 15 μg/kg/min (intermediate dosage): increased renal blood flow, heart rate, inotropic effect with increased cardiac contractility and output
More than 15 μg/kg/min (high dosage): predominant α-adrenergic effect with systemic vasoconstriction

If doses greater than 20 μg/kg/min are needed, and depending on the pathophysiological conditions, vasoconstrictors that are more specific (in case of vasoplegia [epinephrine, norepinephrine, vasopressin, or phenylephrine]) or vasodilators when there is a need to reduce ventricular afterload (nitroprusside, nitroglycerine, phentolamine) should be considered to avoid marked, undesirable side-effects

Neonates: 1 to 20 μg/kg/min; some centers tend to use higher doses as required, up to 50 μg/kg/min, in this age-group[32-34]
Infants/children: 1 to 20 μg/kg/min, maximal dose of 50 μg/kg/min in specific and exceptional scenarios
Adults: 1 to 20 μg/kg/min, maximal dose of 50 μg/kg/min in specific and exceptional scenarios

Pharmacokinetics[38, 39]

Onset of action: 5 minutes
Duration: less than 10 minutes
Protein binding: 30%

Metabolism: 75% in plasma, kidneys, and liver (to inactive metabolites by monoamine oxidase (MAO) and catechol-ortho-methyltransferase) and 25% in sympathetic nerve endings (transformed to norepinephrine)

Half-life: 2 minutes

Clearance: Dopamine clearance seems to be age-and dose-related and varies significantly, particularly in the neonatal period. It may have nonlinear kinetics in children and it may be increased by concomitant administration of dobutamine. A part of the drug may be excreted unchanged by the kidneys. Clearance may also be prolonged by renal and hepatic dysfunction.

Drug Interactions

MAO inhibitors, α-adrenergic agonists, β-adrenergic agonists, and oxytocic drugs may increase dopamine's effect.

Tricyclic antidepressant drugs, β-adrenergic blocking agents, and α-adrenergic blocking agents may decrease dopamine's effect.

Phenytoin may decrease dopamine's effect and cause serious hypotension, seizures, and bradycardia.

Hydrogenated anesthetics may decrease dopamine's effect and cause serious cardiac arrhythmias.

Adverse Effects

Cardiovascular: sinus tachycardia, ectopic beats, peripheral or pulmonary vasoconstriction (*must be used cautiously in patients with elevated pulmonary artery pressure or resistance*), widened QRS complexes, AV conduction abnormalities, ventricular arrhythmias, systemic hypertension (*contraindicated in patients with pheochromocytoma*), palpitations

Respiratory: dyspnea

Central nervous system: headache, anxiety

Gastrointestinal: nausea, vomiting

Genitourinary: decreased urine output (high vasoconstrictive doses)

Renal: azotemia (high vasoconstrictive doses)

Ocular: mydriasis

Cutaneous/peripheral: inflammatory changes, dermal necrosis, gangrene (extravasation), piloerection

Poisoning Information

Adverse effects caused by excessive doses or altered pharmacokinetics of dopamine may be observed. In these circumstances, it is recommended to decrease temporarily or even withdraw the drug and treat symptomatically (significant individual variability). In the case of extravasation, local administration of phentolamine or papaverine should be considered.

Compatible Diluents

Dopamine is to be infused diluted in dextrose with a maximal concentration of 3.2 mg/mL. However, concentrations of up to 6 mg/mL have been used through a central line. It must be administered into a central vein, except in urgent scenarios (using lower concentrations), with an infusion device allowing proper and reliable titration. Administration into an umbilical arterial catheter is not recommended. Dopamine must be protected from light. Solutions that are darker than usual (slightly yellow) should not be used. Dopamine is incompatible with alkaline solutions. It may be administered with other vasoactive drugs, muscle relaxants, and lidocaine.

Dopexamine

Indication

Dopexamine hydrochloride is a catecholamine that is structurally related to dopamine with marked intrinsic agonist activity at β2-adrenoceptors, lesser agonist activity at DA_1- and DA_2-receptors and β1-adrenoceptors, and an inhibitory action on the neuronal catecholamine uptake mechanism. Dopexamine displays beneficial hemodynamic effects in patients with acute heart failure and those requiring hemodynamic support after cardiac surgery, and these effects are substantially maintained during longer-term administration (≤24 h). Dopexamine reduces afterload through pronounced arterial vasodilation, increases renal perfusion by selective renal vasodilation, and evokes mild cardiac stimulation through direct and indirect positive inotropism. It has also been shown to improve gastrointestinal blood flow and to increase oxygen delivery in high-risk surgical patients[40, 41]. Dopexamine may be superior to other dopaminergic agents in patients at risk for splanchnic hypoperfusion[31, 40, 42, 43].

Mechanisms of Action

Dopexamine is an inhibitor of neuronal reuptake of norepinephrine. This pharmacological action results in an increase in cardiac output mediated by afterload reduction (β2, DA_1) and positive inotropism (β2), together with an increase in blood flow to vascular beds (DA_1), such as the renal and mesenteric beds. Dopexamine is not an α-adrenergic agonist and, therefore, does not cause vasoconstriction.

Dosing

Dopexamine is to be used as a continuous infusion and should be titrated within the therapeutic range and to the minimal effective dose until the desired response is achieved. It should be administered under comprehensive hemodynamic monitoring. Dopexamine should be avoided in hypovolemic patients.

> **Neonates, infants, and children:** 0.5 to 6 μg/kg/min, continuous I.V. infusion
> **Adults:** 0.5 to 6 μg/kg/ minute, continuous I.V. infusion

Pharmacokinetics

Onset of action: 10 to 15 minutes
Half-life: 7 to 11 minutes
Metabolism: extensively metabolized in the liver by MAO and catechol-ortho-methyltransferase
Clearance: 20 to 30 mL/kg/min
Elimination: in urine and bile (over 4 d) after methylization and sulfation

Drug Interactions

Dopexamine may enhance the effects of norepinephrine or dopamine.

Its effects may be decreased by MAO inhibitors or dopamine-receptor agonists.

Adverse Effects

Cardiovascular: sinus tachycardia, ventricular ectopic beats, arrhythmogenic potential, angina, chest pain, and palpitations. For this reason, it should be used cautiously in patients with ischemic heart disease
Central nervous system: tremor
Gastrointestinal: nausea, vomiting
Metabolic: hyperglycemia, hypokalemia; *cautious use in patients with hyperglycemia or hypokalemia*
Cutaneous: phlebitis (extravasation)
Other: reversible reduction in neutrophil and platelet counts

Poisoning Information

Adverse effects caused by excessive doses or altered pharmacokinetics of dopexamine may be observed. These effects are likely to be of short duration because of dopexamine's short half-life. In these circumstances, it is recommended to decrease temporarily or even withdraw the drug and treat symptomatically (significant individual variability). In case of extravasation, local administration of phentolamine or papaverine should be considered.

Compatible Diluents

Dopexamine is to be infused diluted in normal saline, dextrose, or Ringer's solutions, with a maximal concentration of 800 μg/mL. It must be administered into a central vein, except in urgent scenarios, with an infusion device allowing proper and reliable titration. It may turn slightly pink in prepared solutions during use. There is no significant loss of potency associated with this change. However, ampules should be discarded if their contents are discolored. Dopexamine should not be added to sodium bicarbonate or any other strongly alkaline solutions. Dopexamine must not be mixed with any other active agents before administration.

Epinephrine (Adrenaline)

Indication

Epinephrine or adrenaline is an α- and β-adrenergic agonist agent with multiple actions: sympathomimetic, hemodynamic, bronchodilator, nasal decongestant, and as an antidote for hypersensitivity reactions. It is, therefore, used to treat bronchospasm, cardiac arrest, situations with compromised cardiac contractility and chronotropy (LCOS, severe hypotension and bradycardia, myocardial dysfunction), anaphylactic reactions and anaphylactic or septic shock, upper airway obstruction and viral croup, open-angle glaucoma, and as a topical nasal decongestant[44-47]. This chapter concentrates on the hemodynamic and respiratory effects of the drug.

Mechanisms of Action

Epinephrine, the end product of endogenous catecholamine synthesis, is a potent stimulator of α1-, β1-, and β2-adrenergic receptors, resulting in relaxation of smooth muscle of the bronchial tree, cardiac stimulation, and dilation of skeletal muscle vasculature. It effects are dose-dependent: at *low doses*, it can cause vasodilation (β2-receptors); at *high doses*, it may produce vasoconstriction (α-receptors) of skeletal and vascular smooth muscle, with a subsequent increase of myocardial oxygen consumption. Moreover, epinephrine has marked metabolic effects, particularly in glucose homeostasis (hyperglycemia), and it may induce leukocytosis. Last, it decreases production of aqueous humor and increases its outflow within the eye.

Dosing

Via parenteral, intraosseous, or intratracheal administration, epinephrine is to be used as a bolus or as a continuous infusion and should be titrated within the therapeutic range to the minimal effective dose until the desired response is achieved[48-51]. Intratracheal administration may require larger doses, up to 10-fold greater than the I.V. doses, to be effective in cases of cardiac arrest. Epinephrine should be administered under comprehensive hemodynamic monitoring. It should be avoided in hypovolemic patients.

Neonates:
>   *I.V. or intratracheal:* 0.01 to 0.03 mg/kg of 1:10,000 solution, to be repeated every 3 minutes as required

Infants/children:
>   *Intramuscular (I.M.) or subcutaneous (S.C.) (anaphylactic reaction, asthma):* 0.01 mg/kg (maximum, 0.3 mg) of a 1:1000 solution
>   *I.V., or intraosseous:*
>   Bradycardia: 0.01 mg/kg (0.1 mL/kg) of a 1:10,000 solution (maximum, 1 mg), to be repeated every 3 to 5 minutes as necessary
>   Asystole: 0.01 mg/kg (0.1 mL/kg) of a 1:10,000 solution, to be repeated as required every 3 to 5 minutes; if intratracheal or ineffective, increase dosage to 0.1 mg/kg (0.1 mL/kg) of a 1:1000 solution and

repeat as required every 3 to 5 minutes; in refractory cases, may try a dose of 0.2 mg/kg (0.2 mL/kg) of a 1:1000 solution

Continuous I.V. infusion (shock): 0.1 to 1 μg/kg/min

Nebulization/inhalation (croup, bronchospasm): 0.25 to 0.5 mL of 2.25% racemic epinephrine solution or equivalent dose of L-epinephrine (10 mg of racemic epinephrine = 5 mg of L-epinephrine) diluted in 3 to 5 mL of normal saline

Adults:

I.M. or S.C. (anaphylactic reaction, asthma): 0.1 to 0.5 mg every 5 to 10 minutes

I.V. or intratracheal:

Asystole: 1 mg every 3 to 5 minutes as required; may escalate to 2 or 5 mg every 3 to 5 minutes if ineffective or if intratracheal

Continuous I.V. infusion: 1 to 10 μg/min

Pharmacokinetics

Onset of action:

I.V.: less than 1 minute

Inhalation: within 1 minute

S.C.: within 5 to 10 minutes

Absorption: active concentrations are not achieved by oral ingestion

Duration: very short, requiring a continuous infusion

Metabolism: hepatic (extensive) and renal (to a lesser degree) metabolism by the enzymes catechol-ortho-methyltransferase and MAO

Half-life: 2 to 3 minutes

Clearance: renal, once metabolized by hepatic glucuronidation and sulfation

Drug Interactions

β-blocking agents (propanolol, atenolol, esmolol), α-blocking agents (phentolamine, phenoxybenzamine, some phenothiazides), α- and β-blocking agents (labetalol), tricyclic antidepressants, and halogenated anesthetic gases may enhance the vasopressor and cardiac effects of epinephrine.

Adverse Effects

Cardiovascular: sinus tachycardia, hypertension, cardiac arrhythmias, angina, sudden death. Use carefully in cases of myocardial ischemia, because epinephrine may increase myocardial oxygen consumption

Respiratory: rebound bronchospasm or laryngospasm, rebound nasal congestion

Central nervous system: headache, anxiety, restlessness, cerebral hemorrhage (rare)

Gastrointestinal: nausea, abdominal pain; mesenteric vasoconstriction at high doses

Genitourinary: acute bladder retention

Renal: decreased renal blood flow

Neuromuscular and skeletal: tremor, weakness
Ocular: exacerbation of acute glaucoma
Metabolic: hyperglycemia (careful use in diabetic patients), thyroid disturbances
Cutaneous: tissue necrosis (extravasation)
Other: leukocytosis

Poisoning Information

Adverse effects caused by excessive doses or altered pharmacokinetics of epinephrine may be observed. In these circumstances, it is recommended to decrease temporarily or even withdraw the drug and treat symptomatically (significant individual variability). In case of extravasation, local administration of phentolamine or papaverine should be considered.

Compatible Diluents

Epinephrine should be protected from light. It is incompatible with alkaline solutions and may be administered with other vasoactive drugs and muscle relaxants. It must be administered into a central vein, except in urgent scenarios, with an infusion device allowing proper and reliable titration.

Dilutions

Inhalation/nebulization: with normal saline to a total of 3 to 5 mL
Intratracheal: with normal saline to a total volume of 3 to 5 mL, followed by several positive pressure ventilations
I.M.: use 1:200 or 1:1000 undiluted solutions
Parenteral:
   I.V. or intraocular (I.O.) injection: maximum concentration of 100 μg/mL (undiluted 1:10,000 solution)
   Continuous I.V. or I.O. infusion: dilute in normal saline or dextrose

Isoproterenol/Isoprenaline

Indication

Isoproterenol is a β1- and β2-adrenergicagonist agent that exerts a sympathomimetic and bronchodilator effect. It has a positive inotropic and chronotropic effect and a nonselective pulmonary and systemic vasodilator effect[52-56]. It is used to treat bronchospasm, ventricular dysrhythmias caused by AV nodal block, bradyarrhythmias and atropine-resistant bradycardia, third-degree AV block (it increases the spontaneous ventricular rate) until insertion of a pacemaker[57], pulmonary hypertension, right ventricular myocardial dysfunction with low cardiac output, and vasoconstrictive shock[46].

Mechanisms of Action

Isoproterenol stimulates β1- and β2-receptors, resulting in relaxation of bronchial, gastrointestinal, and uterine muscle. It increases heart rate and contractility and causes vasodilation of peripheral and pulmonary vasculature.

Dosing

Isoproterenol is to be used as a continuous infusion and should be titrated within the therapeutic range to the minimal effective dose until the desired response is achieved. It should be administered under comprehensive hemodynamic monitoring. Isoproterenol should be avoided in hypovolemic patients. Tachyphylaxis may occur with prolonged use, thus, withdrawal must be slow to prevent rebound phenomenon.

Neonates: 0.05 to 5 µg/kg/min
Infants/children: 0.05 to 5 µg/kg/min
Adults: 2 to 20 µg/min

Pharmacokinetics

Onset of action: immediate
Duration: a few minutes
Metabolism: by catechol-ortho-methyltransferase followed by conjugation in the liver, the kidneys, the lungs and various other tissues
Half-life: 2 to 5 minutes
Clearance: mostly in urine as sulfate conjugates

Drug Interactions

Enhanced effects or cardiotoxicity may be observed when administered with other sympathomimetic drugs.

β-adrenergic blocking agents may decrease isoproterenol effectiveness.
Isoproterenol may increase theophylline elimination.

Adverse Effects

Cardiovascular: flushing, ventricular arrhythmias, sinus tachycardia, hypotension, hypertension, palpitations, chest pain; isoproterenol is *contraindicated in digoxin intoxication and should be avoided in patients with low diastolic pressures caused by "diastolic steal," in patients with unoperated tetralogy of Fallot, and in patients with subaortic obstruction*
Central nervous system: restlessness, anxiety, nervousness, headache, dizziness, insomnia, vertigo
Endocrine and metabolic: parotid gland swelling, careful use in patients with diabetes and hyperthyroidism
Gastrointestinal: heartburn, nausea, vomiting, dyspepsia, dry mouth and throat, xerostomia

Neuromuscular and skeletal: weakness, tremor

Others: diaphoresis, exacerbation of acute glaucoma, urinary retention caused by prostatic hypertrophy

Poisoning Information

Adverse effects caused by excessive doses or altered pharmacokinetics of isoproterenol may be observed. In these circumstances, it is recommended to decrease temporarily or even withdraw isoproterenol and treat symptomatically (with significant individual variability).

Compatible Diluents

Isoproterenol may be diluted in normal saline or in dextrose to a maximal concentration of 20 μg/mL. It should be administered into a central vein whenever possible, with an infusion device allowing proper and reliable titration. Concentrations of 30 μg/mL have been used if infused through a central line.

Norepinephrine (Noradrenaline)

Indication

Norepinephrine or noradrenaline is an adrenergic agonist agent with potent α-adrenergic and weaker sympathomimetic (β1) action. It is used for the treatment of persistent cardiogenic or vasoplegic (distributive) shock in combination with dobutamine, dopamine, or epinephrine and as an alternative to phenylephrine in refractory hypoxic spells in patients with unoperated tetralogy of Fallot[58–62].

Mechanisms of Action

Norepinephrine, a precursor of epinephrine, stimulates α-adrenergic (strong action) and β1-receptors (mild action), inducing significant systemic vasoconstriction that can increase blood pressure and coronary perfusion. α effects are predominant to β effects, with more intense vasoconstriction than inotropic or chronotropic action, which explains why the effect on cardiac contractility and heart rate or on cardiac output is less pronounced.

Dosing

Norepinephrine is to be used as a continuous infusion and should be titrated within the therapeutic range to the minimal effective dose until the desired response is achieved. It should be administered under comprehensive hemodynamic monitoring. Norepinephrine should be avoided in hypovolemic patients.

Neonates: 0.05 to 2.0 μg/kg/min
Infants/children: 0.05 to 2.0 μg/kg/min

Adults: 0.5 to 10.0 µg/min; may be increased up to 30 µg/min in refractory cases

Pharmacokinetics

Onset of action: almost immediate
Duration: very short, requiring a continuous infusion
Metabolism: rapidly metabolized by catechol-ortho-methyltransferase and MAO
Half-life: 1 to 2 minutes
Clearance: by renal excretion (80 to 95% as inactive epinephrine metabolites)

Drug Interactions

Atropine sulphate, tricyclic antidepressant drugs, MAO inhibitors, antihistamines, guanethidine, ergot alkaloids, and methyldopa may enhance the effects of norepinephrine

Adverse Effects

Cardiovascular: palpitations, sinus tachycardia, reflex bradycardia, cardiac arrhythmias, hypertension, chest pain
Respiratory: dyspnea
Central nervous systems: headache, anxiety
Endocrine and metabolic: hyperglycemia, uterine contractions
Gastrointestinal: nausea, vomiting; may induce mesenteric vasoconstriction
Cutaneous and peripheral: inflammatory changes, dermal necrosis (extravasation)
Others: diaphoresis, excessive peripheral vasoconstriction

Poisoning Information

Adverse effects caused by excessive doses or altered pharmacokinetics of norepinephrine may be observed. In these circumstances, it is recommended to decrease temporarily or even withdraw the drug and treat symptomatically (significant individual variability). In case of extravasation, local administration of phentolamine or papaverine should be considered.

Compatible Diluents

Norepinephrine is unstable in alkaline solutions and should, therefore, be diluted in dextrose or at least in a half-saline solution (e.g., a 1:1 mixture of normal saline and 5% dextrose in water) with a maximal concentration between 4 and 16 µg/mL (in case of severe fluid restriction). Concentrations as high as 60 µg/mL have been used if infused through a central line. Norepinephrine must be administered into a central vein, except in urgent scenarios (in which lower concentrations should be used) with an infusion device allowing proper and reliable titration.

Phosphodiesterase Inhibitors

Inamrinone/Amrinone

Indication   Inamrinone (or amrinone) is a type III phosphodiesterase enzyme (PDE) inhibitor used for the treatment of low cardiac output status (myocardial dysfunction after cardiopulmonary bypass, cardiomyopathy) and is particularly useful in patients who have been refractory to conventional inotropic and vasodilator therapies. It is also used as an adjunctive therapy for treatment of pulmonary hypertension[63-66].

Mechanisms of Action   Inamrinone is a bipyridine derivative that inhibits phosphodiesterase III, thus, increasing cyclic AMP (cAMP) by decreasing the breakdown of cAMP to AMP. This potentiates delivery of calcium to myocardial contractile units resulting in a positive inotropic effect; however, it may produce a negative inotropic effect in the neonatal myocardium. PDE III inhibition also results in relaxation of vascular smooth muscle, inducing vasodilation while concomitantly reducing myocardial oxygen consumption.

Dosing   Inamrinone may be used as a bolus followed by a continuous infusion, and should be titrated within the therapeutic range and to the minimal effective dose until the desired response is achieved. It should be administered under comprehensive hemodynamic monitoring. Inamrinone should be avoided in hypovolemic patients.

Hypotension may occur with the loading dose, and many practitioners do not systematically administer the bolus dose, to avoid this complication. If hypotension occurs, treat the patient with 5 to 10 mL/kg of normal saline I.V. and position the patient head down. If hypotension persists, administer a systemic vasopressor and stop the loading dose. Total daily dose should not exceed 10 mg/kg. *Pharmacokinetic studies are not conclusive to define dosing guidelines in pediatric patients[67, 68]. There is no evidence-based data documenting either the safety or effectiveness of long-term treatment (<greater than>48 h) with this drug.*

> **Neonates:** I.V. bolus of 0.75 mg/kg over 3 minutes (may be necessary to repeat the dose after 30 min); loading dose may be increased up to 1 mg/kg over 5 minutes and repeated up to two times; I.V. continuous maintenance dose of 3 to 5 µg/kg/min
> **Infants/children:** I.V. bolus of 0.75 mg/kg over 3 minutes (may be necessary to repeat the dose after 30 min); loading dose may be increased up to 1 mg/kg over 5 minutes and repeated up to two times; I.V. continuous maintenance dose of 5 to 10 µg/kg/min
> **Adults:** I.V. bolus of 0.75 mg/kg over 3 minutes (may be necessary to repeat the dose after 30 min); loading dose may be increased up to 1 mg/kg over

5 minutes and repeated up to two times; I.V. continuous maintenance dose of 5 to 10 µg/kg/min

Pharmacokinetics

Onset of action: 2 to 5 minutes
Maximum effect: within 10 minutes
Duration: 30 minutes to 2 hours (dose-dependent)
Distribution: volume of distribution (Vd):
  Neonates: 1.8 L/kg
  Infants and children: 1.6 L/kg
  Adults: 1.2 L/kg
Protein binding: 10 to 50%
Metabolism: in the liver into several metabolites by glucuronidation, acetylation, or conjugation (glutathione, N-acetate, N-glycolyl, N-glucuronide, O-glucuronide)
Half-life:
  Neonates younger than 1 week: 12 hours
  Neonates 1 to 2 weeks: 22 hours
  Infants younger than 38 weeks: 6.8 hours
  Children: 2.2 to 10 hours
  Adults: 6 hours
Clearance: in urine as metabolites (60 to 90%) and unmodified drug (10 to 40%)

Drug Interactions   Dosage reduction of diuretics (significant hypovolemia) and of disopyramide (hypotension) may be required.

Adverse Effects

Cardiovascular: hypotension, ventricular and supraventricular arrhythmias (reported mostly in adults); inamrinone may exacerbate a preexisting ventricular ectopy or myocardial ischemia
Gastrointestinal: nausea, vomiting, abdominal pain, anorexia
Hematological: reversible, dose-related thrombocytopenia in approximately 2.5% of patients[69]. This is more likely to occur in patients with a higher total dose, longer duration of infusion, high plasma concentrations of N-acetylamrinone (inamrinone metabolite) and higher plasma ratios of N-acetylamrinone to inamrinone. Eosinophilia (idiosyncratic hypersensitivity reaction) may also occur
Hepatic: hepatotoxicity; inamrinone should be discontinued if a significant increase in liver enzymes is documented

Poisoning Information   Adverse effects caused by excessive doses or altered pharmacokinetics of inamrinone may be observed. In these circumstances, it is recommended to decrease temporarily or even withdraw the drug and treat symptomatically (significant individual variability).

Compatible Diluents   Inamrinone should be administered into a central vein, except in urgent scenarios, with an infusion device allowing proper and reliable

titration. It must be diluted only with normal saline or half saline to a concentration of 1 to 3 mg/mL; although incompatible with dextrose-containing solutions, it may be administered into a Y-site with dextrose infusions. It is also incompatible with sodium bicarbonate and furosemide.

Milrinone

Indication   Milrinone is a type III PDE inhibitor used for the short-term parenteral treatment of acutely decompensated cardiac failure and of postoperative LCOS[70], for the prevention of LCOS[71-73] and for long-term infusion therapy in patients awaiting transplantation[74-76]. Milrinone has also been used as an aerosolized drug to treat pulmonary hypertension in pretransplantation patients[77].

Mechanisms of Action   Milrinone is an analog of inamrinone that inhibits phosphodiesterase III, thus, increasing cAMP. This potentiates the delivery of calcium to myocardial contractile units, resulting in a positive inotropic effect, including in newborns, in whom it has been demonstrated to improve cardiac index and to lower filling pressures, systemic and pulmonary arterial pressures, and vascular resistance. It induces an increase in cardiac output and preserves normal myocardial oxygen consumption. Moreover, it results in relaxation of vascular smooth muscle producing vasodilation, predominantly systemic. It may also produce diastolic relaxation and reduce ventricular preload.

Dosing   Milrinone may be used as a bolus or as a continuous infusion and should titrated within the therapeutic range and to the minimal effective dose until the desired response is achieved. It should be administered under comprehensive hemodynamic monitoring. Hypotension may occur with the loading dose, and many practitioners do not systematically administer the bolus dose to avoid this complication. If significant hypotension occurs while administering the loading dose, treat the patient with 5 to 10 mL/kg I.V. of normal saline and reduce the infusion rate. If hypotension persists, suspend the loading bolus and consider administering one dose of a vasopressor[78-81].

> **Neonates, infants, and children:** I.V. loading dose of 50 µg/kg over a period of at least 15 minutes, followed by a continuous maintenance dose of 0.25 to 1 µg/kg/min
>
> **Adults:** I.V. loading dose of 50 µg/kg over a period of 10 to 15 minutes, followed by a continuous maintenance dose of 0.375 to 1 µg/kg/min; maximum daily dose of 1.13 mg/kg
>
> **Renal impairment:** doses must be adjusted to Cl_{cr}, as follows:
>
> Cl_{cr} 50 mL/min/1.73 m²: 0.43 µg/kg/min
> Cl_{cr} 40 mL/min/1.73 m²: 0.38 µg/kg/min
> Cl_{cr} 30 mL/min/1.73 m²: 0.33 µg/kg/min
> Cl_{cr} 20 mL/min/1.73 m²: 0.28 µg/kg/min
> Cl_{cr} 10 mL/min/1.73 m²: 0.23 µg/kg/min
> Cl_{cr} 5 mL/min/1.73 m²: 0.2 µg/kg/min

Pharmacokinetics

Onset of action: 5 to 15 minutes
Maximum effect: within 20 minutes
Half-life: 3 hours
Duration: 30 minutes to 2 hours (dose dependent)
Distribution: V_d β:
  Neonates: unknown
  Infants: 0.9 ± 0.4 L/kg (after cardiac surgery)
  Children: 0.7 ± 0.2 L/kg (after cardiac surgery)
  Adults: 0.3 ± 0.1 L/kg
Protein binding: 70%
Metabolism: Milrinone is excreted unchanged
Half-life (prolonged with of renal impairment):
  Infants: 3.1 ± 2 hours (after cardiac surgery)
  Children: 1.86 ± 2 hours (after cardiac surgery)
  Adults: 1.69 ± 0.18 hours (after cardiac surgery)
Clearance (decreased with renal impairment): excreted in urine as unchanged drug (83%) and glucuronide metabolite (12%). Age-dependent clearance:
  Infants: 3.8 ± 1 mL/kg/min (after cardiac surgery)
  Children: 5.9 ± 2 mL/kg/min (after cardiac surgery)
  Adults: 2 ± 0.7 mL/kg/min (after cardiac surgery)

Drug Interactions   Milrinone interacts with furosemide, producing a precipitate.

Adverse Effects

  Cardiovascular: ventricular and supraventricular arrhythmias (in adult patients), hypotension, angina, chest pain; must be used with caution in patients with background of atrial fibrillation or flutter, ventricular arrhythmia, and right or left outflow tract obstruction
  Respiratory: bronchospasm
  Central nervous system: headache
  Endocrine and metabolic: hypokalemia
  Hematological: thrombocytopenia (0.4%)
  Hepatic: increased liver enzymes
  Neuromuscular and skeletal: tremor
  Renal: careful administration and dosage adjustment in patients with renal dysfunction

Poisoning Information   Adverse effects caused by excessive doses or altered pharmacokinetics of milrinone may be observed. In these circumstances, it is recommended to decrease temporarily or even withdraw the drug and treat symptomatically (significant individual variability).

Compatible Diluents   Milrinone is compatible with normal saline, half-saline, and dextrose solutions, with a maximum recommended concentration of 200 µg/mL. Concentrations as high as 1000 µg/mL have been infused through a central line. It should be administered into a central vein, except in urgent scenarios (in which lower concentrations should be used), with an infusion device allowing proper and reliable titration.

Vasoactive Agents

Vasopressin

Indication

Vasopressin, or 8-arginine vasopressin, is an antidiuretic hormone analog used for the treatment of diabetes insipidus, acute massive hemorrhage of the gastrointestinal tract or esophageal varices, and ventricular fibrillation or tachycardia refractory to initial defibrillation[82, 83] (in adults). Although recommended for severe vasoplegic or distributive shock, there is a lack of adequate randomized, controlled trials providing evidence-based data confirming its usefulness[12, 84–95]. It may be useful to treat refractory hypotension induced by oral hypotensive drugs[96]. This section primarily discusses the two latest indications that are more likely to occur in the pediatric cardiovascular intensive care arena.

Mechanisms of Action

Vasopressin binds to AVPR1 receptors in vascular smooth muscle, inducing the activation of phospholipase C and an increase in intracellular calcium concentration. The Ca^{2+} ions promote interactions between actin and myosin. This produces vascular contraction. In the kidneys, vasopressin increases cAMP, which increases water permeability at the distal convoluted tubule and collecting duct, resulting in decreased urine volume and increased urine osmolality. It also increases peristalsis by direct smooth muscle stimulation. This causes vasoconstriction primarily of small arterioles and capillary vessels. Vasopressin may compromise mesenteric blood flow, and some studies suggest its use concomitantly with dobutamine (with or without norepinephrine) to antagonize this effect. It also stimulates the production of factor VIIIc and Von Willebrand factor.

Dosing

Vasopressin is to be administered exclusively parenterally as a bolus or as a continuous infusion and should be titrated within the therapeutic range and to the minimal effective dose until the desired response is achieved. It should be administered under comprehensive hemodynamic monitoring. Furthermore, fluid intake and output, urine specific gravity, and urine and serum osmolality should be carefully monitored.

Diabetes Insipidus

Children:
  I.M., I.V., or S.C.: 2.5 to 10 units, two to four times a day
  Continuous I.V. infusion: 0.5 milliunits (0.0005 units)/kg/h, double the dose as required to a maximum of 10 milliunits (0.01 units)/kg/h

Adults:
I.M., I.V., or S.C. (maximum 60 units/day): 5 to 10 units, two to four times a day
Continuous I.V. infusion: 0.5 milliunits (0.0005 units)/kg/h, double the dose as required to a maximum of 10 milliunits (0.01 units)/kg/h

Vasoplegic Shock

Children: 0.0002 to 0.003 units/kg/min
Adults: 40 units, I.V

Gastrointestinal Bleeding

Children: 0.002 to 0.005 units/kg/min I.V. continuous infusion, titrate as needed to a maximum dose of 0.01 units/kg/min. After 12 hours of stability, withdraw over 24 to 48 hours
Adults: 0.2 to 0.4 units/min I.V. continuous infusion; titrate as required to a maximum dose of 0.9 units/min. After 12 hours of stability, withdraw over 24 to 48 hours

Ventricular Fibrillation or Tachycardia Unresponsive to Initial Defibrillation

Adults: a single dose of 40 units, I.V.

Pharmacokinetics

Onset of action: 1 hour
Duration: 2 to 8 hours
Metabolism: most of the drug is rapidly metabolized in the liver and kidneys
Protein binding: 10 to 40%
Half-life: 10 to 20 minutes

Drug Interactions

Chlorpropamide, carbamazepine, hydrocortisone, clofibrate, and tricyclic antidepressants may increase vasopressin effect.

Demeclocycline, heparin, lithium, epinephrine, and alcohol may decrease vasopressin effect.

Adverse Effects

Cardiovascular: hypertension, bradycardia, arrhythmia, venous thrombosis, vasoconstriction, angina, heart block, cardiac arrest (all of the above with high doses); pallor
Central nervous system: vertigo, headache, fever, seizures (careful use in case of background of epileptic activity)

Cutaneous: tissue necrosis (extravasation), urticaria

Endocrine and metabolic: water intoxication, hyponatremia

Gastrointestinal: abdominal cramps, nausea, vomiting, diarrhea; vasopressin may induce vasoconstriction of the splanchnic region that may be compensated by dobutamine[97]

Neuromuscular and skeletal: tremor

Respiratory: wheezing, bronchospasm

Renal: careful use in patients with renal dysfunction, chronic nephritis

Hepatic: patients with chronic liver disease might require a downward dose adjustment

Others: diaphoresis

Poisoning Information

Adverse effects caused by excessive doses or altered pharmacokinetics of vasopressin may be observed. In these circumstances, it is recommended to decrease temporarily or even withdraw the drug and treat symptomatically (significant individual variability). In case of extravasation, local administration of phentolamine or papaverine should be considered.

Compatible Diluents

I.V. vasopressin may be diluted in normal saline or in dextrose solutions to a final concentration of 0.1 to 1 units/mL. I.M. and S.C. vasopressin is to be administered without further dilution. It should be administered into a central vein, except in urgent scenarios, with an infusion device allowing proper and reliable titration.

Phenylephrine

Indication

Phenylephrine is an α-adrenergic agonist agent with a sympathomimetic effect in various systems, mainly circulatory, ophthalmic, and nasal. In the cardiovascular patient, it is used as a pure vasoconstrictor drug to treat hypotension and low vascular resistance in distributive shock[98–100], to treat supraventricular arrhythmias[101–103], and it is particularly useful for the treatment of hypoxic spells in tetralogy of Fallot patients unresponsive to sedation, volume loading, and/or β-blockade[104, 105]. It may also be used as a vasoconstrictor in regional anesthesia, for symptomatic relief of nasal and nasopharyngeal mucosal congestion, and as a mydriatic agent for ophthalmic procedures.

Mechanisms of Action

Phenylephrine is a potent α agonist (α-adrenergic stimulator) with a very mild β-adrenergic activity. Therefore, it produces systemic arterial vasoconstriction, causes vasoconstriction of the nasal and conjunctival arterioles, and stimulates the dilator muscle of the pupil producing mydriasis.

Dosing

Phenylephrine is to be used as a bolus or as a continuous infusion and should be titrated within the therapeutic range and to the minimal effective dose until the desired response is achieved. It should be administered under comprehensive hemodynamic monitoring. The following doses are exclusively described for cardiovascular purposes.

Severe Hypotension, Hypoxic Spells in Tetralogy of Fallot, and Vasoplegic Shock

Neonates, infants, and children:
   I.M./S.C.: 0.1 mg/kg/dose (maximum 5 mg) every 1 to 2 hours as required
   I.V. bolus: 5 to 20 μg/kg/dose every 15 to 20 minutes as required
   I.V. continuous infusion: 0.1 to 0.5 μg/kg/min titrated to effect
Adults:
   I.M./S.C.: 2 to 5 mg/dose (maximum 5 mg) every 1 to 2 hours as required
   I.V. bolus: 0.1 to 0.5 mg/dose every 15 to 20 minutes as required
   I.V. continuous infusion: 40 to 180 μg/min titrated to effect

Paroxysmal Supraventricular Tachycardia

Children: 5 to 10 μg/kg I.V., over 30 seconds
Adults: 0.25 to 0.5 mg I.V., over 30 seconds

Pharmacokinetics

Onset of action:
   I.M.: 10 to 15 minutes
   I.V.: immediate
   S.C.: 10 to 15 minutes
Duration:
   I.M.: 30 minutes to 2 hours
   I.V.: 15 to 20 minutes
   S.C.: 1 hour
Metabolism: in the liver and the intestines by MAO
Half-life: 2.5 hours
Elimination: not elucidated

Drug Interactions

Oxytocic drugs, MAO inhibitors, guanethidine, and bretylium may increase the effect of phenylephrine.

   Sympathomimetic agents and halogenated anesthetics may increase the effect of phenylephrine and cause tachycardia or arrhythmia.

α- and β-adrenergic blocking agents may decrease the effect of phenylephrine.

Adverse Effects

Cardiovascular: hypertension, angina, severe reflex sinus bradycardia, arrhythmias, severe peripheral vasoconstriction. Phenylephrine is contraindicated in cases of severe hypertension, pheochromocytoma, ventricular arrhythmias, and myocardial disease

Respiratory: dryness, sneezing, rebound nasal congestion, dyspnea

Central nervous system: restlessness, nervousness, headache, anxiety, dizziness

Cutaneous: dermal necrosis (extravasation), skin blanching, piloerection

Neuromuscular and skeletal: tremor

Ocular: blurred vision, lacrimation, photophobia, stinging. Phenylephrine is contraindicated in cases of narrow-angle glaucoma

Gastrointestinal: Phenylephrine is contraindicated in cases of pancreatitis, hepatitis, and mesenteric vascular disease[106, 107]

Renal: Phenylephrine may reduce renal flow and urine output

Poisoning Information

Adverse effects caused by excessive doses or altered pharmacokinetics of phenylephrine may be observed. In these circumstances, it is recommended to decrease temporarily or even withdraw the drug and treat symptomatically (significant individual variability). In case of extravasation, local administration of phentolamine or papaverine should be considered.

Compatible Diluents

Phenylephrine is compatible with normal saline, dextrose solutions, and Ringer's lactate. For I.V. boluses, dilute 1 mg/mL (add 1 mL to 9 mL of diluting solution); recommended continuous infusion concentrations are 20 to 60 µg/mL. It should be administered into a central vein, except in urgent scenarios, with an infusion device allowing proper and reliable titration.

Metaraminol

Indication

Metaraminol, also called hydroxynorephedrine or metaradrine, is an α-adrenergic agonist with a weak β-receptor stimulating action used for the prevention or treatment of acute hypotension, throughout cardiopulmonary bypass procedures, spinal anesthesia interventions, or in vasoplegic shock states unresponsive to fluid replacement[108–113].

Mechanisms of Action

Metaraminol stimulates α-adrenergic receptors producing systemic arterial vasoconstriction. It also exerts a weak effect on β1-adrenergic receptors, resulting in increased contractility and heart rate. The increased vagal activity occurring as a reflex to increased blood pressure predominates over the chronotropic effect, because bradycardia may occur. Metaraminol also releases norepinephrine from its storage sites.

Dosing

Metaraminol is to be used as a bolus or as a continuous infusion and should be titrated within the therapeutic range and to the minimal effective dose, until the desired response is achieved. It should be administered under comprehensive hemodynamic monitoring.

Treatment of Severe Hypotension or Vasoplegic Shock

Neonates, infants, and children: loading dose of 0.01 mg/kg or 0.3 mg/m² I.V., followed by 0.4 mg/kg or 12 mg/m² infused at a rate titrated to desired results (0.1-1 mcg/kg/min)

Adults: loading dose of 0.5 to 5 mg I.V., followed by 15 to 100 mg infused at a rate titrated to desired results

Prevention of Hypotension

Neonates: not recommended

Infants and children: 0.1 mg/kg or 3 mg/m² I.M. or S.C., repeated as required every 10 minutes

Adults: 2 to 10 mg I.M. or S.C., repeated as required every 10 minutes

Pharmacokinetics

Onset of action:
I.M.: 10 minutes
I.V.: 1 to 2 minutes
S.C.: 5 to 20 minutes
Duration: 20 to 100 minutes
Half-life: 1 to 2 hours
Metabolism: not elucidated
Elimination: not elucidated

Drug Interactions

MAO inhibitors, atropine, tricyclic antidepressants, ergot alkaloids, bretylium, and inhaled anesthetic drugs (halothane, cyclopropane) may increase the effect of metaraminol.

α-adrenergic blocking agents may decrease the metaraminol effect.
Digoxin may decrease the metaraminol effect and ectopic arrhythmias may occur.

Adverse Effects

Cardiovascular: hypertension, tachycardia, bradycardia, palpitations, cardiac arrhythmias, cardiac arrest

Central nervous system: headache, apprehension, dizziness, insomnia

Gastrointestinal: nausea, vomiting; careful use in patients with cirrhosis or mesenteric thrombotic disease

Metabolic: careful use in diabetes mellitus or thyroid disease

Cutaneous: dermal necrosis (extravasation), sloughing or abscess formation at the site of injection

Neuromuscular and skeletal: tremors

Other: diaphoresis, may activate a relapse in patients with a background of malaria and Mediterranean fever (used for provocation tests)

Poisoning Information

Adverse effects caused by excessive doses or altered pharmacokinetics of metaraminol may be observed. In these circumstances, it is recommended to decrease temporarily or even withdraw the drug and treat symptomatically (significant individual variability). Systemic vasodilators and antiarrhythmic drugs might be required. In case of extravasation, local administration of phentolamine or papaverine should be considered.

Compatible Diluents

Metaraminol is stable for 24 hours when diluted in normal saline, dextrose solutions, or Ringer's lactate. Maximal recommended concentration is 1 mg/mL for continuous infusion; it may be administered undiluted as a bolus. It must be administered into a central vein, except in urgent scenarios, with an infusion device allowing proper and reliable titration.

Other

Calcium Chloride

Indication

Calcium chloride is an hypertonic parenteral electrolyte supplement used in the treatment of symptomatic hypocalcemia, hypermagnesemia and severe hyperkalemia, in the treatment of toxicity with calcium channel blocking drugs and tetany, in cardiac arrest states (when associated with electrolyte disturbances, electromechanical dissociation, or calcium channel blockers), and in situations of hemodynamic instability (if the ionized calcium level is low for the patient's age), particularly after cardiac surgery[114, 115]. It is also an important I.V. supplement in cases of persistent bleeding or multiple blood transfusions.

Mechanisms of Action

Calcium is essential for the maintenance of the functional integrity of the nervous, muscular, and skeletal systems and for cell membrane and capillary permeability. This cation is an important activator in many enzymatic reactions and is essential to a number of physiological processes, including the transmission of nerve impulses; contraction of cardiac, smooth, and skeletal muscles; renal function; respiration; and blood coagulation. Calcium also plays a regulatory role in the release and storage of neurotransmitters and hormones, in the uptake and binding of amino acids, in cyanocobalamin (vitamin B_{12}) absorption, and in gastrin secretion. Calcium chloride moderates muscle performance by action potential threshold regulation.

Dosing

Calcium chloride is to be used as a bolus or as a continuous infusion and it should be titrated within the therapeutic range and to the minimal effective dose, until the desired response is achieved. It should be administered under comprehensive hemodynamic monitoring. Furthermore, serum calcium, magnesium, potassium, and phosphate levels should be carefully monitored. Dosage expressed in mg calcium chloride.

Treatment of symptomatic hypocalcemia:
Neonates, infants, and children: 10 to 20 mg/kg/dose slow I.V. (5 to 10 minutes), to be repeated if needed every 4 to 6 hours
Adults: 500 mg to 1 g/dose slow I.V., to be repeated as needed every 6 hours
Treatment of cardiac arrest associated with electrolyte disturbances (hypocalcemia, hypermagnesemia, hyperkalemia), electromechanical dissociation, or calcium-channel blocking agent toxicity:
Neonates, infants, and children: 20 mg/kg slow I.V., to be repeated every 10 minutes as required
Adults: 2 to 4 mg/kg slow I.V., to be repeated every 10 minutes as required
Treatment of tetany:
Neonates, infants, and children: 10 mg/kg slow I.V. (5 to 10 minutes), followed by an I.V. continuous infusion of 200 mg/kg/d
Adults: 1 g slow I.V. (10 to 15 minutes), to be repeated as needed every 6 hours
Treatment of symptomatic hyperkalemia:
Neonates, infants, and children: 25 mg/kg of 7.5% or 10% solution slow I.V.
Adults: 1 g slow I.V. (10 to 15 minutes)

Pharmacokinetics

Onset of action: immediate

Protein binding: Approximately 50% of calcium in plasma is in the physiologically active, ionized form; 45% is bound to protein (principally albumin); and 5% is complexed with phosphates, citrates, and other anions

Excretion: 80% of calcium is excreted via feces and consists of unabsorbed calcium and calcium secreted via bile and pancreatic juice into the lumen of the gastrointestinal tract. The remaining 20% of calcium is excreted by the kidneys

Clearance: 20% of calcium is excreted by the kidney 95% of the calcium filtered by the renal glomeruli is reabsorbed in the kidney. Ascending limb of the loop of Henle and the proximal and distal tubules. Urinary excretion of calcium is decreased by parathyroid hormone, thiazide diuretics, and vitamin D; and increased by calcitonin, other diuretics, and growth hormone

Drug Interactions

Calcium channel blocking agents, nondepolarizing neuromuscular blocking agents, tetracycline, atenolol, iron, quinolones, alendronate, and polystyrene sulfonate may be antagonized by use of calcium chloride.

Calcium chloride may potentiate the effects of digoxin and thiazide diuretics.

Adverse Effects

Cardiovascular: vasodilation, sinus bradycardia, syncope (avoid rapid I.V. administration), hypotension, cardiac arrhythmias, ventricular fibrillation, and cardiac arrhythmias. *In patients receiving digoxin, calcium should be used with caution*

Respiratory: dyspnea, respiratory failure

Central nervous system: headache, dizziness, lethargy, coma

Cutaneous: erythema, dermal necrosis (extravasation)

Endocrine and metabolic: hypercalcemia, hypokalemia, hypomagnesemia, hypercalciuria, hypophosphatemia

Neuromuscular and skeletal: weakness

Gastrointestinal: dry mouth, constipation, nausea, vomiting, hyperamylasemia

Poisoning Information

Adverse effects caused by excessive doses or altered pharmacokinetics of calcium chloride may be observed. Clinical symptoms of intoxication may include thirst, nausea, vomiting, constipation, polyuria, abdominal pain, muscle weakness, mental disturbances, and, in severe cases, cardiac arrhythmia and coma. In these circumstances, it is recommended to decrease temporarily or even withdraw the drug and treat symptomatically (significant individual variability). In severe cases, it is recommended to monitor calcium, potassium, and magnesium blood levels carefully, to rehydrate the patient with a 0.9% sodium chloride infusion, use nonthiazide diuretics to increase calcium excretion, and use β-blockers to prevent cardiac arrhythmias. In some cases, renal replacement therapy might be required. In cases of extravasation, local administration of phentolamine or papaverine should be considered.

Compatible Diluents
Calcium chloride may be administered undiluted or diluted in dextrose or in sodium chloride. In direct I.V. injection, it is to be infused at a maximum rate of 50 to 100 mg/min. In continuous I.V. infusion, it is to be administered with a maximal concentration of 20 mg/mL. Concentrations as high as 100 mg/mL have been infused through a central line in some institutions. It is incompatible with bicarbonates, sulfates, and phosphates, as well as with some antibiotics (tetracyclines). It must be *slowly* administered into a central vein, except and in urgent scenarios (at lower concentrations), with an infusion device allowing proper and reliable titration.

Liothyronine

Indication
Liothyronine, also called T_3 or L-triiodothyronine, is a thyroid product used for replacement or supplemental therapy of hypothyroidism and chronic thyroiditis. Its use has also been proposed in postoperative cardiac surgical patients[116–118]. Adult patients who undergo open-heart surgery and receive thyroid hormone supplementation have demonstrated a dose-dependent increase in cardiac output, which has been associated with an improved clinical outcome. In infants, it may also reduce postoperative morbidity and mortality[119,120]. However, at present, there is a lack of evidence concerning the effects of triiodothyronine supplementation in infants undergoing cardiac surgery, and further randomized, controlled studies are required. This chapter will primarily discuss the properties of this drug when administered parenterally for the last indication.

Mechanisms of Action
The mechanism of action is not well elucidated. However, it is known that T_3 is involved with the metabolism of almost all body organs. It increases basal metabolic rate, oxygen consumption, and metabolism of carbohydrates, lipids, and proteins. Its use in the perioperative course of pediatric cardiac surgery has been based on the theory that cardiopulmonary bypass suppresses circulating thyroid hormone levels, particularly in newborn patients[121].

Dosing

Liothyronine may be used in the perioperative course of pediatric cardiac surgery via parenteral administration as a bolus. It should be administered under comprehensive hemodynamic monitoring. Furthermore, clinical signs of hyperthyroidism and T_3 and thyroid-stimulating hormone (TSH) levels should be carefully monitored.

> **Neonates, infants, and children:** 0.1 to 0.4 µg/kg/dose (maximum of 20 µg,) I.V. every 8 to 12 hours
> **Adults:** 0.8 µg/kg, followed by 0.12 µg/kg/h for 6 hours, I.V.

Pharmacokinetics

> **Onset of action:** a few hours
> **Maximum effect:** 48 to 72 hours
> **Duration:** up to 72 hours
> **Protein binding:** almost nil, which makes it readily available to tissues
> **Metabolism:** in the liver to inactive compounds
> **Elimination:** 75 to 85% in urine

Drug Interactions

Liothyronine increases the effect of oral anticoagulants and decreases the action of digoxin and theophylline.

Cholestyramine and colestipol decrease liothyronine's effects.

Adverse Effects

> **Cardiovascular:** palpitations, sinus tachycardia, cardiac arrhythmias, hypertension, angina, congestive heart failure, chest pain. *Liothyronine should be used cautiously in patients with ischemic disease*
> **Central nervous system:** headache, fever, nervousness, agitation, insomnia
> **Gastrointestinal:** abdominal cramps, diarrhea, vomiting, increased appetite
> **Cutaneous:** alopecia, dermatitis herpetiformis, phlebitis at the site of infusion or injection
> **Neuromuscular and skeletal:** tremor
> **Metabolic:** use with caution in patients with diabetes mellitus or insipidus, thyroid dysfunction, adrenal insufficiency
> **Other:** diaphoresis, heat intolerance, weight loss, fever

Poisoning Information

Adverse effects caused by excessive doses or altered pharmacokinetics of liothyronine may be observed. In these circumstances, it is recommended to decrease temporarily or even withdraw the drug and treat symptomatically (with significant individual variability).

Compatible Diluents

For parenteral administration, it is recommended to dilute a vial of liothyronine in 2 mL of normal saline, shake it until a clear solution is obtained, and draw the required dose. I.V. liothyronine must be administered immediately after preparation in a central or peripheral catheter. It should not be mixed with any other solutions.

Levosimendan

Indication

Levosimendan is a new inodilator used in the treatment of decompensated cardiac failure[122–129] and as an elective drug in patients with perioperative risk of ventricular failure[23, 130–134]. It has also been used in the rescue therapy of patients who have difficulty weaning from cardiopulmonary bypass or from mechanical circulatory support[126, 135]. It has been shown to exert a potent positive inotropic and systemic vasodilator effect, thereby significantly increasing cardiac output and decreasing ventricular filling pressures. There are also reports documenting its favorable effect in reducing pulmonary vascular resistance and endothelin-1 levels and in improving right ventricular failure[126, 136]. Lastly, levosimendan seems to induce a sustained lowering of atrial natriuretic peptide, and it has not shown either an arrhythmogenic effect or a drug-mediated increase in neurohormone levels. Pediatric experience is limited to a few studies to date, but the overall reports are very encouraging. It may be used with conventional inotropic support, has a simple dosing regimen, does not alter diastolic function (neutral or positive lusitropic effect), and demonstrates minimal hemodynamic side effects.

Mechanisms of Action

Levosimendan is a pyridazinone-dinitrate that belongs to a new class of drugs, the calcium sensitizers. In contrast with other inotropic agents, levosimendan is deemed to improve myocardial contractility without increasing intracellular calcium. It acts by binding to myocardial troponin C, causing a conFiguration change in tropomyosin that exposes actin and myosin elements, allowing for a more effective contraction. It offers the advantage of increasing systolic force without compromising coronary perfusion. Moreover, levosimendan opens adenosine triphosphate (ATP)-sensitive vascular potassium channels, causing vascular hyperpolarization and relaxation, coronary artery dilation, and myocyte mitochondrial activation.

Dosing

Levosimendan is to be used as a bolus or as a continuous infusion. It should be administered under comprehensive hemodynamic monitoring.

Neonates, infants, and children: loading dose of 12 µg/kg over 1 hour, followed by a continuous infusion of 0.1 to 0.2 µg/kg/min for 24 hours
Adults: loading dose of 8 to 36 µg/kg over 1 hour, followed by a continuous infusion of 0.2 to 0.3 µg/kg/min for 24 hours

Pharmacokinetics

Onset of action: very rapid (in a dose-proportional manner)
Half-life: 1 hour
Duration: 2 to 4 hours
Protein binding: 97 to 98%
Metabolism: reduced in the gut into an amine metabolite
Clearance: 296 to 368 mL/min; 70% of the unchanged drug is excreted in the urine (30%) and feces (40%)

Drug Interactions

No significant pharmacokinetic interactions have been reported with inotropic drugs, angiotensin-converting enzyme inhibitors, β-blockers, felodipine, digoxin, warfarin, isosorbide mononitrate, or carvedilol.

Adverse Effects

Cardiovascular: palpitations, flushing, symptomatic hypotension (very rare)
Central nervous system: headache, dizziness, vertigo
Gastrointestinal: nausea
Cutaneous: irritation at the injection site

Poisoning Information

Significant adverse effects caused by excessive doses or altered pharmacokinetics of levosimendan have not been described. In case of any adverse reactions, it is recommended to decrease temporarily or even withdraw the drug and treat symptomatically (significant individual variability).

Compatible Diluents

Levosimendan may be diluted in normal saline or in dextrose solutions and administered ideally in a reliable central catheter, except in an emergency situation. It should be administered under comprehensive hemodynamic monitoring.

References

1. Kay JD, Colan SD, Graham TP. Congestive heart failure in pediatric patients. Am Heart J 2001; 142: 923–928.
2. Hoch M, Netz H. Heart failure in pediatric patients. J Thorac Cardiovasc Surg 2005; 53: S129–S134.
3. Balaguru D, Artman M, Auslender M. Management of heart failure in children. Curr Probl Pediatr 2000; 30: 1–35.
4. Parr GVS, Blackstone EH, Kirklin JW. Cardiac performance and mortality early after intracardiac surgery in infants and young children. Circulation 1975; 51: 867–874.
5. Wernovsky G, Wypij D, Jonas RA, et al. Postoperative course and hemodynamic profile after the arterial switch operation in neonates and infants: a comparison of low-flow cardiopulmonary bypass and circulatory arrest. Circulation 1995; 92: 2226–2235.
6. Hoffman TM, Wernovsky G, Atz AM, et al. Efficacy and safety of milrinone in preventing low cardiac output syndrome in infants and children after corrective surgery for congenital heart disease. Circulation 2003; 107: 996–1002.
7. Short BL. Van Meurs K, Evans JR: Cardiology Group. Summary proceedings from the cardiology group on cardiovascular instability in preterm infants. Pediatrics 2006; 117: S34–39.
8. Nissen SE, Cardiovascular and Renal Drugs Advisory Committee. Report from the Cardiovascular and Renal Drugs Advisory Committee: US Food and Drug Administration 2005. Circulation 2005; 112: 2043–2046.
9. Zaristsky A, Chernow B. Use of catecholamines in pediatrics. J Pediatr 1984; 105: 341–350.
10. McGovern JJ, Cheifetz IM, Craig DM, et al. Right ventricular injury in young swine: effects of catecholamines on right ventricular function and pulmonary vascular mechanics. Pediatr Res 2000; 48: 763–769.
11. De Souza RL, de Carvalho WB, Maluf MA, et al. Assessment of splanchnic perfusion with gastric tonometry in the immediate postoperative period of cardiac surgery in children. Arq Bras Cardiol 2001; 77: 509–519.
12. Holmes CL. Vasoactive drugs in the intensive care unit. Curr Opin Crit Care 2005; 11: 413–417.
13. Beale RJ, Hollenberg SM, Vincent JL, et al. Vasopressor and inotropic support in septic shock: an evidence-based review. Crit Care Med 2004; 32: S455–465.
14. Bakir M, Bilgic A. Single daily dose of digoxin for maintenance therapy of infants and children with cardiac disease: is it reliable? Pediatr Cardiol 1994; 15: 229–232.
15. Digitalis Investigation Group. The effect of digoxin on mortality and morbidity in patients with heart failure: N Engl J Med 1997; 336: 525–533.
16. Park MK. Use of digoxin in infants and children with specific emphasis on dosage. J Pediatr 1986; 108: 871–877.
17. Kimball TR, Daniels SR, Meyer RA, et al. Effect of digoxin on contractility and symptoms in infants with a large ventricular septal defect. Am J Cardiol 1991; 168: 377–382.

18. Berman W, Yabek SM, Dillon I, et al. Effects of digoxin in infants with congestive circulatory state due to a ventricular septal defect. N Engl J Med 1983; 308: 363.

19. Seguchi M, Nakazawa M, Momma K. Further evidence suggesting a limited role of digitalis in infants with circulatory congestion secondary to large ventricular septal defect. Am J Cardiol 1999; 83: 1408–1411.

20. Barclay M, Begg E. The practice of digoxin therapeutic drug monitoring. NZ Med J 2003; 116: 704.

21. Bendayan R, McKenzie MW. Digoxin pharmacokinetics and dosage requirements in pediatric patients. Clin Pharm 1983; 2: 224–235.

22. Hussain Z, Swindle J, Hauptman PJ. Digoxin use and digoxin toxicity in the post-DIG trial era. J Card Fail 2006; 12: 343–346.

23. Alvarez J, Bouzada M, Fernandez AL, et al. Hemodynamic effects of levosimendan compared with dobutamine in patients with low cardiac output after cardiac surgery. Rev Esp Cardiol 2006; 59: 338–345.

24. Martikainen TJ, Uusaro A, Tenhunen JJ, et al. Dobutamine compensates deleterious hemodynamic and metabolic effects of vasopressin in the splanchnic region in endotoxin shock. Acta Anaesthesiol Scand 2004; 48: 935–943.

25. Harada K, Tamura M, Ito T, et al. Effects of low-dose dobutamine on left ventricular diastolic filling in children. Pediatr Cardiol 1996; 17: 220–225.

26. Jaccard C, Berner M, Touge JC, et al. Hemodynamic effect of isoprenaline and dobutamine immediately after correction of tetralogy of Fallot: relative importance of inotropic and chronotropic action in supporting cardiac output. J Thorac Cardiovasc Surg 1884; 87: 862–869.

27. Booker PD, Evans C, Franks R. Comparison of the haemodynamic effects of dopamine and dobutamine in young children undergoing cardiac surgery. Br J Anaesth 1995; 74: 419–423.

28. Zaristsky A, Chernow B. Use of catecholamines in pediatrics. J Pediatr 1984; 105: 341–350.

29. McGovern JJ, Cheifetz IM, Craig DM, et al. Right ventricular injury in young swine: effects of catecholamines on right ventricular function and pulmonary vascular mechanics. Pediatr Res 2000; 48: 763–769.

30. Woolsey CA, Coopersmith CM. Vasoactive drugs and the gut: is there anything new? Curr Opin Crit Care 2006; 12: 155–159.

31. De Souza RL, de Carvalho WB, Maluf MA, et al. Assessment of splanchnic perfusion with gastric tonometry in the immediate postoperative period of cardiac surgery in children. Arq Bras Cardiol 2001; 77: 509–519.

32. Miall-Allen VM, Whitelaw AG. Response to dopamine and dobutamine in the preterm infant less than 30 weeks gestation. Crit Care Med 1989; 17: 1166–1169.

33. Short BL. Van Meurs K, Evans JR: Cardiology Group. Summary proceedings from the cardiology group on cardiovascular instability in preterm infants. Pediatrics 2006; 117: S34–39.

34. Osborn D, Paradisis M, Evans N. The effect of inotropes on morbidity and mortality in preterm infants with low systemic or organ blood flow. Cochrane Database Syst Rev 2007 24; 1: CD005090.

35. Li J, Zhang G, Holtby H, Humpl T, Caldarone CA, Van Arsdell GS, Redington AN. Adverse effects of dopamine on systemic hemodynamic status and oxygen transport in neonates after the Norwood procedure. J Am Coll Cardiol 2006; 48: 1859–1864.

36. Woo EB, Tang AT, el-Gamel A, Keevil B, Greenhalgh D, Patrick M, Jones MT, Hooper TL. Dopamine therapy for patients at risk of renal dysfunction following cardiac surgery: science or fiction? Eur J Cardiothorac Surg 2002; 22: 106–111.

37. Schenarts PJ, Sagraves SG, Bard MR, Toschlog EA, Goettler CE, Newell MA, Rotondo MF. Low-dose dopamine: a physiologically based review. Curr Surg 2006; 63: 219–225.

38. Eldadah MK, Schwartz PH, Harrison R, et al. Pharmacokinetics of dopamine in infants and children. Crit Care Med 1991; 19: 1008–1011.

39. Banner W, Vermon DD, Dean JM, et al. Nonlinear dopamine pharmacokinetics in pediatric patients. J Pharmacol Exp Ther 1989; 249: 131–133.

40. Renton MC, Snowden CP. Dopexamine and its role in the protection of hepatosplanchnic and renal perfusion in high-risk surgical and critically ill patients. Br J Anaesth 2005; 94: 459–467.

41. Fitton A, Benfield P. Dopexamine hydrochloride. A review of its pharmacodynamic and pharmacokinetic properties and therapeutic potential in acute cardiac insufficiency. Drugs 1990; 39: 308–330.

42. Seguin P, Laviolle B, Guinet P, et al. Dopamine and norepinephrine versus epinephrine on gastric perfusion in patients with septic shock: a randomized study. Crit Care 2006; 10: 32.

43. Schmoelz M, Schelling G, Dunker M, et al. Comparison of systemic and renal effects of dopexamine and dopamine in norepinephrine-treated septic shock. J Cardiothorac Vasc Anesth 2006; 20: 173–178.

44. Rachelefsky GS, Siegel SC. Asthma in infants and children. Treatment of childhood asthma. Part I. J Allergy Clin Immunol 1985; 76: 409–425.

45. Waisman Y, Klein BL, Boenning DA, et al. Prospective randomized double-blind study comparing L-epinephrine and racemic epinephrine in the treatment of laryngotracheitis (croup). Pediatrics 1992; 89: 302–306.

46. American Heart Association. 2005 American Heart Association (AHA) guidelines for cardiopulmonary resuscitation (CPR) and emergency cardiovascular care (ECC) of pediatric and neonatal patients: pediatric basic life support. Pediatrics 2006; 117: e989–1004.

47. International Liaison Committee on Resuscitation. The International Liaison Committee on Resuscitation (ILCOR) consensus on science with treatment recommendations for pediatric and neonatal patients: pediatric basic and advanced life support. Pediatrics. 2006; 117(5): e955–977.

48. American College of Cardiology, American Heart Association Task Force. Adult Advanced Cardiac Life Support. JAMA 1992; 268: 2199–2241.

49. American College of Cardiology, American Heart Association Task Force. Pediatric Advanced Life Support Guidelines. JAMA 1992; 268: 2262–2275.

50. American Heart Association in collaboration with the International Liaison Committee on Resuscitation. Guidelines 2000 for Cardiopulmonary Resuscitation

and Emergency Cardiovascular Care. Part 10: Pediatric Advanced Life Support. Circulation 2000; 102: 1291–1342.

51. American Heart Association in collaboration with the International Liaison Committee on Resuscitation. Guidelines 2000 for Cardiopulmonary Resuscitation and Emergency Cardiovascular Care. Part 11: Neonatal Resuscitation. Circulation 2000; 102: 1343–1357.

52. Jaccard C, Berner M, Touge JC, et al. Hemodynamic effect of isoprenaline and dobutamine immediately after correction of tetralogy of Fallot: relative importance of inotropic and chronotropic action in supporting cardiac output. J Thorac Cardiovasc Surg 1884; 87: 862–869.

53. Fujino H, Nakazawa M, Momma K, Imai Y. Long-term results after surgical repair of total anomalous pulmonary venous connection-hemodynamic evaluation of pulmonary venous obstruction with isoproterenol infusion. Jpn Circ J 1995; 59: 198–204.

54. Friedman M, Wang SY, Stahl GL, Johnson RG, Sellke FW. Altered beta-adrenergic and cholinergic pulmonary vascular responses after total cardiopulmonary bypass. J Appl Physiol 1995; 79: 1998–2006.

55. Fullerton DA, Mitchell MB, Jones DN, Maki A, McIntyre RC Jr. Pulmonary vasomotor dysfunction is produced with chronically high pulmonary blood flow. J Thorac Cardiovasc Surg 1996; 111: 190–197.

56. Durandy Y, Batisse A, Lecompte Y. Postoperative inotropic treatment in cardiac surgery of the newborn infant and infant. Ann Fr Anesth Reanim 1988; 7: 105–109.

57. Batmaz G, Villain E, Bonnet D, Iserin L, Fraisse A, Kachaner J. Therapy and prognosis of infectious complete atrioventricular block in children. Arch Mal Coeur Vaiss 2000; 93: 553–557.

58. Carcillo JA, Fields AI; American College of Critical Care Medicine Task Force Committee Members. Clinical practice parameters for hemodynamic support of pediatric and neonatal patients in septic shock. Crit Care Med 2002; 30: 1365–1378.

59. Seguin P, Laviolle B, Guinet P, et al. Dopexamine and norepinephrine versus epinephrine on gastric perfusion in patients with septic shock: a randomized study. Crit Care 2006; 10: 32.

60. Schmoelz M, Schelling G, Dunker M, et al. Comparison of systemic and renal effects of dopexamine and dopamine in norepinephrine-treated septic shock. J Cardiothorac Vasc Anesth 2006; 20: 173–178.

61. Waisman Y, Klein BL, Boenning DA, et al. Prospective randomized double-blind study comparing l-epinephrine and racemic epinephrine in the treatment of laryngotracheitis (croup). Pediatrics 1992; 89: 302–306.

62. Nygren A, Thoren A, Ricksten SE. Vasopressors and intestinal mucosal perfusion after cardiac surgery: Norepinephrine vs. phenylephrine. Crit Care Med 2006; 34: 722–729.

63. Wilmshurst PT, Thompson DS, Juul SM, et al. Comparison of the effects of amrinone and sodium nitroprusside on haemodynamics, contractility and myocardial metabolism in patients with cardiac failure due to coronary artery disease and dilated cardiomyopathy. Br Heart J 1984; 52: 38–48.

64. Allen-Webb EM, Ross MP, Pappas JB, et al. Age-related amrinone pharmacokinetics in a pediatric population. Crit Care Med 1994; 22: 1016–1024.

65. Lawless S, Burckart G, Diven W, et al. Amrinone in neonates and infants after cardiac surgery. Crit Care Med 1989; 17: 751–754.

66. Lynn AM, Sorensen GK, Williams GD. Hemodynamic effects of amrinone and colloid administration in children following cardiac surgery. J Cardiothorac Vasc Anesth 1993; 7: 560–565.

67. Allen-Webb EM, Ross MP, Pappas JB, et al. Age-related amrinone pharmacokinetics in a pediatric population. Crit Care Med 1994; 22: 1016–1024.

68. Honerjager P. Pharmacology of bipyridine phosphodiesterase III inhibitors. Am Heart J 1991; 121: 1939–1944.

69. Ross MP, Allen-Webb EM, Pappas JB, et al. Amrinone-associated thrombocytopenia: pharmacokinetic analysis. Clin Pharmacol Ther 1993; 53: 661–667.

70. Hausdorf G. Experience with phosphodiesterase inhibitors in paediatric cardiac surgery. Eur J Anaesth 1993; 8: 25–30.

71. Hoffman TM, Wernovsky G, Atz AM, et al. Efficacy and safety of milrinone in preventing low cardiac output syndrome in infants and children after corrective surgery for congenital heart disease. Circulation 2003; 107: 996–1002.

72. Hoffman TM, Wernovsky G, Atz AM, et al. Prophylactic intravenous use of milrinone after cardiac operation in pediatrics (PRIMACORP) study. Prophylactic intravenous use of milrinone after cardiac operation in pediatrics. Am Heart J 2002; 143: 15–21.

73. Chang AC, Atz AM, Wernovsky G, et al. Milrinone: systemic and pulmonary hemodynamic effects in neonates after cardiac surgery. Crit Care Med 1995; 23: 1907–1914.

74. Bhat G. Predictors of clinical outcome in advanced heart failure patients on continuous intravenous milrinone therapy. ASAIO J 2006; 52: 677–681.

75. Price JF, Towbin JA, Dreyer WJ, Moffett BS, Kertesz NJ, Clunie SK, Denfield SW. Outpatient continuous parenteral inotropic therapy as bridge to transplantation in children with advanced heart failure. J Card Fail 2006; 12: 139–143.

76. Brozena SC, Twomey C, Goldberg LR, Desai SS, Drachman B, Kao A, Popjes E, Zimmer R, Jessup M. A prospective study of continuous intravenous milrinone therapy for status IB patients awaiting heart transplant at home. J Heart Lung Transplant 2004; 23: 1082–1086.

77. Sablotzki A, Starzmann W, Scheubel R, Grond S, Czeslick EG. Selective pulmonary vasodilation with inhaled aerosolized milrinone in heart transplant candidates. Can J Anaesth 2006; 52: 1076–1082.

78. Ramamoorthy C, Anderson GD, Williams GD, et al. Pharmacokinetics and side-effects of milrinone in infants and children after open heart surgery. Anesth Analg 1998; 86: 283–289.

79. Lindsay CA, Barton P, Lawless S, et al. Pharmacokinetics and pharmacodynamics of milrinone lactate in pediatric patients with septic shock. J Pediatr 1998; 132: 329–334.

80. Barton P, Garcia J, Kouatli A, et al. Hemodynamic effects of IV milrinone lactate in pediatric patients with septic shock. A prospective, double-blinded, randomized, placebo-controlled interventional study. Chest 1996; 109: 1302–1312.

81. Honerjager P. Pharmacology of bipyridine phosphodiesterase III inhibitors. Am Heart J 1991; 121: 1939–1944.

82. Xavier LC, Kern KB. Cardiopulmonary resuscitation guidelines 2000 update: what's happened since? Curr Opin Crit Care 2003; 9: 218–221.

83. Klingenheben T. Resuscitation in ventricular fibrillation: what is essential? Herzschrittmacherther Elektrophysiol 2005; 16: 78–83.

84. Carcillo JA, Fields AI; American College of Critical Care Medicine task force committee members. Clinical practice parameters for hemodynamic support of pediatric and neonatal patients in septic shock. Crit Care Med 2002; 30: 1365–1378.

85. Rosenzweig EB, Starc TJ, Chen JM, et al. Intravenous arginine-vasopressin in children with vasodilatory shock after cardiac surgery. Circulation 1999; 100: II182–186.

86. Beale RJ, Hollenberg SM, Vincent JL, et al. Vasopressor and inotropic support in septic shock: an evidence-based review. Crit Care Med 2004; 32: S455–465.

87. Rivers E, Nguyen B, Havstad S, et al. Early-goal directed therapy in the treatment of severe sepsis and septic shock. N Engl J Med 2001; 345: 1368–1377.

88. Rhodes A, Bennett ED. Early goal-directed therapy: an evidence-based review. Crit Care Med 2004; 32: S448–S450.

89. Holmes CL, Walley KR. Vasopressine in the ICU. Curr Opin Crit Care 2004; 10: 442–444.

90. Sharshar T, Blanchard A, Paillard M, Raphael JC, Gajdos P, Annane D. Circulating vasopressin levels in septic shock. Crit Care Med 2003; 31: 1752–1758.

91. Mullner M, Urbanek B, Havel C, et al. Vasopressors for shock. Edited by The Cochrane Database Systematic Reviews 2004; CD003709.

92. Landry DW, Oliver JA. The pathogenesis of vasodilatory shock. N Engl J Med 2001; 345: 588–595.

93. Zimmerman MA, Albright TN, Raeburn CD, et al. Vasopressin in cardiovascular patients: therapeutic implications. Expert Opin Pharmacother 2002; 3: 505–512.

94. Leone M, Martin C. Rescue therapy in septic shock—is terlipressin the last frontier? Crit Care 2006; 10: 131.

95. Jochberger S, Mayr VD, Luckner G, et al. Serum vasopressin concentrations in critically ill patients. Crit Care Med 2006; 34: 293–299.

96. McNamee JJ, Trainor D, Michalek P. Terlipressin for refractory hypotension following angiotensin-II receptor antagonist overdose. Anaesthesia 2006; 61: 408–409.

97. Martikainen TJ, Uusaro A, Tenhunen JJ, et al. Dobutamine compensates deleterious hemodynamic and metabolic effects of vasopressin in the splanchnic region in endotoxin shock. Acta Anaesthesiol Scand 2004; 48: 935–943.

98. Heytman M, Rainbird A. Use of alpha-agonists for management of anaphylaxis occurring under anaesthesia: case studies and review. Anaesthesia 2004; 59: 1210–1215.

99. Mullner M, Urbanek B, Havel C, et al. Vasopressors for shock. Edited by The Cochrane Database Systematic Reviews 2004; CD003709.

100. Landry DW, Oliver JA. The pathogenesis of vasodilatory shock. N Engl J Med 2001; 345: 588–595.

101. Gajraj NM, Wallace DH, Pace NA. Supraventricular tachycardia in a parturient under spinal anesthesia. Reg Anesth 1993; 18: 261–263.

102. Strasburger JF. Cardiac arrhythmias in childhood. Diagnostic considerations and treatment. Drugs 1991; 42: 974–983.

103. Garson A Jr, Gillette PC, McNamara DG. Supraventricular tachycardia in children: clinical features, response to treatment, and long-term follow-up in 217 patients. J Pediatr 1981; 98: 875–882.

104. Shaddy RE, Viney J, Judd VE, et al. Continuous intravenous phenylephrine infusion for treatment of hypoxemic spells in tetralogy of Fallot. J Pediatr 1989; 114: 468–470.

105. Tanaka T, Kitahata H, Kawahito S, et al. Phenylephrine increases pulmonary blood flow in children with tetralogy of Fallot. Can J Anaesth 2003; 50: 926–929.

106. Nygren A, Thoren A, Ricksten SE. Vasopressors and intestinal mucosal perfusion after cardiac surgery: Norepinephrine vs. phenylephrine. Crit Care Med 2006; 34: 722–729.

107. Krejci V, Hiltebrand LB, Sigurdsson GH. Effects of epinephrine, norepinephrine, and phenylephrine on microcirculatory blood flow in the gastrointestinal tract in sepsis. Crit Care Med 2006; 34:1456–1463.

108. Heytman M, Rainbird A. Use of alpha-agonists for management of anaphylaxis occurring under anaesthesia: case studies and review. Anaesthesia 2004; 59: 1210–1215.

109. Natalini G, Schivalocchi V, Rosano A, Taranto M, Pletti C, Bernardini A. Norepinephrine and metaraminol in septic shock: a comparison of the hemodynamic effects. Intensive Care Med 2005; 31: 634–637.

110. Brown SG. Cardiovascular aspects of anaphylaxis: implications for treatment and diagnosis. Curr Opin Allergy Clin Immunol 2005; 5: 359–362.

111. Wood DM, Wright KD, Jones AL, Dargan PI. Metaraminol (Aramine) in the management of a significant amlodipine overdose. Hum Exp Toxicol 2005; 24: 377–381.

112. Kapur S, Mutagi H, Raphael J. Use of metaraminol in patients with Familial Mediterranean Fever. Anaesthesia 2006; 61: 815.

113. Ford SA, Kam PC, Baldo BA, Fisher MM. Anaphylactic or anaphylactoid reactions in patients undergoing cardiac surgery. J Cardiothorac Vasc Anesth 2001; 15: 684–688.

114. Murdoch JA, Qureshi SA, Huggon IC. Perioperative haemodynamic effects of an intravenous infusion of calcium chloride in children following cardiac surgery. Acta Paediatr 1994; 83: 658–661.

115. Urban MK, Hines R. The effect of calcium on pulmonary vascular resistance and right ventricular function. J Thorac Cardiovasc Surg 1992; 104: 327–332.

116. Bennett-Guerrero E, Jimenez JL, White WD, et al. Cardiovascular effects of intravenous triiodothyronine in patients undergoing coronary artery bypass graft surgery. A randomized, double-blind, placebo-controlled trial. Duke T3 study group. JAMA 1996; 275: 687–692.

117. Boylston BF. Triiodothyronine and cardiac surgery. JAMA 1996; 276: 100–101.

118. Klemperer JD. Thyroid hormone and cardiac surgery. Thyroid 2002; 12: 517–521.

119. Dimmick S, Badawi N, Randell T. Thyroid hormone supplementation for the prevention of morbidity and mortality in infants undergoing cardiac surgery. The Cochrane Database of Systematic Reviews 2004; 3: CD004220.

120. Mainwaring RD, Nelson JC. Supplementation of thyroid hormone in children undergoing cardiac surgery. Cardiol Young 2002; 12: 211–217.

121. Portman MA, Fearneyhough C, Ning XH, et al. Triiodothyronine repletion in infants during cardiopulmonary bypass for congenital heart disease. J Thorac Cardiovasc Surg 2000; 120: 604–608.

122. Toller WG, Stranz C. Levosimendan, a new inotropic and vasodilator agent. Anesthesiology 2006; 104: 556–569.

123. Huang L, Weil MH, Tang W, et al. Comparison between dobutamine and levosimendan for management of postresuscitation myocardial dysfunction. Crit Care Med 2005; 33: 487–491.

124. Morelli A, Teboul JL, Maggiore SM, Vieillard-Baron A, Rocco M, Conti G, De Gaetano A, Picchini U, Orecchioni A, Carbone I, Tritapepe L, Pietropaoli P, Wesrphal M. Effects of levosimendan on right ventricular afterload in patients with acute respiratory distress. Crit Care Med 2006; 34: 2287–2293.

125. Lilleberg J, Laine M, Palkama T, Kivikko M, Pohjanjousi P, Kupari M. Duration of haemodynamic action of a 24-h infusion in patients with congestive heart failure. Eur J Heart Fail 2007; 9: 75–82.

126. Parissis JT, Adamopoulos S, Farmakis D, Filippatos G, Paraskevaidis I, Panou F, Iliodromitis E, Kremastinos DT. Effects of serial levosimendan infusions on left ventricular performance and plasma biomarkers of myocardial injury and neuro-hormonal and immune activation in patients with advanced heart failure. Heart 2006; 92: 1768–1772.

127. Missant C, Rex S, Segers P, Wouters PF. Missant C, Rex S, Segers P, Wouters PF. Levosimendan improves right ventriculovascular coupling in a porcine model of right ventricular dysfunction. Crit Care Med 2007; 35: 707–715.

128. Parissis JT, Farmakis D, Bistola V, Adamopoulos S, Kremastinos DT. Levosimendan for the treatment of acute heart failure syndromes: time to identify subpopulations of responding patients. Am J Cardiol 2007; 99: 146–147.

129. Namachivayam P, Crossland DS, Butt W, Shekerdemian LS. Early experience with levosimendan in children with ventricular dysfunction. Pediatr Crit Care Med 2006; 7: 445–448.

130. Tritapepe L, De Santis V, Vitale D, Santulli M, Morelli A, Nufroni I, Puddu PE, Singer M, Pietropaoli P. Preconditioning effects of levosimendan in coronary artery bypass-grafting—a pilot study. Br J Anaesth 2006; 96: 694–700.

131. Egan JR, Clarke AJ, Williams S, et al. Levosimendan for low cardiac output: a pediatric experience. J Intensive Care Med 2006; 21: 183–187.

132. Raja SG, Rayen BS. Levosimendan in cardiac surgery: current best available evidence. Ann Thorac Surg 2006; 81: 1536–1546.

133. Siirila-Waris K, Suojaranta-Ylinen R, Harjola VP. Levosimendan in cardiac surgery. J Cardiothorac Vasc Anesth 2005; 19: 345–349.

134. Kumar S, Kumar A, Santis V. The preconditioning effects of levosimendan. Br J Anaesth 2006; 97: 425.

135. Lechner E, Moosbauer W, Pinter M, Mair R, Tulzer G. Use of levosimendan, a new inodilator, for postoperative myocardial stunning in a premature neonate. Pediatr Crit Care Med 2007; 8: 61–63.

136. Turanlahti M, Boldt T, Palkama T, et al. Pharmacokinetics of levosimendan in pediatric patients evaluated for cardiac surgery. Pediatr Crit Care Med 2004; 5: 457–462.

4. Vasodilators

*Stephen J. Roth, Ricardo Munoz, Carol G. Schmitt,
Eduardo da Cruz, Jonathan Kaufman, and Cécile Tissot*

Pharmacological manipulation of afterload or systemic vascular resistance
(SVR) has become increasingly important in the management of pediatric cardiac patients, just as it has for adult cardiac patients. Specifically, the principal
groups of pediatric patients with cardiovascular disease who may benefit from
afterload reduction therapies include the following:

1. Patients with normal cardiac anatomy and myocardial function who have systemic hypertension.
2. Patients with normal cardiac anatomy but impaired myocardial function, either
   caused by primary myocardial disease (e.g., familial cardiomyopathy), or
   acquired myocardial disease (e.g., dilated cardiomyopathy secondary to viral
   myocarditis).
3. Patients with congenital heart disease (CHD) who have undergone palliative (e.g.,
   the modified Norwood procedure for hypoplastic left heart syndrome) or repara-
   tive surgery and developed myocardial dysfunction.
4. Patients with CHD immediately or early after cardiac surgery, especially cardiopulmonary bypass surgery.

The vasodilators are pharmacological agents that produce relaxation of
smooth muscle in the wall of blood vessels, leading to reduced vascular
resistance and the potential for increased blood flow. Some vasodilators
act on arterial vessels, others on venous vessels, and a third group on both
arteries and veins. The vasodilators can be classified according to their
predominant site of action or by their mechanism of action. In this chapter,
these agents are classified by their mechanism of action (see Table 4-1).

The types of vasodilators discussed include the following: angiotensin-
converting enzyme (ACE) inhibitors, angiotensin II receptor blockers, calcium
channel blockers, nitrates and nitrate-like agents, α-adrenoceptor antagonists,
dopaminergic receptor antagonists, prostaglandins, and the direct arteriolar
vasodilator, hydralazine (Table 4-1).

Table 4-1. Vasodilators classified according to mechanism of action

Agent	Mechanism of Action
ACE Inhibitors Captopril Enalapril Lisinopril	Inhibit ACE, which promotes the conversion of angiotensin I to the potent vasoconstrictor, angiotensin II
Angiotensin II receptor blockers Losartan	Competitive binding to angiotensin II receptors
Calcium channel blockers Nifedipine Amlodipine Nicardipine	Block entry of calcium into vascular smooth muscle cells, thereby causing relaxation
Nitrates and nitrate-like agents Nitroglycerin Nitroprusside	NO donors. NO promotes the production of cGMP, which promotes relaxation of vascular smooth muscle
Adrenoceptor antagonists Phentolamine Phenoxybenzamine	Competitive inhibition of $\alpha 1$ adrenoceptors
Dopaminergic receptor agonists Fenoldopam	Bind to vascular dopaminergic Type 1 and 2 (DA_1 and DA_2) receptors
Prostaglandins Alprostadil (PGE_1)	Bind to prostaglandin receptors, resulting in elevated intracellular cAMP levels
Hydralazine	Direct arteriolar vasodilator by unknown mechanism

Individual Agents

ACE Inhibitors: Captopril

Indication

Captopril is used in adults primarily to treat systemic hypertension, congestive heart failure (CHF), and left ventricular dysfunction in stable patients after a myocardial infarction.[1] In pediatric patients, it is also used to treat systemic hypertension and CHF; additionally, it is used in CHD patients who have single ventricle anatomy, atrioventricular valve (AVV) regurgitation, and aortic valve regurgitation.

Mechanism of Action

Captopril is a competitive inhibitor of ACE; it, therefore, blocks the conversion of angiotensin I to angiotensin II. Angiotensin II is a strong vasoconstrictor, therefore, reducing its blood level leads to less vasoconstriction. In addition, plasma renin levels are increased and aldosterone secretion reduced.

Dosing

Neonates, premature:
   Oral: initial or "test" dose 0.01 mg/kg/dose by mouth (P.O.) or nasogastric (N.G.). Dose every 8 to 12 hours and titrate dose for response

Neonates:
   Oral: initial or "test" dose 0.05 to 0.1 mg/kg/dose P.O./N.G. Dose every 8 to 24 hours. Titrate dose to maximum of 0.5 mg/kg/dose and administer every 6 to 24 hours

Infants/children:
   Oral: initial or "test" dose 0.15 to 0.5 mg/kg/dose P.O./N.G. Dose every 8 to 24 hours. Titrate dose to maximum of 6 mg/kg/day in one to four divided doses. Usual dose is 2.5 to 6 mg/kg/day. For older children, initial dose is usually 6.25 to 12.5 mg/dose P.O./N.G. Dose every 12 to 24 hours. Titrate dose to maximum of 6 mg/kg/day in two to four divided doses

Adults:
   Oral: initial dose 12.5 to 25 mg/dose P.O./N.G. Dose every 8 to 12 hours. Titrate dose upward by 25 mg/dose at 1- to 2-week intervals to a maximum dose of 450 mg/day. Usual dose range is 25 to 100 mg/day in two divided doses

Note: Dosing for all age groups should be titrated to an individual patient's response, and the lowest dose that achieves this response should be chosen. Lower doses are appropriate for patients who are also being treated with diuretics and are water and sodium depleted.

Dosing adjustment for renal impairment:
   Creatinine clearance (Cl_{cr}) 10 to 50 mL/min/1.73 m^2: administer 75% of dose
   Cl_{cr} less than 10 mL/min/1.73 m^2: administer 50% of dose

Pharmacokinetics

Onset of action: decrease in blood pressure typically observed within 15 to 60 minutes
Absorption: 60 to 75%
Distribution: 7 L/kg
Maximum effect: hypotensive effect at 60 to 90 minutes; the full hypotensive effect may take weeks to occur

Half-life:
  Infants with CHF: 3.3 hours (1.2 to 12.4 h)
  Children: 1.5 hours (1 to 2.3 h)
  Normal adults (dependent on renal and cardiac function): 1.9 hours
  Adults with CHF: 2.1 hours
  Anuria: 20 to 40 hours
Duration: dose-related
Protein binding: 25 to 30%
Metabolism: 50% metabolized
Clearance: time to peak serum concentration: 1 to 2 hours
Elimination: 95% excreted in urine in 24 hours

Monitoring Parameters

Blood pressure, blood urea nitrogen (BUN), creatinine, urine dipstick for protein, white blood cell count (WBC) with differential, and serum potassium. Monitoring for blood pressure effect should focus on the period 1 to 3 hours after dosing.

Contraindications

Hypersensitivity to captopril (any component) or other ACE inhibitors.

Adverse Effects

  Cardiovascular: hypotension, tachycardia
  Respiratory: cough, dyspnea. An isolated, dry cough has been reported in 7 (17%) of 42 pediatric patients[2]
  Central nervous system: headache, dizziness, fatigue, insomnia
  Gastrointestinal: loss of taste perception (related to zinc deficiency with long-term use)
  Hepatic: cholestatic jaundice, fulminant hepatic necrosis (rare, but potentially fatal)
  Renal: elevated BUN and serum creatinine, proteinuria, oliguria
  Endocrine/metabolic: hyperkalemia
  Hematological: neutropenia, agranulocytosis, eosinophilia. The risk of neutropenia is increased by approximately 15-fold in patients with renal dysfunction
  Cutaneous/peripheral: rash, angioedema
  Other: fever, anaphylactoid reaction

Precautions

Dosing should be adjusted downward in patients with renal impairment, collagen vascular disease, or obstruction to systemic arterial flow (e.g., aortic coarctation, renal artery stenosis). Monitor renal function closely in patients with known renal impairment, low cardiac output, or volume depletion (e.g., coadministration of diuretic medications).

Drug-Drug Interactions
In patients who are also receiving potassium supplements or a potassium-sparing diuretic (e.g., spironolactone), an additive hyperkalemic effect may occur. In patients who are also receiving indomethacin or a nonsteroidal anti-inflammatory drug (NSAID), the antihypertensive effect of captopril may be diminished.

Compatible Diluents/Administration
Captopril is only available for oral/enteral administration. Administer either on an empty stomach 1 hour before meals or 2 hours after meals. Absorption may be reduced by presence of food in the gastrointestinal tract.

References

1. Chobarian AV, Bakris GL, Black HR, et al. The Seventh Report of the Joint National Committee on Prevention, Detection, Evaluation, and Treatment of High Blood Pressure: The JNC 7 Report. JAMA 2003; 289:2560–2572.
2. von Vigier RO, Mozzetti S, Truttmann AC, et al. Cough is Common in Children Prescribed Converting Enzyme Inhibitors. Nephron 2000; 84:98.

ACE Inhibitors: Enalapril and Enalaprilat

Indication
Enalapril (oral/enteral administration) is used in adults primarily to treat systemic hypertension, CHF, asymptomatic left ventricular dysfunction, and proteinuria in steroid-resistant nephrotic syndrome.[1] In pediatric patients, enalapril is also used to treat systemic hypertension and CHF; additionally, it is used in CHD patients who have single ventricle anatomy, AVV regurgitation, and aortic valve regurgitation.[2] Enalaprilat (intravenous [I.V.] administration) is used in hospital settings to treat systemic hypertension.[3]

Mechanism of Action
Enalapril/enalaprilat is a competitive inhibitor of ACE; therefore, it blocks the conversion of angiotensin I to angiotensin II. Angiotensin II is a strong vasoconstrictor, therefore, reducing its blood level leads to less vasoconstriction. In addition, plasma renin levels are increased and aldosterone secretion reduced.

Dosing

Neonates:

Oral, enalapril: initial or "test" dose 0.1 mg/kg/dose P.O./N.G. Dose once every 24 hours. Titrate dose and interval (up to every 12 h) every 3 to 5 days

I.V., enalaprilat: initial or "test" dose 5 to 10 μg/kg/dose I.V. Dose every 8 to 24 hours and titrate for response. Administer via an infusion over 5 minutes

Infants/children:

Oral, enalapril: initial or "test" dose 0.05 to 0.1 mg/kg/dose P.O./N.G. Dose once every 12 to 24 hours. Titrate dose over 2 weeks to maximum of 0.5 mg/kg/day

I.V., enalaprilat: initial or "test" dose 5 to 10 μg/kg/dose I.V. Dose every 8 to 24 hours and titrate for response. Administer via an infusion over 5 minutes

Adults:

Oral, enalapril: initial or "test" dose 2.5 to 5.0 mg/dose P.O./N.G. Dose every 12 to 24 hours. Titrate dose upward by 2.5 mg/dose increments. Usual dose for hypertension is 10 to 40 mg/dose administered every 12 to 24 hours. Usual dose for CHF is 5 to 20 mg/dose in two divided doses. Maximum dose, 40 mg/day

I.V., enalaprilat: initial or "test" dose, 0.625 mg/dose I.V. Usual dosing, 0.625 to 1.25 mg/dose I.V. administered every 6 hours. Maximum dose, 5 mg/dose every 6 hours (20 mg/day)

Note: Dosing for all age groups should be titrated to an individual patient's response, and the lowest dose that achieves this response should be chosen. Lower doses are appropriate for patients who are also being treated with diuretics and are water and sodium depleted, those with renal impairment and severe CHF, and patients with systemic arterial obstruction (e.g., coarctation of the aorta, renal artery stenosis). For additional dosing precautions in neonates, see "Poisoning Information"

Dosing adjustment for renal impairment:

Cl_{cr} 10 to 50 mL/min/1.73 m²: administer 75 to 100% of dose
Cl_{cr} less than 10 mL/min/1.73 m²: administer 50% of dose

No data exist for neonates and children 16 years or younger with a glomerular filtration rate less than 30 mL/min/1.73 m², and use in these patients is not recommended

Pharmacokinetics

Onset of action:

Oral: within 1 hour
I.V.: within 15 minutes

Absorption: Oral: 55 to 75%
Maximum effect:
  Oral: 4 to 8 hours
  I.V.: 1 to 4 hours
Half-life:
  Enalapril:
    Neonates 10 to 19 days of age with CHF (n = 3): 10.3 hours (4.2–13.4h)
    Infants/children (≤ 6.5 years) with CHF (n = 11): 2.7 hours (1.3–6.3h)
    Adults: healthy, 2 hours; with CHF, 3.4 to 5.8 hours
  Enalaprilat:
    Neonates 10 to 19 days of age with CHF (n = 3): 11.9 hours (5.9–15.6h)
    Infants 6 weeks to 8 months: 6 to 10 hours
    Infants/children (≤ 6.5 years) with CHF (n = 11): 11.1 hours (5.1–20.8h)
    Adults: 35 to 38 hours
Duration:
  Oral: 12 to 24 hours
  I.V.: 4 to 6 hours (dose dependent)
Protein binding: 50 to 60%
Metabolism: enalapril is a prodrug (inactive) that is transformed in the
  liver to enalaprilat (active)
Clearance: time to peak serum concentration:
  Enalapril: 0.5 to 1.5 hours
  Enalaprilat: 3 to 4.5 hours
Elimination: 60 to 80% in urine, with some in feces

Monitoring Parameters

Blood pressure, BUN, creatinine, WBC, serum potassium, serum glucose. Monitoring for blood pressure effect should focus on the period 1 to 3 hours (enalapril) or 15 to 60 minutes (enalaprilat) after dosing.

Contraindications

Hypersensitivity to enalapril, enalaprilat, any component, or other ACE inhibitors. In addition, patients with idiopathic or hereditary angioedema or a history of angioedema with administration of ACE inhibitors should not receive these drugs.

Adverse Effects

  Cardiovascular: hypotension, tachycardia, syncope
  Respiratory: cough, dyspnea, eosinophilic pneumonitis. An isolated, dry
    cough has been reported in 7 (17%) of 42 pediatric patients receiving
    ACE inhibitors[4]

Central nervous system: fatigue, vertigo, dizziness, headache, insomnia

Gastrointestinal: nausea, diarrhea, loss of taste perception

Hepatic: cholestatic jaundice, fulminant hepatic necrosis (rare, but potentially fatal)

Renal: diminished renal function

Genitourinary: impotence

Neuromuscular and skeletal: muscle cramps

Endocrine/metabolic: hypoglycemia, hyperkalemia

Hematological: agranulocytosis, neutropenia, anemia

Cutaneous/peripheral: rash, angioedema. The risk of angioedema is higher in the first 30 days of use and for enalapril and lisinopril as compared with captopril

Drug-Drug Interactions

In patients who are also receiving potassium supplements or a potassium-sparing diuretic (e.g., spironolactone), an additive hyperkalemic effect may occur. In patients who are also receiving indomethacin or a NSAID, the antihypertensive effect of enalapril may be diminished, and renal dysfunction may be exacerbated (usually reversible). Enalapril may increase serum lithium levels.

Poisoning Information

Enalaprilat contains benzyl alcohol (9 mg/mL), which may cause allergic reactions and a potentially fatal toxicity in neonates, called "gasping syndrome" at high doses ($\geq$ 99 mg/kg/d). Gasping syndrome is manifested by metabolic acidosis, respiratory distress with gasping respirations, central nervous system dysfunction (seizures, hemorrhage), hypotension, and cardiovascular collapse. Therefore, enalaprilat should be used with caution and close monitoring in neonates.

Compatible Diluents/Administration

Enalapril is available for oral/enteral administration. It may be administered without regard to the ingestion of food. Enalaprilat can be administered undiluted or diluted with normal saline; infuse over 5 minutes.

References

1. Chobarian AV, Bakris GL, Black HR, et al. The Seventh Report of the Joint National Committee on Prevention, Detection, Evaluation, and Treatment of High Blood Pressure: The JNC 7 Report. JAMA 2003; 289:2560–2572.
2. Leversha AM, Wilson NJ, Clarkson PM, et al. Efficacy and Dosage of Enalapril in Congenital and Acquired Heart Disease. Arch Dis Child 1994; 70:35.
3. Marcadis ML, Kraus DM, Hatzopoulos FK, et al. Use of Enalaprilat for Neonatal Hypertension. J Pediatr 1991; 119:505.
4. von Vigier RO, Mozzetti S, Truttmann AC, et al. Cough is Common in Children Prescribed Converting Enzyme Inhibitors. Nephron 2000; 84:98.

ACE Inhibitor: Lisinopril

Indication
Lisinopril is used in adults to treat systemic hypertension and as an adjunctive therapy in patients with CHF and left ventricular dysfunction after a myocardial infarction.[1] In pediatric patients, it is also used to treat systemic hypertension and CHF; additionally, it is used in CHD patients who have single ventricle anatomy, AVV regurgitation, and aortic valve regurgitation.

Mechanism of Action
Lisinopril is a competitive inhibitor of ACE; therefore, it blocks the conversion of angiotensin I to angiotensin II. Angiotensin II is a strong vasoconstrictor, therefore, reducing its blood level leads to less vasoconstriction. In addition, plasma renin levels are increased and aldosterone secretion reduced.

Dosing
> Neonates (premature and full term), infants, and children younger than 6 years: no dosing information is available; because of this, the manufacturer recommends not using lisinopril in patients younger than 6 years of age
>
> Children older than 6 years: initial or "test" dose 0.07 mg/kg/dose P.O./N.G. Dose once per 24 hours. Maximum initial dose, 5 mg once daily. Increase dose at 1- to 2-week intervals for desired effect. No data are available on doses greater than 0.61 mg/kg or greater than 40 mg
>
> Adults:
>> *Oral:* initial or "test" dose, 10 mg/dose P.O./N.G. administered once daily. Increase dose by 5 to 10 mg/day at 1- to 2-week intervals for desired

effect. Usual dose, 20 to 40 mg/dose administered once daily. Maximum daily dose reported is 80 mg/day

For adults with CHF: initial or "test" dose, 5 mg/dose P.O./N.G. administered once daily. Increase dose by at most 10 mg/dose by at least 2-week intervals based on clinical response. Usual dose is 5 to 10 mg/dose administered once daily. Maximum dose is 40 mg/day

Note: Dosing for all age groups should be titrated to an individual patient's response, and the lowest dose that achieves this response should be chosen. Lower doses are appropriate for patients who are also being treated with diuretics and are water and sodium depleted, those with renal impairment and severe CHF, and patients with systemic arterial obstruction (e.g., coarctation of the aorta, renal artery stenosis). For additional dosing precautions in neonates, see "Poisoning Information"

Dosing adjustment for renal impairment:

Cl_{cr} *greater than 30 mL/min/1.73 m²:* usual dose, 10 mg once daily
Cl_{cr} *10 to 30 mL/min/1.73 m²:* initial dose, 5 mg once daily
Cl_{cr} *less than 10 mL/min/1.73 m²:* initial dose, 2.5 mg once daily

In adults with renal impairment, dose titration should be performed cautiously. In addition, lower doses (e.g., one-half those listed) should be used for patients with hyponatremia, hypovolemia, severe CHF, reduced renal function, or if receiving diuretics. Use is not recommended in children who have a Cl_{cr} less than 30 mL/min/1.73 m².

Pharmacokinetics

Onset of action: 1 hour (blood pressure lowered)
Absorption:
Children (6–16 years): 28%
Adults: 25% (6–60%)
Maximum effect: 6 to 8 hours
Half-life: 11 to 13 hours; increased with renal dysfunction
Duration: 24 hours
Protein binding: 25%
Clearance: time to peak serum concentration:
Children (6–16 years): 6 hours
Adults: 7 hours
Elimination: in urine as unchanged drug. Can be removed by hemodialysis

Monitoring Parameters

Blood pressure, BUN, serum creatinine, WBC, and serum potassium. Monitoring for blood pressure should be conducted with knowledge that the maximum effect is 6 to 8 hours after dosing.

Contraindications

Hypersensitivity to lisinopril (any component) or other ACE inhibitors. Also contraindicated in patients with a history of idiopathic or hereditary angioedema or angioedema with previous ACE use.

Adverse Effects

Cardiovascular: hypotension, chest discomfort, orthostatic hypotension, tachycardia, syncope

Respiratory: cough, dyspnea, eosinophilic pneumonitis

Central nervous system: headache, dizziness, fatigue

Gastrointestinal: diarrhea, nausea, vomiting, loss of taste perception, intestinal angioedema (rare)

Hepatic: cholestatic jaundice, hepatitis, fulminant hepatic necrosis (rare, but potentially fatal)

Renal: elevated BUN and serum creatinine

Endocrine/metabolic: hyperkalemia

Hematological: neutropenia, agranulocytosis, eosinophilia. The risk of neutropenia is increased in patients with renal dysfunction

Cutaneous/peripheral: rash, angioedema. The risk of angioedema is higher in the first 30 days of use and is greater for lisinopril and enalapril than captopril

Other: anaphylactoid reactions

Precautions

Note: Dosing for all age groups should be titrated to an individual patient's response, and the lowest dose that achieves this response chosen. Lower doses are appropriate for patients who are also being treated with diuretics and are water and sodium depleted, those with renal impairment and severe CHF, and patients with systemic arterial obstruction (e.g., coarctation of the aorta, renal artery stenosis).

Angioedema may occur in the head, neck, extremities, or intestines (rare). Airway obstruction can occur with swelling of the tongue, larynx, or glottis, especially in patients who have a history of airway surgery. For patients at higher risk of airway obstruction, equipment to establish airway patency and medications to relieve airway swelling (e.g., epinephrine) should be available.

Drug-Drug Interactions

In patients who are also receiving potassium supplements or a potassium-sparing diuretic (e.g., spironolactone), an additive hyperkalemic effect may occur. In patients who are also receiving indomethacin or a NSAID, the antihypertensive effect of enalapril may be diminished, and renal dysfunction may be exacerbated (usually reversible). Enalapril may increase serum lithium levels.

Compatible Diluents/Administration

Only available for oral/enteral administration. Lisinopril may be administered without regard to ingestion of food.

References

1. Chase SL, Sutton JD. Lisinopril: A New Angiotensin-Converting Enzyme Inhibitor. Pharmacotherapy 1989; 9:120.

Angiotensin II Receptor Antagonists: Losartan

Indication

Losartan is used in adults to treat systemic hypertension, diabetic nephropathy in patients with Type 2 (noninsulin dependent) diabetes mellitus, and hypertension, and to reduce the risk of stroke in patients with hypertension and left ventricular hypertrophy.[1] Losartan is commonly combined with a thiazide diuretic in adults to treat hypertension. For adult patients with CHF who develop persistent cough on an ACE inhibitor, losartan is often used to replace the ACE inhibitor. In pediatric patients, it is used predominantly to treat systemic hypertension, and it seems to have a protective effect on the kidneys in children with renal insufficiency and hypertension.[2]

Mechanism of Action

Losartan (and its principal active metabolite, E-3174) selectively blocks the binding of the potent vasoconstrictor angiotensin II to the AT_1 receptor. AT_1 receptors exist in many tissues, including vascular smooth muscle and the adrenal glands. By inhibiting angiotensin II binding to these receptors, losartan reduces vasoconstriction and aldosterone secretion, which lowers systemic blood pressure. Angiotensin II receptor antagonists may be more inhibitory than ACE inhibitors on the renin-angiotensin system, and, in addition, they do not affect the vascular response to bradykinin (a potent vasodilator) or induce as much cough or angioedema as ACE inhibitors. Losartan is also a natriuretic and kaliuretic and increases urine output.

Dosing

Neonates (premature and full term) and infants: no data are available to guide dosing in neonates, infants, and children younger than 6 years of age

Children 6 to 16 years:

Oral: data from a single trial of pediatric patients (n = 177) aged 6 to 16 years forms the basis of pediatric dosing recommendations.[3] 0.7 mg/kg P.O./N.G. once daily. Titrate dose based on response. Maximum dose, 50 mg/d

Adults:

Oral: usual starting dose is 50 mg P.O./N.G. once daily. Total daily doses range from 25 to 100 mg. May be administered in one or two doses per day

Dosing adjustments:

1. Patients receiving diuretics or with low intravascular volume: initial dose, 25 mg once daily.
2. Renal impairment:
   Children: Use not recommended if Cl_{cr} is less than 30 mL/min/1.73 m^2
   Adults: No adjustment necessary
3. Hepatic impairment: reduce initial dose in adults to 25 mg/d and administer in two versus one dose per day.
4. No adjustment required for food.

Pharmacokinetics

Onset of action: 6 hours

Absorption: well absorbed; bioavailability, 25 to 33%

Distribution: volume of distribution—losartan, 34 L; E-3174, 12 L

Maximum effect: peak concentrations—losartan, 1 hour; E-3174, 3 to 4 hours

Half-life: losartan, 1.5 to 2 hours; E-3174, 6 to 9 hours

Protein binding: greater than 98%

Metabolism: extensive first-pass effect. Metabolized in liver (14%) via the cytochrome P450 isoenzymes, CYP2C9 and CYP3A4, to the active metabolite, E-3174

Clearance: losartan, 600 mL/min; E-3174, 50 mL/min

Elimination: via the urine, 4% as unchanged drug and 6% as E-3174. Biliary secretion also occurs

Monitoring Parameters

Blood pressure (while supine), serum electrolytes, BUN, serum creatinine, complete blood cell count (CBC), and urinalysis

Contraindications

Hypersensitivity to losartan or any component in its formulation or to other angiotensin II receptor antagonists, bilateral renal artery stenosis, pregnancy (particularly the second and third trimesters).

Adverse Effects

> **Cardiovascular:** chest pain, hypotension, orthostatic hypotension, first-dose hypotension, tachycardia
>
> **Respiratory:** cough, bronchitis, upper respiratory infection, nasal congestion, sinusitis
>
> **Central nervous system:** fatigue, dizziness, hypoesthesia, insomnia
>
> **Gastrointestinal:** diarrhea, gastritis, weight gain, dyspepsia, abdominal pain, nausea
>
> **Genitourinary:** urinary tract infection (patients with diabetic nephropathy)
>
> **Neuromuscular and skeletal:** weakness, back pain, knee pain, leg pain, muscle cramps, myalgia
>
> **Endocrine/metabolic:** hypoglycemia, hyperkalemia
>
> **Hematological:** anemia
>
> **Cutaneous/peripheral:** cellulitis (patients with diabetic nephropathy)
>
> **Other:** fever, infections, flu-like syndrome

Precautions

Drugs that affect the angiotensin system in humans can cause injury or death to a fetus during the second or third trimester; therefore, losartan should be discontinued as soon as possible once pregnancy is detected. Avoid use in nursing mothers because excretion in breast milk occurs. Because losartan can cause hypotension, especially with the initial dose, particular care should be used in patients who have low intravascular volume. Use with caution in patients who have baseline hepatic or renal dysfunction. Consider discontinuing potassium supplementation or potassium-sparing diuretics because of risk of hyperkalemia. Patients with unilateral renal artery stenosis or significant aortic or mitral stenosis are at risk for inadequate systemic blood flow.

Drug-Drug Interactions

Because losartan is metabolized in the liver by the cytochrome P450 system as a substrate of isoenzymes CYP3A4 and CYP2C9, it has multiple interactions with other drugs. The most significant interactions reported are as follows:

1. Losartan and E-3174 levels are decreased by concomitant administration of phenobarbital and rifampin.
2. Fluconazole decreases E3174 levels but increases losartan levels.
3. Losartan may increase the levels or effects of CYP2C8 (e.g., amiodarone) and CYP2C9 (e.g., warfarin, phenytoin, and fluoxetine) substrates and lithium levels.
4. NSAIDs may reduce the effectiveness of losartan.

Compatible Diluents/Administration

Losartan may be taken with or without food.

References

1. Epstein BJ, Gums JG. Angiotensin Receptor Blockers Versus ACE Inhibitors: Prevention of Death And Myocardial Infarction in High-Risk Populations. Ann Pharmacother 2005; 39:470–480.
2. Ellis D, Moritz ML, Vats A, Janosky JE. Antihypertensive and Renoprotective Efficacy and Safety of Losartan. A Long-Term Study in Children with Renal Disorders. Am J Hypertens 2004; 7:928–935.
3. Cozaar® (Losartan potassium). In Physicians' Desk Reference. 60th Edition. Thomson PDR, Montvale, New Jersey. 2006. pp. 1213–1918.

Calcium Channel Blockers: Nifedipine

Indication

Nifedipine is used in adults for the treatment of angina, hypertrophic cardiomyopathy, and hypertension (extended-release forms of the drug). In pediatric patients, it is predominantly used to treat systemic hypertension and hypertrophic cardiomyopathy.[1]

Mechanism of Action

Nifedipine prevents calcium ions from entering both vascular smooth muscle cells and myocardial cells via specific slow calcium channels. Thus, it decreases the intracellular concentration of calcium such that less calcium is available to bind to contractile proteins in these cells. This results in vasodilation, including the coronary arteries, and a negative inotropic effect. The negative inotropic effect of nifedipine is less clinically significant than its vasodilatory effect.

Dosing

Neonates (premature and full term) and infants: specific dosing information has not been obtained for neonates and infants

Children:

Oral or sublingual (S.L.): hypertensive emergencies, 0.25 to 0.5 mg/kg/dose P.O./S.L. every 4 to 6 hours, as needed. Maximum single dose is 10 mg/dose; and the daily dose is 1 to 2 mg/kg/day

Hypertrophic cardiomyopathy: 0.6 to 0.9 mg/kg/24 hours in three to four divided doses

Hypertension (chronic treatment) extended-release forms: initial, 0.25 to 0.5 mg/kg/day P.O./S.L. in one to two doses per day. Titrate to desired effect. Maximum dose is 3 mg/kg/day, up to 180 mg/day

Adults:

Oral or S.L:

Capsules: initial, 10 mg three times per day. Maintenance, 10 to 30 mg, three to four times per day

Extended-release tablets: initial, 30 to 60 mg once daily. Usual dosage for hypertension is 30 to 60 mg once daily. Maximum dose is 120 mg/day

Note: Doses are typically titrated to achieve the desired effect (e.g., reduce hypertension) over 1 to 2 weeks.

Pharmacokinetics

Onset of action:

S.L. or "bite and swallow": within 1 to 5 minutes

Oral:

Immediate release: within 20 to 30 minutes

Extended release: 2 to 2.5 hours

Absorption: bioavailability:

Capsules: 45 to 75%

Extended release: 65 to 85%

Half-life:

Healthy adults: 2 to 5 hours

Adults with cirrhosis: 7 hours

Duration:
 Immediate release: 4 to 8 hours
 Extended release: 24 hours
Protein binding: 92 to 98%
Metabolism: in the liver, to inactive metabolites
Elimination: in urine, with greater than 90% excreted as inactive metabolites

Monitoring Parameters
Blood pressure, CBC, and liver enzymes.

Contraindications
Hypersensitivity to nifedipine (any component) and recent myocardial infarction.

Adverse Effects

Cardiovascular: hypotension, tachycardia, flushing, palpitations, syncope, peripheral edema
Respiratory: shortness of breath
Central nervous system: headache, dizziness
Gastrointestinal: nausea, diarrhea, constipation, gingival hyperplasia
Hepatic: elevated liver enzymes, cholestasis, jaundice, allergic hepatitis (rare)
Neuromuscular and skeletal: joint stiffness, arthritis with an elevated antinuclear antibody (ANA)
Hematological: thrombocytopenia, leukopenia, anemia
Ophthalmological: blurred vision, transient blindness
Cutaneous/peripheral: dermatitis, urticaria, purpura, photosensitivity (rare)
Other: fever, chills, diaphoresis

Precautions
Initiation of antihypertensive therapy with nifedipine should be performed cautiously and with close blood pressure monitoring, because significant hypotension can occur. Upward titrations of dosing should be monitored similarly. Patients receiving concomitant treatment with β-blockers are at increased risk of hypotension. Angina and acute myocardial infarction in adults has been reported with initiation of nifedipine therapy. Patients with either CHF or aortic stenosis are also at increased risk.

Drug-Drug Interactions

Concomitant use of β-blockers may increase cardiovascular adverse events. Hypotension may be accentuated with anesthetic doses of fentanyl. Nifedipine may increase the serum concentrations of phenytoin, cyclosporin, and possibly digoxin. It may decrease serum quinidine concentration. Cimetidine and saquinavir may increase serum nifedipine concentration. Combined administration with cyclosporin in transplant patients seems to increase significantly the incidence of gingival hyperplasia. Delavirdine may decrease nifedipine metabolism and, thus, increase serum level. Administration of calcium typically reduces the effects of a calcium channel-blocking agent.

Compatible Diluents/Administration

Administer tablets with food. Avoid coadministration with grapefruit juice, because this may increase oral bioavailability. Sustained-release tablets should be swallowed whole. Nifedipine from liquid-filled capsules can be removed and administered either S.L. or swallowed (only a small amount of a S.L. dose is absorbed in the mouth).

References

1. Flynn JT, Pasko DA. Calcium Channel Blockers: Pharmacology and Place in Therapy of Pediatric Hypertension. Pediatr Nephrol 2000; 15:302.

Calcium Channel Blockers: Amlodipine

Indication

Amlodipine is used in adults for the treatment of angina pectoris and also for hypertension. In pediatric patients, it is used to treat systemic hypertension.[1,2]

Mechanism of Action

Amtopidine prevents calcium ions from entering both vascular smooth muscle cells and myocardial cells via specific slow calcium channels during depolarization. Thus, it decreases the intracellular concentration of calcium such that less calcium is available to contractile proteins in these cells. As a result, vasodilation occurs. Relaxation of the coronary vascular smooth muscle specifically treats anginal pain by increasing myocardial oxygen delivery.

Dosing

Neonates and infants:
Specific dosing information has not been obtained for neonates and infants

Oral, hypertension: for children ages 6 to 17 years, the manufacturer's recommended dose is 2.5 to 5 mg P.O./N.G. once daily. Initial doses reported in the literature have varied from 0.05 to 0.13 mg/kg/day. Doses are typically titrated by 25 to 50% every 5 to 7 days. Required doses reported in the literature have varied from 0.12 to 0.5 mg/kg/day, and younger patients tend to need higher doses for effect. Insufficient data exist on doses greater than 5 mg/day in pediatrics

Adults:
Oral:
Hypertension: initial, 2.5 to 5 mg P.O./N.G. once daily, with a 2.5 mg/dose recommended for smaller, less stable patients. Titrate dose to a maximum of 10 mg/dose once daily over 7 to 24 days. Usual dose is 5 mg/dose once daily

Angina: 5 to 10 mg/dose P.O./N.G. once daily. Lower doses are appropriate for patients with hepatic impairment; no adjustment for renal impairment is required

Pharmacokinetics

Onset of action: 30 to 50 minutes
Absorption: well absorbed orally
Distribution: mean volume of distribution:
Children older than 6 years: similar to adults on a per-kilogram basis
Adults: 21 L/kg
Maximum effect: peak serum concentration at 6 to 12 hours
Half-life: terminal half-life 30 to 50 hours
Duration: ≥ 24 hours with routine dosing
Protein binding: 93%
Metabolism: in the liver, with 90% metabolized to inactive metabolites
Clearance: in children older than 6 years of age, weight-adjusted clearance is similar to adults

Elimination: 10% of unchanged drug and 60% of metabolites are excreted in the urine. Amlodipine is not removed by dialysis

Monitoring Parameters
Blood pressure and liver enzymes.

Contraindications
Hypersensitivity to amlodipine or any of its components.

Adverse Effects

Cardiovascular:
More common: flushing, palpitations, peripheral edema
Rare: hypotension, dysrhythmia, chest pain, syncope, peripheral ischemia, vasculitis, myocardial infarction
Respiratory: dyspnea, pulmonary edema, epistaxis
Central nervous system:
More common: headache, dizziness, somnolence, fatigue
Less common: insomnia, vertigo, depression, anxiety
Gastrointestinal: nausea, abdominal pain, dyspepsia, anorexia, constipation, diarrhea, dysphagia, pancreatitis, vomiting, xerostomia, gingival hyperplasia
Hepatic: jaundice, elevated liver enzymes
Genitourinary: sexual dysfunction
Neuromuscular and skeletal: muscle cramps, asthenia, arthralgia, myalgia, paresthesia, peripheral neuropathy, hypoesthesia, tremor
Endocrine/metabolic: weight gain or loss, gynecomastia, hyperglycemia
Hematological: thrombocytopenia, leukopenia, purpura
Ophthalmological: diplopia, abnormal vision, eye pain, and conjunctivitis
Cutaneous/peripheral: rash, pruritus, erythema multiforme, angioedema
Other: tinnitus, diaphoresis, increased thirst

Precautions
In adult patients with severe coronary artery disease, both initiation of amlodipine therapy and increased dosing have been associated with increased severity and frequency of angina as well as acute myocardial infarction. Acute hypotension is more common in patients with CHF and left ventricular outflow tract obstruction (e.g., aortic stenosis).

Increased caution should be used in patients with impaired hepatic function because of amlodipine's hepatic metabolism. Do not discontinue amlodipine abruptly in patients with angina or significant coronary artery disease.

Drug-Drug Interactions

Concomitant administration of rifampin may decrease serum amlodipine concentration. Azole antifungal agents (e.g., ketoconazole) may inhibit metabolism in the liver and increase serum amlodipine concentration. Amlodipine may increase serum cyclosporine level (uncertain). As for all calcium channel-blocking agents, administration of calcium may mitigate the drug's effect.

Compatible Diluents/Administration

Amlodipine tablets may be administered without regard to food, because food does not affect its bioavailability. Concomitant ingestion of grapefruit juice increased amlodipine peak serum concentration in some reports but not others.

References

1. Flynn JT, Smoyer WE, Bunchman TE. Treatment of Hypertensive Children with Amlodipine. Am J Hypertens 2000; 13:1061–1066.
2. Tallian KB, Nahata MC, Turman MA, et. al. Efficacy of Amlodipine in Pediatric Patients with Hypertension. Pediatr Nephrol 1999; 13:304–310.

Calcium Channel Blockers: Nicardipine

Indication

Nicardipine is used in adults for the treatment of angina pectoris and hypertension. In pediatric patients, it is used predominantly to treat hypertension. Both oral and I.V. preparations of the drug are available. The I.V. preparation is typically used in monitored inpatient settings (e.g., an intensive care unit) when oral dosing is either not possible or tighter blood pressure control is desired (e.g., early after cardiovascular surgery).[1]

Mechanism of Action

Nicardipine prevents calcium ions from entering both vascular smooth muscle cells and myocardial cells via specific slow calcium channels. Thus, it decreases the intracellular concentration of calcium such that less calcium is available to contractile proteins in these cells. This results in vasodilation. Relaxation of coronary vascular smooth muscle specifically treats anginal pain by increasing myocardial oxygen delivery.

Dosing

Neonates (premature and full term):
Oral: no information
I.V. continuous infusion: dosing data from two studies (n = 28 patients) suggested an initial dose of 0.5 µg/kg/min I.V.[2,3] Doses were titrated by blood pressure over the first day to a mean maximal dose of 0.74 ± 0.41 µg/kg/min (range, 0.5–2 µg/kg/min)

Infants/children: data for infants and children are also limited, and dosing is not well established.
Oral: case reports only. Doses of 20 to 30 mg/dose P.O. every 8 hours in two 14-year-old children have been reported
I.V. continuous infusion: initial, 0.5 to 1 µg/kg/min I.V., then titrate dose to achieve the desired blood pressure. Dosing changes can be made every 15 to 30 minutes. Maximum dose 4 to 5 µg/kg/min

Adults:
Oral:
Immediate release: initial, 20 mg P.O., three times per day. Titrate to response allowing at least 3 days between dose increases. Usual dose, 20 to 40 mg, three times per day
Sustained release: initial, 30 mg P.O. twice daily. Usual dosage range, 30 to 60 mg, twice daily
I.V. continuous infusion: hypertension (patients not receiving oral nicardipine): initial, 5 mg/h I.V. Titrate dose by increasing infusion by 2.5 mg/h every 5 to 15 minutes until target achieved or maximum dose of 15 mg/h reached. Once target blood pressure is achieved, decrease infusion rate to 3 mg/h or lowest rate to achieve desired blood pressure

Pharmacokinetics

Onset of action:
Oral: 0.5 to 2 hours
I.V.: within minutes
Absorption: oral dose, 100%; but large first-pass effect. Bioavailability, oral dose, 35%
Distribution: volume of distribution in adults, 8.3 L/kg
Maximum effect:
Immediate-release capsules: 1 to 2 hours
Sustained-release capsules: sustained 2 to 7 hours after dose
I.V. continuous infusion: 50% of maximum effect within 45 minutes, and final effect by 50 hours
Half-life: Dose-dependent (nonlinear) pharmacokinetics, therefore, apparent half-life depends on serum concentration
Oral dose: 2 to 4 hours over first 8 hours; terminal half-life, 8.6 hours

I. V. infusion: serum concentration decreases exponentially in 3 phases—
α (2.7 minutes), β (44.8 minutes), and terminal (14.4 h)
Duration:
Immediate-release capsules: less than 8 hours
Sustained-release capsules: 12 hours
I.V. single dose: 3 hours
I.V. continuous infusion: 50% decrease in 30 minutes with gradual loss of
antihypertensive effect over 50 hours
Protein binding: 95%
Metabolism: saturable first-pass effect with dose-dependent pharma-
cokinetics. Extensive hepatic metabolism by cytochrome P450 isoenzyme,
CYP3A4
Clearance: decreased in patients with hepatic dysfunction, and may be
decreased with renal dysfunction
Elimination: 60% of an oral dose is excreted in the urine, with less than 1%
as unchanged drug; 35% excreted in the feces. Not removed by dialysis

Monitoring Parameters

Blood pressure, heart rate, liver function, and renal function. Monitor blood
pressure carefully, especially with I.V. infusion and dosing changes.

Contraindications

Hypersensitivity to nicardipine or any component, and significant aortic stenosis.

Adverse Effects

Cardiovascular: vasodilation/flushing, tachycardia, palpitations, hypotension (6% with I.V. form), orthostasis, syncope, peripheral and facial
edema, increased angina, electrocardiographic changes, myocardial inf-
arction
Respiratory: dyspnea
Central nervous system: headache, dizziness, somnolence, paresthesias,
anxiety, insomnia, intracranial hemorrhage (0.7% with I.V. form)
Gastrointestinal: nausea, vomiting, dyspepsia, xerostomia, diarrhea, con-
stipation, abdominal pain
Genitourinary: polyuria, nocturia, hematuria (0.7% with I.V. form).
Neuromuscular and skeletal: asthenia, myalgia, malaise, tremor, hypoesthesia
Endocrine/metabolic: hypokalemia (0.7% with I.V. form)
Ophthalmological: blurred vision
Cutaneous/peripheral: rash
Other: diaphoresis, injection site reaction or pain (I.V. form)

Precautions

In adult patients with severe coronary artery disease, both initiation of nicardipine therapy and increased dosing have been associated with increased severity and frequency of angina. Abrupt withdrawal may cause rebound angina in patients with coronary artery disease.

Negative inotropic effects may occur in those patients with CHF and left ventricular dysfunction, resulting in low cardiac output. Symptomatic hypotension may occur, especially with the I.V. form. Because vessel irritation is common, infusion sites for the I.V. form should be changed every 12 hours on therapy.

Drug-Drug Interactions

Nicardipine affects several cytochrome P450 isoenzymes and, thus, has numerous drug interactions. Serum concentrations of the following drugs may be increased by nicardipine: cyclosporine, metoprolol, vecuronium (I.V. nicardipine), and digoxin. Either serum concentrations or the effects of multiple other drugs that are substrates for various cytochrome P450 enzymes may be affected, including CYP2C8/9 substrates (e.g., amiodarone, warfarin), CYP2C19 substrates (e.g., phenytoin, propranolol), CYP2D6 substrates (e.g., selected β-blockers, lidocaine, risperidone), and CYP3A4 substrates (e.g., benzodiazepines, other calcium channel blockers, and tacrolimus).

Drugs that are strong inhibitors of the cytochrome P450 isoenzyme, CYP3A4, such as azole antifungals, clarithromycin, propofol, and protease inhibitors, may all increase serum concentrations or effects of nicardipine, whereas drugs that induce isoenzyme CYP3A4, such as carbamazepine, phenytoin, phenobarbital, and rifampin, may decrease the concentration or effects of nicardipine. Lastly, nicardipine may decrease the serum concentration or effects of common narcotic agents (e.g., codeine, hydrocodone, and oxycodone) that are prodrug substrates for isoenzyme CYP2D6.

Compatible Diluents/Administration

For oral forms of nicardipine, administration of the drug with high-fat meals may decrease peak concentrations. Concurrent use of grapefruit juice may increase serum concentration. The I.V. form should be protected from light. It can be diluted in either dextrose- (e.g., 5% dextrose in water [D5W]) or saline-based I.V. fluid, but not in lactated Ringer's solution. Nicardipine is not compatible with 5% sodium bicarbonate, furosemide, heparin, or thiopental.

References

1. Tobias JD. Nicardipine to Control Mean Arterial Pressure After Cardiothoracic Surgery in Infants and Children. Am J Ther 2001; 8:3–6.
2. Milou C, Debuche-Benouachkou V, Semama DS, et al. Intravenous Nicardipine as a First-Line Antihypertensive Drug in Neonates. Intensive Care Med 2000; 26:956–958.
3. Gouyon JB, Geneste B, Semama DS, et al. Intravenous Nicardipine in Hypertensive Preterm Infants. Arch Dis Child Fetal Neonatal Ed 1997; 76:F126–127.

Nitrates: Nitroglycerin

Indication
Nitroglycerin is used in adult patients for both the acute treatment and prophylaxis of angina pectoris[1] and the acute treatment of CHF (e.g., associated with acute myocardial infarction). Other indications include hypertensive emergencies, pulmonary hypertension, and to improve coronary blood flow after cardiovascular surgery or transcatheter coronary revascularization. In pediatric patients, it is used primarily for treatment of hypertensive emergencies and after cardiovascular surgery (especially with cardiopulmonary bypass) to improve coronary blood flow and myocardial perfusion.

Mechanism of Action
Nitroglycerin is a nitric oxide (NO) donor that causes relaxation of vascular smooth muscle and, thus, vasodilation by increasing the intracellular concentration of cyclic guanosine monophosphate (cGMP). Increased cGMP leads to an increased intracellular calcium concentration, which causes smooth muscle cells to relax. Nitroglycerin seems to dilate veins more than arteries, although the coronary arteries respond well, resulting in improved myocardial oxygen delivery. Systemic venous dilation results in lower atrial filling pressures (preload) and ventricular end diastolic pressures; this effect reduces myocardial oxygen demand. Systemic arterial dilation also reduces myocardial oxygen demand by reducing afterload.

Dosing

Children:
  I.V. continuous infusion: initial, 0.25 to 0.5 µg/kg/min I.V. Dose is titrated to achieve desired effect by 0.5 to 1 µg/kg/min increments every 3 to 5 minutes. Usual maximum dose is 5 µg/kg/min, but doses to 20 µg/kg/min have been described
Adults:
  Oral: 2.5 to 9 mg every 8 to 12 hours

S.L.: 0.2 to 0.6 mg every 5 minutes for maximum of three doses in 15 minutes

Lingual: one to two sprays into mouth or under tongue every 3 to 5 minutes for maximum of three sprays in 15 minutes. Can be used before activities that cause angina

Ointment: 1 inch to 2 inches every 8 hours

Patch: initial, 0.2 to 0.4 mg/h and titrate 0.4 to 0.8 mg/h. To minimize tolerance, have patch in place for only 12 to 14 h/day

I.V. continuous infusion: initial, 5 μg/min I.V.; increase by 5 μg/min every 3 to 5 minutes to 20 μg/min, then increase as needed by 10 μg/min every 3 to 5 minutes up to a maximum dose of 200 μg/min

Note: Diminished efficacy of nitroglycerin, termed tolerance, typically occurs in 24 to 48 hours of ongoing use.[2] Both the hemodynamic and antianginal effects of the drug are reduced. To minimize tolerance, a daily drug-free interval of 10 to 12 h/day is recommended, along with the lowest effective dose possible. Tolerance may also be reversed with the administration of *N*-acetylcysteine

Pharmacokinetics (Table 4-2)

Distribution: volume of distribution in adults, 3 L/kg

Half-life: 1 to 4 minutes

Protein binding: 60%

Metabolism: extensive first-pass; metabolized by red blood cells, blood vessel walls, and the liver

Clearance: approximately 1 L/kg/min

Elimination: inactive metabolites are excreted in the urine

Table 4-2. Pharmacodynamics of various forms of nitroglycerin

Dosage Form	Onset (min)	Duration
I.V.	1–2	3–5 min
S.L.	1–3	30–60 min
Translingual spray	2	30–60 min
Buccal, extended release	2–3	3–5 h
Oral, sustained release	40	4–8 h
Topical ointment	20–60	2–12 h
Transdermal	40–60	12–24 h

Source: Nitroglycerin, in Lexi-Comp's Pediatric Dosage Handbook, 12th Edition, 2005, p 916.

Monitoring Parameters

Blood pressure, heart rate (with I.V. infusion).

Contraindications

Hypersensitivity to nitroglycerin and organic nitrates (rare) or any component (adhesive in transdermal patches included); glaucoma; severe anemia; increased intracranial pressure; concurrent use of sildenafil; the I.V. form is contraindicated in patients with hypotension, uncontrolled hypokalemia, pericardial tamponade, constrictive pericarditis, or obstructive hypertrophic cardiomyopathy.

Adverse Effects

Cardiovascular: hypotension, reflex tachycardia, pallor, flushing, and cardiovascular collapse; acute cessation of therapy may cause severe hypotension, bradycardia, and acute coronary insufficiency

Central nervous system: headache (most commonly reported side effect), dizziness, restlessness

Gastrointestinal: nausea, vomiting

Endocrine/metabolic: one I.V. formulation contains alcohol and may cause alcohol intoxication

Cutaneous/peripheral: allergic contact dermatitis and exfoliative dermatitis (occur with patches and ointment)

Other: perspiration

Precautions

An excessive vasodilatory effect of nitroglycerin may cause severe hypotension, so caution should be used in treating any patient who is either hypovolemic or hypotensive, including those with an acute myocardial infarction.

Drug-Drug Interactions

Nitroglycerin may antagonize the anticoagulant effect of heparin; thus, when nitroglycerin is discontinued, a reduction in heparin dose may be required. Alcohol and drugs that lower blood pressure, such as β-blockers and calcium channel blockers, may potentiate nitroglycerin's hypotensive effect. Concomitant use of sildenafil may cause severe hypotension from excessive vasodilation.

Compatible Diluents/Administration

The I.V. form of nitroglycerin can be mixed in D5W. Because it attaches to plastics, nitroglycerin for I.V. infusion must be prepared in glass bottles and run through nonpolyvinyl chloride tubing sets. I.V. nitroglycerin should not be mixed with other drugs. Multiple additional forms of nitroglycerin exist for oral (tablet, capsule, and aerosol) and topical (ointment and transdermal patch) administration (see, for example, Lexi-Comp's Pediatric Dosage Handbook, 13th Edition, 2006[3] for additional details on these multiple formulations).

References

1. Corwin S, Reiffel JA. Nitrate Therapy for Angina Pectoris. Arch Int Med 1985; 145:538.
2. Elkayam V. Tolerance to Organic Nitrates: Mechanisms, Clinical Relevance, and Strategies for Prevention. Ann Int Med 1991; 114:667–677.
3. Taketomo CK, Hodding JH, Kraus DM. Lexi-Comp's Pediatric Dosage Handbook, 13th Edition, 2006.

Nitrates: Nitroprusside

Indication

Nitroprusside (also known as sodium nitroprusside) is used in adults to treat hypertensive crises, CHF, and to reduce SVR to generate controlled hypotension during anesthesia.[1] In pediatric patients, it is used to treat hypertension in inpatient settings (e.g., the intensive care unit), in which minute-to-minute control of blood pressure is desired. It is also used to reduce SVR (afterload) after cardiopulmonary bypass surgery.

Mechanism of Action

Like nitroglycerin, nitroprusside is an NO donor that induces vascular smooth muscle relaxation and, thus, vasodilation. Nitroprusside seems to cause more systemic arterial (at the arteriolar level) dilation than systemic venous dilation. Therefore, it causes more reduction of afterload than preload. Cardiac output increases and aortic and left ventricular impedance are decreased.

Dosing

> **Neonates (premature and full term) and infants:** insufficient data on dosing exist for neonates and infants. In clinical practice, dosing guidelines developed for children are typically followed for infants

Children:
> *I.V. continuous infusion:* initial, 0.5 to 1 μg/kg/min by continuous I.V. infusion. The dose is titrated to achieve the desired reduction in blood pressure by increasing in increments of 1 μg/kg/min every 20 to 60 minutes. Usual dose is 3 μg/kg/min; maximum dose is 5 μg/kg/min

Adults:
> *I.V. continuous infusion:* initial, 0.3 to 0.5 μg/kg/min by continuous I.V. infusion. The dose is titrated to achieve the desired effect or until headache or nausea appear by increasing in increments of 0.5 μg/kg/min. Usual dose is 3 μg/kg/min; maximum dose, 10 μg/kg/min

Pharmacokinetics

Onset of action: less than 2 minutes (hypotensive effect)
Half-life: parent drug, less than 10 minutes; thiocyanate, 2.7 to 7 days
Duration: effects cease within 10 minutes of discontinuation of administration
Metabolism: converted by erythrocytes and tissue sulfhydryl group interactions to cyanide, which is then converted to thiocyanate in the liver by the enzyme rhodanase
Elimination: thiocyanate is excreted in the urine

Monitoring Parameters

Blood pressure and heart rate (reflex tachycardia with hypotension) should be monitored continuously. Monitor closely for signs of cyanide and thiocyanate oxicity (see Poisoning Information), including acid-base status, blood cyanide level (especially patients with hepatic dysfunction), and blood thiocyanate level.

Contraindications

Hypersensitivity to nitroprusside or any component, decreased cerebral perfusion, arteriovenous shunt, unrepaired coarctation of the aorta, high-output CHF, and congenital optic atrophy.

Adverse Effects

Cardiovascular: excessive hypotensive response, palpitations, reflex tachycardia, substernal chest pain
Respiratory: tachypnea or respiratory distress (from metabolic acidosis caused by cyanide toxicity), hypoxemia
Central nervous system: disorientation, restlessness, headache, psychosis, elevated intracranial pressure
Gastrointestinal: nausea, vomiting

Neuromuscular and skeletal: weakness, muscle spasm
Endocrine/metabolic: thyroid suppression
Hematological: thiocyanate toxicity
Other: diaphoresis, tinnitus

Precautions

Because both the liver and kidney contribute to removal of nitroprusside's breakdown products, use with caution in patients with either hepatic or renal dysfunction. Patients with renal dysfunction are at increased risk of thiocyanate toxicity, and patients with hepatic dysfunction are at increased risk of cyanide toxicity. See also Poisoning Information.

Drug-Drug Interactions

The addition of nitroprusside to treatment regimens that include other agents that reduce blood pressure can lead to excessive hypotension.

Poisoning Information

Toxicity from nitroprusside can occur either by cyanide toxicity or thiocyanate toxicity.[2] Signs and symptoms of excessive cyanide levels include metabolic acidosis (with increased blood lactate), increased mixed venous oxygen saturation, tachycardia, altered consciousness, coma, convulsions, and an almond-like smell on the breath. Thiocyanate toxicity is manifested by psychosis, hyperreflexia, confusion, weakness, tinnitus, dilated pupils, seizures, and coma. Patients with hepatic dysfunction or anemia should have blood cyanide levels measured. Patients receiving nitroprusside doses of at least 4 µg/kg/min I.V. lasting longer than 3 days, or with renal dysfunction, should have blood thiocyanate levels measured. Reference ranges are given in Table 4-3.

If toxicity develops, in addition to discontinuing nitroprusside administration, therapies include:

Table 4-3. Reference ranges for blood thiocyanate and cyanide levels

Thiocyanate	Cyanide
Therapeutic: 6–29 µg/mL	Normal: < 0.2 µg/mL
Toxic: 35–100 µg/mL	Normal (smoker): < 0.4 µg/mL
Fatal: > 200 µg/mL	Toxic: > 2 µg/mL
	Potentially lethal: > 3 µg/mL

1. Support respiration and supply oxygen.
2. Antidotal therapy with sodium nitrate 300 mg I.V. and sodium thiosulfate 12.5 grams I.V. (adult doses), and, if needed:
3. Dialysis (thiocyanate is removed by dialysis).

Compatible Diluents/Administration

Nitroprusside should be prepared for I.V. administration by dilution in D5W. Because light causes nitroprusside to break down to form cyanide, it must be protected from light (e.g., by wrapping mixture in aluminum foil). Use only if the mixed solution remains clear; slight discoloration (e.g., brownish, light orange) is common, but blue discoloration suggests break down to cyanide. Discard any solution suspected of degradation and prepare a fresh mixture. The solution is stable at room temperature for up to 24 hours if protected from light.

References

1. Palmer RF, Lasseter KC. Drug Therapy: Sodium Nitroprusside. N Engl J Med 1975; 292:294–297.
2. Vessey CJ, Cole PV. Blood Cyanide and Thiocyanate Concentrations Produced by Long-Term Therapy with Sodium Nitroprusside. Br J Anaesth 1985; 57:148–155.

Systemic Vasodilators: Phenoxybenzamine and Phentolamine

Phenoxybenzamine

Indication   Phenoxybenzamine is a nonspecific, long-acting, α-adrenergic antagonist used in pediatric patients for the treatment of arterial hypertension, particularly when secondary to pheochromocytoma,[1] and in the acute postoperative course of congenital or acquired cardiac anomalies. It is a potent systemic and mild pulmonary vasodilator. In some pediatric cardiac centers, it is considered to be an essential drug in the armamentarium for the treatment of low cardiac output state after weaning from cardiopulmonary bypass.[2] It may also be useful in treating radial artery grafts before surgical coronary revascularization procedures,[3] and it may be used in combination with other vasodilators.[4,5] Phenoxybenzamine can maintain organ perfusion on cardiopulmonary bypass and improve peripheral blood flow, as demonstrated by smaller base deficits and temperature gradients intraoperatively and in the intensive care unit as compared with nitroprusside.[6–8]

It has efficacy in decreasing the incidence of sudden circulatory collapse after the first-stage Norwood operation.[9–11] Lastly, it may also be beneficial in establishing more uniform rewarming after bypass and as a nonselective pulmonary vasodilator.[12]

Mechanism of Action Phenoxybenzamine forms a permanent and irreversible covalent bond with nitrogen atoms on the surface of α-adrenoceptors, thereby blocking epinephrine and norepinephrine from binding with these receptors. This causes systemic vasodilation, and to some extent, pulmonary vasodilation because of a reduction in vascular resistances. These activities are beneficial in controlling the effects of endogenously released catecholamines in the perioperative stress response.

By affecting postsynaptic membrane adrenoceptors in the sympathetic nervous pathway, phenoxybenzamine also acts on $\alpha1$ and $\alpha2$ receptors, reducing sympathetic activity. This resulting "chemical sympathectomy" induces further general vasodilation, miosis, an increase in gastrointestinal tract motility, secretions, and glycogen synthesis.

In addition to the α-blockade effect, phenoxybenzamine irreversibly inhibits responses to 5-hydroxytryptamine (serotonin), histamine, and acetylcholine.

There is no effect on the parasympathetic nervous system.

Phenoxybenzamine is a noncompetitive (irreversible) antagonist, meaning that receptor blockade cannot be overcome by addition of agonist drugs.

Dosing Phenoxybenzamine should be slowly titrated to the desired effect after a small initial dose and under close hemodynamic monitoring. It may be infused in D5W or in 0.9% NaCl.

Neonates, infants, and children:

> *Oral:* 0.2 to 1 mg/kg P.O./N.G. every 12 to 24 hours
>
> *I.V.:* 1 mg/kg I.V. over 2 hours, followed by 0.5 mg/kg/dose every 6 to 12 hours administered over 2 hours. It may be progressively increased to 2 mg/kg once or twice a day in patients younger than 12 years, or 1 mg/kg once or twice a day in patients older than 12 years

Adults:

> *Oral:* 5 to 10 mg P.O./N.G twice a day; dose may be increased every other day to 20 to 80 mg two or three times a day

Note: In patients with pheochromocytoma, if persistent or excessive tachycardia occurs, the use of a concomitant β-blocker may be necessary

Pharmacokinetics

> **Onset of action:** rapid
>
> **Absorption:** when administered orally, 20 to 30% of the drug is absorbed in the active form[13]
>
> **Duration:** 3 to 4 days
>
> **Metabolism:** hepatic
>
> **Half-life:** the half-life of oral phenoxybenzamine is not well known; intravenously, the half-life is approximately 24 hours, and effects may persist for 3 to 4 days. Effects of daily administration are cumulative for nearly a week. The duration of action is dependent not only on the presence of the drug, but also on the rate of synthesis of α-receptors
>
> **Elimination:** renal and biliary

Contraindications Phenoxybenzamine is contraindicated in patients with hypersensitivity to the drug or any of its components. The induction of α-adrenergic blockade leaves β-adrenergic receptors unopposed. Compounds that stimulate both types of receptors may produce an exaggerated hypotensive response with reflex tachycardia.

Adverse Effects

> **Cardiovascular:** tachycardia, arrhythmias, hypotension (mostly in patients with intravascular volume depletion), shock
> **Gastrointestinal:** vomiting
> **Metabolic:** water and sodium retention
> **Central nervous system:** dizziness, drowsiness, postural hypotension
> **Neuromuscular and skeletal:** weakness
> **Ophthalmological:** miosis
> **Other:** nasal congestion, irritation, fatigue, lethargy

Drug-Drug Interactions Phenoxybenzamine interacts with compounds that stimulate both α- and β-adrenergic receptors to produce severe hypotension and tachycardia. Phenoxybenzamine blocks the hyperthermia produced by norepinephrine and blocks the hypothermia produced by reserpine.

Poisoning Information Overdosage of phenoxybenzamine produces symptoms of sympathetic nervous system blockade; symptoms and signs include hypotension, tachycardia, dizziness or fainting, vomiting, lethargy, and shock. Treatment of overdosage consists of the following:

- Drug withdrawal
- Recumbent position with leg elevation
- I.V. volume
- Infusion of norepinephrine in cases of severe hypotension. *Note:* usual inotropic agents are not effective. **Epinephrine is contraindicated** because it stimulates both α- and β-receptors, and, because α-receptors are blocked, epinephrine may produce further hypotension via β-receptor stimulation
- Antagonism with vasopressin has been described as effective, particularly for the treatment of phenoxybenzamine-induced side effects in patients after the Norwood procedure[14]

References

1. Tobias JD. Preoperative blood pressure management of children with cathecholamine-secreting tumors: time for a change. Pediatr Anesth 2005; 15:537–540.
2. Kawamura M, Minamikawa O, Yokochi H, Maki S, Yasuda T, Mizukawa Y. Combined use of phenoxybenzamine and dopamine for low cardiac output syndrome in children at withdrawal from cardiopulmonary bypass. Br Heart J 1980; 43:388–392.

3. Kulik A, Rubens FD, Gunning D, Bourke ME, Mesana TG, Ruel M. Radial artery graft treatment with phenoxybenzamine is clinically safe and may reduce perioperative myocardial injury. Ann Thorac Surg 2007; 83:502–509.

4. Kiran U, Zuber K, Kakani M. Combination of low-dose phenoxybenzamine and sodium nitroprusside in children undergoing cardiac surgery. J Cardiothorac Vasc Anesth 2006; 20:291–292.

5. Kiran U, Makhija N, Das SN, Bhan A, Airan B. Combination of phenoxybenzamine and nitroglycerin: effective control of pulmonary artery pressures in children undergoing cardiac surgery. J Cardiothorac Vasc Anesth 2005; 19:274–275.

6. Motta P, Mossad E, Toscaca D, Zestos M, Mee R. Comparison of phenoxybenzamine to sodium nitroprusside in infants undergoing surgery. J Cardiothorac Vasc Anesth 2006; 20:291–292.

7. Motta P, Mossad E, Toscana D, Zestos M, Mee R. Comparison of phenoxybenzamine to sodium nitroprusside in infants undergoing surgery. J Cardiothorac Vasc Anesth 2005; 19: 54–59.

8. Li DM, Mullaly R, Ewer P, Bell B, Eyres RL, Brawn WJ, Mee RB. Effects of vasodilators on rates of change of nasopharyngeal temperature and systemic vascular resistance during cardiopulmonary bypass in anaesthetized dogs. Aust N Z J Surg 1988; 58:327–333.

9. De Oliveira NC, Ashburn DA, Khalid F, Burkhart HM, Adatia IT, Holtby HM, Williams WG, Van Arsdell GS. Prevention of early sudden circulatory collapse after the Norwood operation. Circulation 2004; 110(Suppl 1):II133–138.

10. De Oliveira NC, Van Arsdell GS. Practical use of alpha blockade strategy in the management of hypoplastic left heart syndrome following stage one palliation with a Blalock-Taussig shunt. Semin Thorac Cardiovasc Surg Pediatr Card Surg Annu 2004: 7:11–15.

11. O'Blenes SB, Roy N, Konstantinov I, Bohn D, Van Arsdell GS. Vasopressin reversal of phenoxybenzamine-induced hypotension after the Norwood procedure. J Thorac Cardiovasc Surg 2002; 123:1012–1013.

12. Kiran U, Makhija N, Das SN, Bhan A, Airan B. Combination of phenoxybenzamine and nitroglycerin: effective control of pulmonary artery pressures in children undergoing cardiac surgery. J Cardiothorac Vasc Anesth 2005; 19:274–275.

13. Weiner N: Drugs that inhibit adrenergic nerves and block adrenergic receptors. In: Goodman & Gillman, The Pharmacological Basis of Therapeutics, 6th Edition, New York, MacMillan Publishing Co, 1980. pp. 179–182.

14. O'Blenes SB, Roy N, Konstantinov I, Bohn D, Van Arsdell GS. Vasopressin reversal of phenoxybenzamine-induced hypotension after the Norwood procedure. J Thorac Cardiovasc Surg 2002; 123:1012–1013.

Phentolamine

Indication   Phentolamine is a reversible, competitive, nonselective, α-adrenergic antagonist that has similar affinities for α1 and α2 receptors. Its effects on the cardiovascular system are very similar to those of phenoxybenzamine, and, therefore, its primary action is systemic vasodilation. It may also have a positive inotropic and chronotropic effect on the heart.

The primary application for phentolamine is for the control of hypertensive emergencies, most notably caused by pheochromocytoma.[1] It may also be used for the treatment of cocaine-induced hypertension,[2] when one would generally avoid β-blockers and, in which case, calcium channel blockers are not effective. It has also been used to treat hypertensive crises secondary to monoamine oxidase inhibitor-sympathomimetic amine interactions and for withdrawal of clonidine, propranolol, or other antihypertensives.

In patients with congenital or acquired cardiac defects, phentolamine is used to induce peripheral vasodilation and afterload reduction after cardiopulmonary bypass surgery. Similar to phenoxybenzamine, the use of phentolamine during bypass is associated with reduced systemic anaerobic metabolism and more uniform body perfusion.[3]

Phentolamine can be used locally to prevent dermal necrosis after extravasation of an α-agonist or to relieve arterial spasms caused by intra-arterial catheters.[4]

There have been anecdotal reports regarding the usefulness of phentolamine in improving mixing in newborns with transposition of the great arteries. Presumably, improved mixing of blood would be caused by both a reduction in afterload and an alteration in the diastolic function of the right ventricle, allowing more left-to-right shunting across the atrial septal defect.[5]

Phentolamine also has a diagnostic role in cases of pheochromocytoma and complex regional pain syndromes (e.g., reflex sympathetic dystrophy).

Interestingly, although widely used in the pediatric patients, literature describing its use is scant.

Mechanism of Action Phentolamine is a long-acting, α-receptor blocking agent that can produce and maintain a "chemical sympathectomy" by oral administration. It increases blood flow to the skin, mucosa, and abdominal viscera, and lowers both supine and erect blood pressures. It has no effect on the parasympathetic nervous system. Phentolamine works by blocking α-receptors present in vascular smooth muscle, thereby inducing vasodilation. It also blocks receptors for serotonin, and it causes release of histamine from mast cells. Phentolamine also blocks potassium channels,[6] which can accentuate vasodilation.

Phentolamine is a competitive antagonist, meaning that blockade can be surmounted by increasing the concentration of agonist drugs.

Dosing Phentolamine should be slowly titrated to the desired effect after a small initial dose and with rigorous hemodynamic monitoring. It may be infused in D5W or in 0.9% NaCl.

Neonates, infants, and children:

Treatment of hypertension or to achieve afterload reduction: 0.02 to 0.1 mg/kg (maximum 10 mg) I.V. to be administered over 10 to 30 minutes, followed by a continuous infusion at 5 to 50 mcg/kg/min. I.V.

Treatment of extravasation: subcutaneous infiltration of the affected area with 0.1 to 0.2 mg/kg (maximum 10 mg) in up to 5 mL of sterile water for injection within 12 hours of the event

Diagnosis of pheochromocytoma: single dose of 1 mg I.V.
Adults:
Diagnosis of pheochromocytoma: single dose of 5 mg I.V.
Treatment of hypertension: 2.5 to 5 mg I.V. single doses as required to control blood pressure

Pharmacokinetics

Onset of action: immediate
Duration: 30 to 45 minutes
Maximum effect: 2 minutes
Metabolism: extensively metabolized in the liver
Half-life: 19 minutes (adults)
Elimination: 10% excreted in the urine as unchanged drug

Contraindications   Phentolamine is contraindicated in patients with ischemic myocardial disease or cerebral ischemic disease and in cases of hypersensitivity to the drug or any of its components. Phentolamine should be used with additional care in patients with impairment of renal function, gastritis, peptic ulcer disease, or a history of arrhythmia or angina.

Adverse Effects

Cardiovascular: hypotension (mostly in patients with intravascular volume depletion), tachycardia, arrhythmias, shock, ischemic cardiac events
Gastrointestinal: vomiting, nausea, abdominal pain, diarrhea, exacerbation of peptic ulcer
Neuromuscular and skeletal: weakness
Central nervous system: dizziness
Other: flushing, nasal congestion

Drug-Drug Interactions   Vasoconstrictive and hypertensive effects of epinephrine and ephedrine are antagonized by phentolamine.

Poisoning Information   Similar to phenoxybenzamine, overdosage is suspected in cases of excessive tachycardia, shock, vomiting, and dizziness (symptoms of sympathetic nervous system blockade and of increased circulating epinephrine). Treatment of overdosage consists of the following:

- Drug withdrawal
- Recumbent position with leg elevation
- I.V. fluid administration
- Because this drug binds competitively as opposed to phenoxybenzamine, inotropic agents with α-agonist effects may be effective. Nevertheless, **epinephrine is contraindicated,** because epinephrine stimulates both α- and β-receptors, and because α-receptors are blocked, epinephrine may produce further hypotension.

References

1. Tuncel M, Ram VC. Hypertensive emergencies. Etiology and management. Am J Cardiovasc Drugs 2003; 3:21–31.
2. Murphy DJ, Walker ME, Culp DA, Francomacaro DV. Effects of adrenergic antagonists on cocaine-induced changes in respiratory function. Pulm Pharmacol 1991; 4:127–134.
3. Koner O, Tekin S, Koner A, Soybir N, Seren S, Karaoglu K. Effects of phentolamine on tissue perfusion in pediatric cardiac surgery. J Cardiothorac Vasc Anesth 1999; 13:191–197.
4. Molony D. Adrenaline-induced digital ischaemia reversed with phentolamine. ANZ J Surg. 2006; 76:1125–1126.
5. Galal MO, El-Naggar WI, Sharfi MH. Phentolamine as a treatment for poor mixing in transposition of the great arteries with adequate intra atrial communication. Pediatr Cardiol 2005; 26:444–445.
6. McPherson GA. Current trends in the study of potassium channel openers. Gen Pharmacol 1993; 24:275–281.

Dopaminergic Receptor Agonist: Fenoldapam

Indication

Treatment of significant systemic hypertension. I.V. fenoldopam may have advantages over sodium nitroprusside because it causes both a diuresis and natriuresis, is not associated with cyanide toxicity, and is not sensitive to light. In addition, rebound hypertension has not occurred after discontinuation of fenoldopam administered via continuous infusion.[1]

Mechanism of Action

Fenoldopam is a direct-acting vasodilator that binds to postsynaptic dopaminergic Type 1 (DA_1) receptors in the renal, coronary, cerebral, and splanchnic vasculature, resulting in arterial dilation and lower mean arterial pressure (MAP). Through its selective receptor binding, fenoldopam reduces systemic blood pressure by decreasing peripheral vascular resistance and improves renal blood flow and diuresis.[1] Fenoldopam is six times as potent as dopamine in producing renal vasodilation.

Dosing

Infants/children:
I.V. continuous infusion, hypertension (severe), short-term treatment: initial, 0.2 µg/kg/min I.V.; increase in increments of up to 0.3 to 0.5 µg/

kg/min every 20 to 30 minutes; dosages greater than 0.8 µg/kg/min have resulted in tachycardia with no additional benefit; administer for up to 4 hours

Adults:

Hypertension (severe), short-term treatment:

Initial, 0.03 to 0.1 µg/kg/min I.V.; increase every 15 min by 0.05 to 0.1 µg/kg/min based on response; maximum rate 1.6 µg/kg/min; administer for up to 48 hours

Usual treatment length of 1 to 6 hours, with dose tapering of 12% every 15 to 30 minutes

No dosage adjustment required in renal or hepatic impairment

Pharmacokinetics

Onset of action: 10 minutes with peak response in 30 minutes to 2 hours
Distribution: volume of distribution is approximately 0.6 L/kg
Half-life: elimination half-life is approximately 10 minutes
Metabolism: fenoldopam has an extensive first-pass effect. It is metabolized in the liver to multiple metabolites, which may have some activity
Elimination: 80% is excreted in the urine and 20% is excreted in feces

Monitoring Parameters

Blood pressure, heart rate, electrocardiogram, and renal and liver function tests.

Contraindications

Hypersensitivity to fenoldopam or sulfites.

Adverse Effects

Cardiovascular: angina, flattening of T-waves (asymptomatic)[2], atrial fibrillation, atrial flutter, chest pain, edema, hypotension, tachycardia
Central nervous system: headache, dizziness[3]
Gastrointestinal: diarrhea, nausea, vomiting, dry mouth
Ophthalmological: increased intraocular pressure, blurred vision
Hepatic: increased portal pressure in patients with cirrhosis

Drug-Drug Interactions

β-blockers increase the risk of hypotension, and acetaminophen may increase fenoldopam levels by 30 to 70%.

Compatible Diluents/Administration

I.V., dilute in 0.9% NaCl or 5% dextrose to a final concentration of 40 µg/mL. Administer by continuous I.V. infusion; do not use a bolus dose.

References

1. Post JB 4th, Frishman WH. Fenoldopam: a new dopamine agonist for the treatment of hypertensive urgencies and emergencies. J Clin Pharmacol 1998; 38(1):2–13.

2. White WB, Radfod MJ, Gonzales FM, et al. Selective dopamine-1 agonist therapy in severe hypertension: effects of intravenous fenoldopam. J Am Coll Cardiology 1988; 11:1118–1121.

3. Bednzarczyk EM, White WB, Munger MA, et al. Comparative acute blood pressure reduction from intravenous fenoldopam mesylate versus sodium nitroprusside in severe systemic hypertension. Am J Cardiology 1989; 63:993–996.

Prostaglandins: Prostaglandin E$_1$/Alprostadil

Indication

Prostaglandin E$_1$ is used for the temporary maintenance of patency of the ductus arteriosus in neonates with ductal-dependant CHD until the patient can undergo an interventional procedure. Congenital heart defects that create ductal-dependent circulations include pulmonary atresia, critical pulmonary stenosis, tricuspid atresia, tetralogy of Fallot and pulmonary atresia without major aortopulmonary collaterals, transposition of the great arteries, hypoplastic left heart syndrome, critical aortic stenosis, critical coarctation of the aorta, and interrupted aortic arch.

Patients with severe pulmonary hypertension that is refractory to pulmonary antihypertensive drugs may benefit from a prostaglandin E$_1$ infusion. This drug will maintain patency of the ductus arteriosus, which may decompress the pulmonary circulation while maintaining an adequate systemic cardiac output, albeit at the expense of systemic oxygen desaturation.

Mechanism of Action

Prostaglandin E$_1$ causes vasodilation by exerting direct effects on vascular and ductus arteriosus smooth muscle.

Dosing

Neonates and infants:
I.V. continuous infusion: 0.05 to 0.1 µg/kg/min I.V. Infusion rate may be slowly increased; the lowest effective dose should be used. Maintenance

dose range, 0.01 to 0.4 µg/kg/min. The usual infusion rate is 0.1 µg/kg/min, but is often possible to reduce the dose to 1/2 or 1/10 of this dose and maintain ductal patency

Pharmacokinetics

Onset of action: rapid; dilation of ductus arteriosus typically occurs within 30 minutes of I.V. infusion[1]

Duration: ductus arteriosus will begin to close within 1 to 2 hours after infusion is discontinued

Maximum effect: in acyanotic CHD, the maximal effect is seen in 1.5 to 3 hours, with a range of 15 minutes to 11 hours. In cyanotic CHD, the usual maximal effect is seen within 30 minutes

Half-life: The half-life is 5 to 10 minutes, therefore, prostaglandin E_1 must be administered by continuous infusion

Metabolism: 70 to 80% of prostaglandin E_1 is metabolized by oxidation during one pass through the lungs. One active metabolite (13–14 dihydro-PGE_1) has been identified in neonates

Elimination: 90% of prostaglandin E_1 is excreted in the urine as metabolites within 24 hours

Monitoring Parameters

Arterial blood pressure, heart rate, respiratory rate, and temperature. Patients receiving an infusion for longer than 5 days should be monitored for the development of gastric outlet obstruction.[2]

Contraindications

Respiratory distress syndrome without ductal-dependant CHD. Prostaglandin E_1 may cause hypotension and worsen ventilation/perfusion matching in the lungs. In addition, it may worsen hypoxemia because of increased right-to-left shunting across either a patent foramen ovale and/or the ductus arteriosus.

Adverse Effects

Cardiovascular: flushing, bradycardia, systemic hypotension, tachycardia, edema

Respiratory: apnea may occur in about 10% of neonates, with greater risk in those weighing less than 2 kg at birth; usually occurs during the first hour of the infusion

Central nervous system: seizures, headache, fever

Gastrointestinal: gastric outlet obstruction secondary to antral hyperplasia[3]

Neuromuscular and skeletal: cortical hyperostosis has been seen with long-term infusions and is related to duration of therapy and cumulative dose.[3] Most cases have occurred after 4 to 6 weeks of therapy, however, there is one report of it developing after 11 days[4]

Endocrine/metabolic: hypocalcemia, hypokalemia, hyperkalemia, hypoglycemia

Hematological: may cause inhibition of platelet aggregation

Drug-Drug Interactions

Use with antihypertensive agents may increase the risk of hypotension.

Compatible Diluents/Administration

Compatible with 5% dextrose, 10% dextrose, and 0.9% NaCl solutions. Infuse into a large vein or an umbilical arterial catheter placed at the ductal opening. Maximum concentration for I.V. infusion is 20 μg/mL.

Concentrations as high as 30 μg/mL have been infused through a central line in some institutions.

References

1. Zahka KG, Roland MA, Cutilletta AF, et al. Management of aortic arch interruption with prostaglandin E₁ infusion and microporous expanded polytetrafluoroethylene grafts. Am J Cardiol 1980; 46:1001–1005.

2. Peled N, Dagan O, Babyn P, et al. Gastric-outlet obstruction induced by prostaglandin therapy in neonates. N Engl J Med 1992; 327:505–510.

3. Woo K, Emery J, & Peabody J. Cortical hyperostosis: a complication of prolonged prostaglandin infusion in infants awaiting cardiac transplantation. Pediatrics 1994; 93: 417–420.

4. Kalloghlian AK, Frayha HH, deMoor MM. Cortical hyperostosis simulating osteomyelitis after short-term prostaglandin E1 infusion. Eur J Pediatr 1996; 155(3):173–174.

Miscellaneous Agents: Hydralazine

Indication

Management of moderate to severe hypertension.

Mechanism of Action

Hydralazine is a direct-acting vasodilator that exerts its effect on arterioles with little effect on veins and decreases systemic resistance. The precise mechanism of action is unknown.

Dosing

Infants/children:

Oral: initial, 0.75 to 1 mg/kg/day P.O./N.G. in two to four divided doses, not to exceed 25 mg/dose. Increase over 3 to 4 weeks to a maximum of 5 mg/kg/day in infants and 7.5 mg/kg/day in children administered in two to four divided doses. Maximum daily dose, 200 mg/day

I.M., I.V.: initial, 0.1 to 0.2 mg/kg/dose I.V. (not to exceed 20 mg) every 4 to 6 hours as needed; up to 1.7 to 3.5 mg/kg/day may be administered in four to six divided doses

Adults:

Oral: initial, 10 mg four times per day P.O./N.G. Dose may be increased by 10 to 25 mg/dose every 2 to 5 days to a maximum of 300 mg/d. Usual dose range for hypertension, 25 to 100 mg/dose in two divided doses

I.M., I.V., hypertension: initial, 10 to 20 mg I.V. per dose every 4 to 6 hours as needed. May increase to a maximum of 40 mg/dose

Dosing in renal impairment:[1]

Cl_{cr} *10 to 50 mL/min/1.73 m²:* administer every 8 hours

Cl_{cr} *less than 10 mL/min/1.73 m²:* administer every 8 to 16 hours in fast acetylators and every 12 to 24 hours in slow acetylators

Pharmacokinetics

Onset of action:

Oral: 30 minutes

I.V.: 5 to 20 minutes

Distribution: hydralazine crosses the placenta and is found in breast milk

Half-life: in adults with normal renal function, the range is 2 to 8 hours; however, it may vary depending on individual acetylation rates

Duration:

Oral: 2 to 4 hours

I.V.: 2 to 6 hours

Protein binding: 85 to 95% protein bound

Metabolism: metabolized in the liver with an extensive first-pass effect with oral administration

Elimination: 14% is excreted unchanged in the urine

Monitoring Parameters

Blood pressure should be closely monitored with I.V. administration, heart rate, and ANA (antinuclear antibody) titers (see Adverse Effects, and Other).

Contraindications

Hydralazine is contraindicated in patients with dissecting aortic aneurysms, mitral valve rheumatic heart disease, and significant coronary artery disease.

Precautions
Hydralazine may cause a drug-induced, lupus-like syndrome, especially with large doses administered over a long period. Discontinue therapy if patient develops this syndrome. Hydralazine is usually administered together with a diuretic and a β-blocker to counteract the side effects of sodium and water retention and reflex tachycardia.

Adverse Effects

Cardiovascular: tachycardia, palpitations, flushing, edema
Central nervous system: headache, dizziness
Gastrointestinal: nausea, vomiting, diarrhea
Neuromuscular and skeletal: arthralgias, weakness
Other: drug-induced lupus-like syndrome.[2] Dose-related findings include fever, arthralgia, lymphadenopathy, splenomegaly, positive ANA, maculopapular facial rash, positive direct Coombs' test, pericarditis

Drug-Drug Interactions
The use of hydralazine concomitantly with monoamine oxidase inhibitors may cause a significant decrease in blood pressure. Hydrazine may cause an increase in the levels of metoprolol and propranolol (β-blockers that are not extensively metabolized in the liver are less affected). Indomethacin may decrease the hypotensive effect of hydralazine.[3]

Compatible Diluents/Administration
Usually administered by slow I.V. push over 3 to 5 minutes. Do not exceed an administration rate of 0.2 mg/kg/min. The maximum concentration for I.V. administration is 20 mg/mL.

References

1. Bennett WM, Aronoff GR, Golper TA, et al. Drug Prescribing in Renal Failure. American College of Physicians, Philadelphia, PA, 1994.
2. Russell GI, Bing RF, Jones JA, et al. Hydralazine sensitivity: clinical features, autoantibody changes and HLA-DR phenotype. Q J Med *1987*; 65:845–852.
3. Cinquegrani MP, Liang CS. Indomethacin attenuates the hypotensive action of hydralazine. Clin Pharmacol Ther 1986; 39:564–570.

5. Diuretic Medications

Donald Berry and Traci M. Kazmerski

Loop Diuretics

Furosemide

Indication
Furosemide is most commonly used in the management of edema during congestive heart failure (CHF) and hepatic or renal disease. Frequently, it is the diuretic of choice to treat postoperative edema after cardiac surgery. It may also be used in the treatment of hypertensive patients[1] alone or in combination with other antihypertensive medications.

Mechanism of Action
Furosemide is a loop diuretic and functions through inhibition of reabsorption of sodium and chloride from the ascending loop of Henle. It interferes with the chloride-binding cotransport system (Na^+-K^+-$2Cl^-$ symporter) and halts salt transport in this segment. This action causes increased excretion of water, sodium, chloride, and potassium. The drug also inhibits calcium and magnesium reabsorption in the ascending limb by eliminating the transepithelial potential difference.

Dosing

Neonates, premature:
: *Oral (poor bioavailability):* doses of 1 to 4 mg/kg/dose once or twice daily have been used
: *Intramuscular (I.M.), intravenous (I.V.):* 0.25 to 2 mg/kg/dose administered every 12 to 24 hours

Infants and children:
: *Oral:* 1 to 6 mg/kg/day divided every 6 to 12 hours
: *I.M., I.V.:* 0.25 to 2 mg/kg/dose every 6 to 12 hours
: *I.V. continuous infusion:* 0.05 mg/kg/h initially, titrate to clinical effect. Usual dosage range, 0.1 to 0.4 mg/kg/h.

Adults:
: *Oral:* initial, 20 to 80 mg/dose; increase in increments of 20 to 40 mg/dose at intervals of 6 to 8 hours; usual maintenance dose interval is once or twice daily; may be titrated up to 600 mg/day for severe edematous states
: *I.M., I.V.:* 20 to 40 mg/dose; repeat in 1 to 2 hours as needed and increase by 20 mg/dose until the desired effect has been obtained; usual dosing

interval, 6 to 12 hours; for acute pulmonary edema, the usual dose is 40 mg I.V.; if not adequate, may increase dose to 80 mg
Continuous I.V. infusion: initial I.V. bolus dose of 20 to 40 mg followed by continuous I.V. infusion doses of 0.1 mg/kg/h doubled every 2 hours to a maximum of 0.4 mg/kg/h

Pharmacokinetics

The onset of action of furosemide after oral administration is 30 to 60 minutes after administration. The peak effects occur within 1 to 2 hours and the duration of action is 6 to 8 hours. After I.V. injection, diuresis begins after 5 minutes and lasts for 2 hours. After oral dosing, 45 to 65% of the drug is absorbed and the protein binding is 98%. The hepatic metabolism of the drug is minimal and the half-life is approximately 30 minutes.

> **Monitoring parameters:** serum electrolytes (sodium, potassium, chloride, and bicarbonate), renal function (blood urea nitrogen [BUN] and creatinine [Cr]), blood pressure
> **Contraindications:** Anuria

Precautions/Adverse Effects

Warning: loop diuretics are potent agents. Excess amounts may lead to profound diuresis with fluid and electrolyte loss. Close medical supervision and dose evaluation is required.

Adverse effects of furosemide use include serious depletion of total body Na^+ manifesting in hyponatremia or extracellular fluid volume depletion associated with hypotension, reduced glomerular filtration rate (GFR), or circulatory collapse. Also reported are dizziness, urticaria, hypokalemia, nausea, pancreatitis, headaches, photosensitivity, diarrhea, dehydration, and anemia. Ototoxicity is possible, as is appearance of the Sweet syndrome.[3] Other effects may include hypochloremia, metabolic alkalosis, hypercalciuria, agranulocytosis, thrombocytopenia, nephrocalcinosis, prerenal azotemia, hyperuricemia, and interstitial nephritis. Oral solutions contain sorbitol, which may cause diarrhea.

Drug-Drug Interactions

Nonsteroidal anti-inflammatory drugs (NSAIDs) decrease the effect of furosemide. There is increased ototoxicity with aminoglycosides and ethacrynic acid; and drugs affected by potassium depletion, such as digoxin. There is increased anticoagulation by warfarin; decreased glucose tolerance may increase requirements of oral antidiabetic agents; and there is decreased lithium excretion with furosemide administration.

Poisoning Information

Symptoms of furosemide overdose may include weakness, muscle cramps, fatigue, dizziness, fainting, confusion, irregular pulse, dry mouth, dehydration, nausea, and vomiting. Decontamination using activated charcoal is recommended and other treatment is supportive and symptomatic.

Compatible Diluents/Administration

Injection can be administered undiluted or can be diluted in normal saline (NS) or 5% dextrose in water (D5W) to a concentration of 1 to 2 mg/mL and will be stable for 24 hours at room temperature. Administration is by direct I.V. injection at a maximum rate of 0.5 mg/kg/min.

Bumetanide

Indication

Bumetanide is commonly used in the management of edema secondary to CHF and hepatic or renal disease. It may also be used in the treatment of hypertensive patients.[1]

Mechanism of Action

Bumetanide is a loop diuretic that is 40 times more potent than furosemide.[4] Bumetanide functions through inhibition of reabsorption of sodium and chloride from the ascending loop of Henle. It interferes with the chloride-binding cotransport system (Na^+-K^+-$2Cl^-$ symporter) and halts salt transport in this segment. This action causes increased excretion of water, sodium, chloride, and potassium. The drug also inhibits calcium and magnesium reabsorption in the ascending limb by eliminating the transepithelial potential difference.

Dosing

Neonates:
 Oral, I.M., I.V.: 0.01 to 0.05 mg/kg/dose every 24 to 48 hours
Infants and children:
 Oral, I.M., I.V.: 0.015 to 0.1 mg/kg/dose every 6 to 24 hours (maximum, 10 mg/day)
 Continuous I.V. infusion: the total daily I.V. intermittent dose can be administered as a continuous infusion over 24 hours (5–50 µg/kg/h)
Adults:
 Oral: 0.5 to 2 mg/dose (maximum, 10 mg/day) once or twice daily
 I.M., I.V.: 0.5 to 1 mg/dose (maximum, 10 mg/day)
 Continuous I.V. infusion: 0.9 to 1 mg/hr

Pharmacokinetics

Bumetanide has an onset of action for oral or I.M. administration within 30 to 60 minutes after the initial dose and within a few minutes after the I.V. injection. The duration of action after a usual dose of the drug is 4 to 6 hours.

Bumetanide is almost completely absorbed from the gastrointestinal (GI)tract, with protein binding at 95%. The drug undergoes partial hepatic metabolism, with the majority of the drug eliminated as the parent molecule or as a metabolite in the urine. The half-life of bumetanide is 1 to 1.5 hours in adults and 2.5 hours in infants younger than 6 months of age.

> **Monitoring parameters:** serum electrolytes, renal function, blood pressure
> **Contraindications:** anuria or increasing azotemia

Warnings/Adverse Effects

Warning: loop diuretics are potent agents. Excess amounts may lead to profound diuresis with fluid and electrolyte loss. Close medical supervision and dose evaluation is required. The injectable formulation of this drug contains benzyl alcohol and large amounts (>99 mg/kg/d) have been associated with a potentially fatal toxicity ("gasping syndrome") in neonates. This syndrome consists of metabolic acidosis, respiratory distress, gasping respirations, central nervous system (CNS) dysfunction, hypotension, and cardiovascular collapse. In vitro animal studies have shown that benzoate, a metabolite of benzyl alcohol, displaces bilirubin from protein binding sites. Avoid or use injection cautiously in neonates. In vitro studies using pooled sera from critically ill neonates have also shown bumetanide to be a potent displacer of bilirubin. Avoid use in neonates at risk for kernicterus. There is an increased risk of ototoxicity with rapid I.V. administration, renal impairment, excessive doses, and concurrent use with other ototoxins. Use with caution in patients with previous hypersensitivity reactions to sulfonamides or thiazides.

Adverse effects that may occur with bumetanide use include hypotension, chest pain, dizziness, headache, encephalopathy, vertigo, and potential rashes. Other effects may include urticaria, hypokalemia, nausea, pancreatitis, photosensitivity, diarrhea, dehydration, and decreased uric acid excretion. Hyponatremia, hypochloremia, arthritic pain, metabolic alkalosis, hypercalciuria, agranulocytosis, thrombocytopenia, hyperuricemia, and cramps have also been reported.

Drug-Drug Interactions

Hypotension may occur when bumetanide is used with other antihypertensive medications and angiotensin-converting enzyme (ACE) inhibitors. NSAIDs decrease the effect of bumetanide. There is increased ototoxicity when bumetanide is used with aminoglycosides and ethacrynic acid; and drugs affected by potassium depletion, such as digoxin. With bumetanide administration, there is decreased glucose tolerance with antidiabetic agents; and decreased lithium excretion.

Poisoning Information

Symptoms of bumetanide overdose may include acute and profound water loss, volume and electrolyte depletion, dehydration, reduction of blood volume, and circulatory collapse with a possibility of vascular thrombosis and embolism. Electrolyte depletion may be manifested by weakness, dizziness, mental confusion, anorexia, lethargy, vomiting, and cramps. Decontamination using activated charcoal is recommended and other treatment is supportive and symptomatic. Replacement of fluid and electrolyte losses may be necessary.

Compatible Diluents/Administration
Administer undiluted by direct I.V. injection over 1 to 2 minutes; may be diluted in D5W or NS and infused over 5 minutes; dilute in D5W to 0.024 mg/mL for continuous infusion.

Torsemide

Indication
Torsemide is most commonly used in the management of edema during CHF and hepatic or renal disease. It may also be used in the treatment of hypertensive patients[1] alone or in combination with other antihypertensive medications.

Mechanism of Action
Torsemide is a loop diuretic and functions through inhibition of reabsorption of sodium and chloride from the ascending loop of Henle. It interferes with the chloride-binding cotransport system (Na^+-K^+-$2Cl^-$ symporter) and halts salt transport in this segment. This action causes increased excretion of water, sodium, chloride, and potassium. The drug also inhibits calcium and magnesium reabsorption in the ascending limb by eliminating the transepithelial potential difference.

Dosing
> **Neonates, infants, and children:** no data is available
> **Adults:**
> > *Oral, I.V.:*
> > > Edema: 10 to 20 mg once daily. Titrate up to maximum dose of 200 mg/day
> > > Hypertension: 5 mg once daily initially, then increase to 10 mg once daily, if needed, after 4 to 6 weeks

Pharmacokinetics
Rapidly absorbed; bioavailability, 80 to 90%. Peak serum concentrations are reached in 1 hour. Torsemide is metabolized by cytochrome P450. The half-life of torsemide is normally 2 to 4 hours, but is increased to 7 to 8 hours in cirrhosis. Of the total dose, 20% is excreted unchanged in the urine.

> **Monitoring parameters:** serum electrolytes, renal function, blood pressure
> **Contraindications:** anuria

Precautions/Adverse Effects

Warning: loop diuretics are potent agents. Excess amounts may lead to profound diuresis with fluid and electrolyte loss. Close medical supervision and dose evaluation is required.

Adverse effects that may occur with torsemide use include hypotension, chest pain, dizziness, headache, prerenal azotemia, and rashes. Other effects may include hypokalemia, nausea, pancreatitis, photosensitivity, diarrhea, dehydration, and decreased uric acid excretion. Hyponatremia, hypochloremia, arthritic pain, metabolic alkalosis, hypercalciuria, agranulocytosis, anemia, hyperuricemia, and cramps have also been reported.

Drug-Drug Interactions

Increased potassium losses with torsemide increase the risk of digoxin toxicity. Use of torsemide with aminoglycosides or ethacrynic acid increases risk of ototoxicity. Torsemide use increases the anticoagulant effects of warfarin. NSAIDs decrease the diuretic effect of torsemide. Torsemide decreases lithium excretion; and decreased glucose tolerance with torsemide may increase requirements of oral antidiabetic agents.

Poisoning Information

Symptoms of torsemide overdose may include acute and profound water loss, volume and electrolyte depletion, dehydration, reduction of blood volume, and circulatory collapse. Electrolyte depletion may be manifested by weakness, dizziness, mental confusion, anorexia, lethargy, vomiting, and cramps. Decontamination using activated charcoal is recommended and other treatment is supportive and symptomatic. Replacement of fluid and electrolyte losses may be necessary.

Compatible Diluents/Administration

Administer torsemide undiluted by direct I.V. injection over at least 2 minutes; torsemide may be diluted in D5W or NS to concentrations of 0.1, 0.2, 0.4, or 0.8 mg/mL for continuous infusion, and is stable for 24 hours at room temperature.

Ethacrynic Acid

Indication

Ethacrynic acid is commonly used in the management of edema secondary to CHF and hepatic or renal disease. It may also be used in the treatment of hypertensive patients.[1]

Mechanism of Action

Ethacrynic acid is a loop diuretic that functions through inhibition of reabsorption of sodium and chloride from the ascending loop of Henle.

It interferes with the chloride-binding cotransport system (Na^+-K^+-$2Cl^-$ symporter) and halts salt transport in these segments. This action causes increased excretion of water, sodium, potassium, and chloride. The drug also inhibits calcium and magnesium reabsorption in the ascending limb by eliminating the transepithelial potential difference.

Dosing

Children:
    Oral: 1 mg/kg/dose every 24 to 48 hours; adjust dose as needed at 2- to 3-day intervals to a maximum of 3 mg/kg/day
    I.V.: 0.5 to 1 mg/kg/dose (maximum, 50 mg/dose); repeated doses not routinely recommended but may be administered every 8 to 12 hours

Adults:
    Oral: 25 to 400 mg/day in one to two divided doses
    I.V.: 0.5 to 1 mg/kg/dose (maximum, 100 mg/dose); repeat doses not routinely recommended but may be administered every 8 to 12 hours

Note: Avoid use in patients with a Cr clearance (Cl_{Cr}) less than 10 mL/min

Pharmacokinetics

Ethacrynic acid has an onset of action within 30 minutes of administration of oral doses and within 5 minutes of I.V. injection. The duration of diuresis is approximately 6 to 8 hours after oral and 2 hours after I.V. administration. The drug is rapidly absorbed and hepatically metabolized to an active cysteine conjugate. The half-life ranges from 30 to 70 minutes, and the drug and metabolites are eliminated in the bile and urine.

    Monitoring parameters: serum electrolytes, renal function, blood pressure, hearing
    Contraindications: anuria, hypotension, metabolic alkalosis with hypokalemia, hyponatremic dehydration

Precautions/Adverse Effects

Warning: loop diuretics are potent agents. Excess amounts may lead to profound diuresis with fluid and electrolyte loss. Close medical supervision and dose evaluation is required. Use with corticosteroids may increase risk of GI hemorrhage. Avoid use in patients with severe renal impairment ($Cl_{Cr} < 10$ mL/min).

Adverse effects of ethacrynic acid include hypotension, fluid and electrolyte imbalances (hypokalemia, hyponatremia, hypomagnesemia, hypocalcemia), hyperglycemia, thrombocytopenia, neutropenia, agranulocytosis, abnormal liver function test results, GI irritation or bleeding, ototoxicity (higher risk than other loop diuretics), hyperuricemia, phlebitis, headache, rash, and hematuria.

Drug-Drug Interactions

Ethacrynic acid administration causes increased potassium losses with amphotericin and steroids. Use of ethacrynic acid with aminoglycosides increases the risk of ototoxicity; increases the anticoagulant affects of warfarin; and decreases lithium excretion. Decreased glucose tolerance with ethacrynic acid may increase requirements of oral antidiabetic agents.

Poisoning Information

Symptoms of ethacrynic acid overdose may include acute and profound water loss, volume and electrolyte depletion, dehydration, reduction of blood volume, and circulatory collapse. Electrolyte depletion may be manifested by weakness, dizziness, mental confusion, anorexia, lethargy, vomiting, and cramps. Treatment is supportive and symptomatic, and replacement of fluid and electrolyte losses may be necessary.

Compatible Diluents/Administration

Ethacrynic acid is stable for 24 hours at room temperature when mixed at 1 mg/mL in D5W or NS; inject slowly over 20 to 30 minutes. Ethacrynic acid is a tissue irritant and is not to be administered I.M. or subcutaneously.

Thiazide and Thiazide-Like Diuretics

Chlorothiazide

Indication

Chlorothiazide is used in the treatment of mild to moderate hypertension. Additionally, chlorothiazide is used for the treatment of edema caused by CHF, pregnancy, bronchopulmonary dysplasia, nephrotic syndrome, or after cardiac surgery.

Mechanism of Action

Chlorothiazide is a thiazide diuretic whose primary site of action is the distal convoluted tubule and whose secondary site of action is the proximal tubule.[6] In these regions, chlorothiazide inhibits sodium reabsorption causing increased excretion of sodium and water as well as potassium, bicarbonate, magnesium, phosphate, and calcium (transiently).

Dosing

Note: I.V. dosage in infants and children has not been established. The following dosages in infants and children are based on anecdotal reports. Lower dosing regimens have been extrapolated from oral dosing recommendations, because 10 to 20% of an oral dose is absorbed.

Neonates and infants younger than 6 months:
   Oral: 20 mg/kg/day in two divided doses; maximum, 375 mg/day
   I.V.: 2 to 8 mg/kg/day in two divided doses; doses up to 20 mg/kg/day
   have been used
Infants older than 6 months and children:
   Oral: 20 mg/kg/day in two divided doses; maximum, 1 g/day
   I.V.: 4 mg/kg/day divided in one to two doses; doses up to 20 mg/kg/day
   have been used
Adults:
   Hypertension:
      Oral: 125 to 500 mg once daily
   Edema:
      Oral: 500 mg to 2 g/day divided in one to two doses
      I.V.: 100 to 500 mg/day divided in one to two doses

Pharmacokinetics

Chlorothiazide has an onset of action of 2 hours after oral administration and a duration of action of 6 to 12 hours. The duration of action is approximately 2 hours after I.V. injection. Oral absorption of the drug is only 10 to 20%, and protein binding ranges from 20 to 80%. Chlorothiazide is not metabolized, and its half-life is 1 to 3 hours. Almost all of the I.V. dose is eliminated unchanged in the urine within 3 to 6 hours, and 35 to 60% of the oral dose is excreted within 24 hours.

   Monitoring parameters: serum electrolytes, renal function, blood glucose, triglycerides, uric acid, blood pressure
   Contraindications: anuria, sulfonamide allergy

Precautions/Adverse Effects

Warning: do not administer the injectable formulation I.M. or subcutaneously. Use cautiously in patients with severe renal disease, reduced hepatic function, and in patients with high triglyceride or cholesterol levels.

   Side effects of chlorothiazide use include hypotension, rashes, hypokalemia, hypochloremic metabolic alkalosis, hyperglycemia, hyperlipidemia, hyperuricemia, prerenal azotemia, thrombocytopenia, cholestasis, photosensitivity, arrhythmias, nausea, vomiting, diarrhea, pancreatitis, and fevers. Rarely, blood dyscrasias may also occur.

Poisoning Information

Chlorothiazide overdose is characterized by lethargy, dizziness, drowsiness, muscle weakness, arrhythmias, cramps, and fainting. On onset of these symptoms, drug administration should be stopped and symptomatic treatment should be initiated.

Drug-Drug Interactions

NSAIDs may decrease the antihypertensive effect of chlorothiazide. Steroids, loop diuretics, and amphotericin B will cause additive potassium losses. With chlorothiazide use, there is a decreased clearance of lithium; there is increased hyperglycemia with diazoxide; there are increased hypersensitivity reactions to allopurinol; and there is an increased risk of renal toxicity with cyclosporine.

Compatible Diluents/Administration

Do not administer chlorothiazide I.M. or subcutaneously; avoid extravasation; administer chlorothiazide by I.V. injection over 3 to 5 minutes or by I.V. infusion over 30 minutes at a maximum concentration of 25 mg/mL in D5W or NS; reconstituted injectable formulation is stable for 24 hours at room temperature.

Hydrochlorothiazide

Indication

Hydrochlorothiazide is used in the treatment of mild to moderate hypertension. Additionally, hydrochlorothiazide is used for the treatment of edema caused by CHF, bronchopulmonary dysplasia, or nephrotic syndrome.

Mechanism of Action

Hydrochlorothiazide is a thiazide diuretic whose primary site of action is the distal convoluted tubule and secondary site of action is the proximal tubule.[6] In these regions, the drug inhibits sodium reabsorption, causing increased excretion of sodium and water as well as potassium, bicarbonate, magnesium, phosphate, and calcium (transiently).

Dosing

>**Neonates and infants younger than 6 months:**
>*Oral:* 2 to 4 mg/kg/day in one to two doses; maximum daily dose, 37.5 mg
>**Infants older than 6 months and children:**
>*Oral:* 2 mg/kg/day in one to two doses; maximum daily dose, 200 mg
>**Adults:**
>*Oral:* 12.5 to 100 mg/day in one to two doses; maximum, 200 mg/day
>**Note:** Daily dosages should be decreased if used with other antihypertensive agents

Pharmacokinetics

Hydrochlorothiazide has an onset of action within 2 hours of oral administration, with a duration of action of 6 to 12 hours. The oral absorption in the

GI tract is approximately 60 to 80%. The half-life of hydrochlorothiazide is 5 to 15 hours, and hydrochlorothiazide is eliminated almost completely via the kidneys as unchanged drug.

> **Monitoring parameters:** serum electrolytes, blood pressure, BUN, Cr, fluid balance
> **Contraindications:** anuria; thiazide or sulfonamide allergy

Precautions/Adverse Effects
Use cautiously in patients with severe renal disease, reduced hepatic function, diabetes mellitus, systemic lupus erythematosus, and gout.

Adverse side effects of hydrochlorothiazide may include drowsiness, paresthesia, hypokalemia, hyponatremia, hypochloremic metabolic alkalosis, hyperglycemia, nausea, vomiting, anorexia, pancreatitis, cholestasis, hypotension, agranulocytosis, thrombocytopenia, leukopenia, prerenal azotemia, polyuria, and photosensitivity.

Poisoning Information
The most likely manifestations of hydrochlorothiazide overdose are lethargy, confusion, hypermotility, and muscle weakness. Treatment is supportive and symptomatic.

Drug-Drug Interactions
With hydrochlorothiazide use, there is a decreased antihypertensive effect with NSAIDS. With hydrochlorothiazide use, there are increased potassium losses with steroids and amphotericin B; and increased hypersensitivity reactions to allopurinol. With hydrochlorothiazide use, there is increased hyperglycemia with diazoxide; a decreased effectiveness of antidiabetic agents; a decreased clearance of lithium; increased hypotension with ACE inhibitors; and increased renal toxicity with cyclosporine.

Metolazone

Indication
Metolazone is used in the treatment of mild to moderate hypertension. It is also commonly used in conjunction with a loop diuretic in the management of edema secondary to CHF.[5] Additionally, metolazone is used for the treatment of edema caused by nephrotic syndrome and in postoperative cardiac surgical patients.

Mechanism of Action
Metolazone is a thiazide-type diuretic whose primary site of action is the distal convoluted tubule and whose secondary site of action is the proximal tubule.[6] In

these regions, metolazone inhibits sodium reabsorption, causing increased excretion of sodium and water as well as potassium and hydrogen ions.

Dosing
Metolazone is only available for oral/enteral administration.

> **Children:** 0.2 to 0.4 mg/kg/day divided every 12 to 24 hours
> **Adults:**
> *Edema:* 5 to 20 mg/dose every 24 hours
> *Hypertension:* 2.5 to 5 mg/dose every 24 hours

Pharmacokinetics
Metolazone has an onset of action of approximately 1 hour and a duration of action of 12 to 24 hours. Oral absorption of the drug is dependent on the preparation used, and protein binding is 95%. The half-life is 6 to 20 hours and 70 to 95% of the drug is eliminated unchanged in the urine.

> **Monitoring parameters:** serum electrolytes, blood pressure, BUN, Cr, fluid balance
> **Contraindications:** anuria, allergy to thiazide diuretics or sulfonamides, hepatic coma

Precautions/Adverse Effects
Use cautiously in patients with severe renal disease, reduced hepatic function, diabetes mellitus, systemic lupus erythematosus, gout, and in patients with high triglyceride or cholesterol levels.

Common adverse reactions with metolazone use include palpitations, chest pain, hypotension, headaches, drowsiness, rash, and GI irritation. Hypokalemia, hyponatremia, hypochloremia, metabolic alkalosis, hyperglycemia, thrombocytopenia, leukopenia, aplastic anemia, and hyperuricemia have also been reported. Patients may experience sensitivity to light, chills, and abdominal bloating.

Poisoning Information
Metolazone overdose is commonly characterized by orthostatic hypotension, dizziness, drowsiness, fainting, and volume depletion. Treatment is supportive and symptomatic and replacement of fluid and electrolyte losses may be necessary.

Drug-Drug Interactions
With metolazone use, there is a decreased antihypertensive effect with NSAIDs. There are also increased potassium losses with steroids and amphotericin B; and increased hypersensitivity reactions to allopurinol. There is increased incidence of digoxin toxicity caused by hypokalemia and hypomagnesemia.

Potassium-Sparing Diuretics

Spironolactone

Indication
Spironolactone is used in the management of edema associated with CHF, hepatic cirrhosis, and nephrotic syndrome. It is also used to treat hypertension, hypokalemia, and primary aldosteronism. Spironolactone has also been associated with increased success in the treatment of patients with CHF who undergo antialdosterone therapy.[9]

Mechanism of Action
Spironolactone is a potassium-sparing diuretic that competes with aldosterone for binding to receptor sites in the distal tubule of the kidneys. It increases the excretion of sodium, chloride, and water and inhibits the excretion of potassium and hydrogen. The effect of aldosterone on arteriolar smooth muscle may also be blocked.

Dosing
Spironolactone is only available for oral/enteral administration.

> **Neonates:**
> *Diuretic:* 1 to 3 mg/kg/day divided every 12 to 24 hours
> **Children:**
> *Diuretic, hypertension:* 1.5 to 3.5 mg/kg/day or 60 mg/m^2/day in one to four divided doses daily
> **Adults:**
> *Edema, hypokalemia:* 25 to 200 mg/day in one to two divided doses
> *Hypertension:* 25 to 50 mg/day in one to two doses daily

Pharmacokinetics
Spironolactone is well absorbed after oral administration, with bioavailability at approximately 90%. The protein binding of the drug ranges from 91 to 98%, with hepatic metabolism to multiple metabolites, including the active agent, canrenone. The half-life of spironolactone is 78 to 84 minutes and the half-life of canrenone is 13 to 24 hours. The duration of action is 2 to 3 days.

> **Monitoring parameters:** potassium, sodium, renal function
> **Contraindications:** anuria, hyperkalemia, renal failure

Precautions/Adverse Effects
Warning: severe hyperkalemia may result when used with ACE inhibitors, potassium supplements, and NSAIDs; monitor potassium levels and renal function closely.

Use with caution in patients with decreased renal function, hyponatremia, dehydration, or reduced hepatic function.

Adverse reactions associated with spironolactone include hyperkalemia, dehydration, hyponatremia, hyperchloremic metabolic alkalosis, headaches, fever, diarrhea, vomiting, nausea, lethargy, rash, anorexia, gynecomastia (in males), amenorrhea, agranulocytosis, and decreased renal function.

Poisoning Information
Symptoms of spironolactone overdose include lethargy, fatigue, drowsiness, dizziness, confusion, nausea, and vomiting. Dehydration, electrolyte imbalance, and severe hyperkalemia may occur with large doses. Treatment of the hyperkalemia is with I.V. glucose and insulin, and possibly sodium bicarbonate.

Drug-Drug Interactions
Hyperkalemia may occur when spironolactone is used with ACE inhibitors, NSAIDs, potassium supplements, or other potassium-sparing diuretics. Spironolactone use may decrease clearance of digoxin; may cause a decreased response to norepinephrine; and may decrease the effects of oral anticoagulants.

Amiloride

Indication
Amiloride reduces potassium loss caused by other diuretics used in the management of hypertension or edema associated with CHF, hepatic cirrhosis, and hyperaldosteronism. Amiloride is usually used with other diuretics.

Mechanism of Action
Amiloride inhibits sodium-potassium ion exchange in the distal convoluted tubule by inhibiting cellular sodium transport mechanisms and inhibits hydrogen ion secretion; its diuretic activity is not dependent on aldosterone.

Dosing
Amiloride is only available for oral/enteral administration.

Children 6 to 20 kg: 0.625 mg/kg/day administered once daily (maximum dose, 10 mg/day)

Children heavier than 20 kg and adults: 5 to 10 mg/day (maximum dose, 20 mg/day)

In patients with renal impairment: reduce dose 50% for Cl_{Cr} 10 to 50 mL/min. Avoid use if Cl_{Cr} is less than 10 mL/min

Pharmacokinetics

Amiloride has an onset of action of 2 hours and a duration of 24 hours. Oral bioavailability is 15 to 25%. The half-life in normal renal function is 6 to 9 hours and up to 144 hours in severe renal disease. Amiloride is eliminated in the urine and feces.

> **Monitoring parameters:** serum potassium, blood pressure, BUN, Cr, fluid balance
>
> **Contraindications:** anuria, hyperkalemia

Precautions/Adverse Effects

Use amiloride with caution with potassium supplements or other potassium-sparing diuretics; reduce dosage in patients with renal insufficiency; use cautiously in patients with diabetic nephropathy, hyponatremia, dehydration, electrolyte imbalance, or decreased hepatic function.

Adverse effects include hypotension, arrhythmias, hyperkalemia, hyponatremia, dehydration, hyperchloremic metabolic acidosis, nausea, vomiting, diarrhea, GI bleeding, liver function abnormalities, muscular weakness, paresthesias, neutropenia, aplastic anemia, headache, dizziness, confusion, insomnia, skin rash, and bladder spasms.

Poisoning Information

Symptoms include dehydration and electrolyte imbalances. Large doses can produce life-threatening hyperkalemia. Treatment is with I.V. glucose and insulin along with I.V. sodium bicarbonate. Dialysis may be necessary.

Drug-Drug Interactions

Amiloride increases serum potassium when used with potassium supplements, potassium-sparing diuretics, ACE inhibitors, angiotensin receptor blockers, tacrolimus, and cyclosporine. Amiloride use decreases digoxin clearance, and decreases lithium clearance. NSAIDs decrease the effects of amiloride.

Carbonic Anhydrase Inhibitors

Acetazolamide

Indication

Acetazolamide is used to reduce intraocular pressure in glaucoma and as a diuretic.[7] Acetazolamide may also be used in the treatment of hydrocephalus, refractory seizures, epilepsy, and altitude sickness.[8] It is also use to treat secondary metabolic alkalosis.

Mechanism of Action

As a diuretic, acetazolamide initiates competitive, reversible inhibition of carbonic anhydrase, which results in increased renal excretion of sodium, potassium, bicarbonate, and water. Acetazolamide also inhibits carbonic anhydrase in the CNS, thus, reducing discharges from CNS neurons.

Dosing

Children:
Edema:
Oral, I.V.: 5 mg/kg/dose or 150 mg/m^2/dose once every day
Secondary metabolic alkalosis:
Oral, I.V.: 3 to 5 mg/kg/dose every 6 hours for four doses
Adults:
Edema:
Oral, I.V.: 250 to 375 mg once daily
Urine alkalinization:
Oral: 5 mg/kg/dose repeated two to three times over 24 hours
In patients with renal impairment:
Cl_{Cr} 10 to 50 mL/min: administer every 12 hours
Cl_{Cr} less than 10 mL/min: avoid use

Pharmacokinetics

Acetazolamide has an onset of action of 2 minutes after I.V. injection, 1 to 2 hours after tablet ingestion, and 2 hours after extended-release capsule administration. The duration of action of the drug is 4 to 5 hours if administered I.V., 8 to 12 hours after a tablet, and 18 to 24 hours after an extended-release capsule. Absorption of acetazolamide is dose dependent, and acetazolamide distributes into erythrocytes and the kidneys. The half-life ranges from 2.4 to 5.8 hours, with 70 to 100% of the I.V. or tablet dose eliminated unchanged in the urine within 1 day.

Monitoring parameters: CBC, platelets, serum electrolytes
Contraindications: allergy to sulfonamides, hyperchloremic acidosis, severe renal disease, hepatic insufficiency, low serum sodium or potassium

Precautions/Adverse Effects

Warning: sulfonamides have caused fatalities caused by toxic epidermal necrolysis, Stevens-Johnson syndrome, hepatic necrosis, aplastic anemia, and other blood dyscrasias. Discontinue use at the first sign of rash or adverse reaction.

Use with caution in patients with chronic obstructive pulmonary disease, respiratory acidosis, gout, and diabetes mellitus; reduce dosage in patients with renal dysfunction.

Common side effects of acetazolamide include cyanosis, drowsiness, fever, seizures, dizziness, depression, rash, photosensitivity, vertigo, hypokalemia, hyperchloremic metabolic acidosis, hyperglycemia, nausea, vomiting, black stools, polyuria, muscle weakness, anorexia, cholestatic jaundice, hepatic insufficiency, and hyperpnea.

Poisoning Information

Symptoms of acetazolamide overdose include drowsiness, nausea, vomiting, confusion, tachycardia, sweating, dizziness, convulsions, tingling of lips and tongue, and low blood sugar. Treat hypoglycemia with dextrose I.V. if necessary.

Drug-Drug Interactions

Acetazolamide may decrease the rate of excretion of other drugs, such as procainamide, flecainide, quinidine, and tricyclic antidepressants; and it may increase the excretion of salicylates and phenobarbital. Acetazolamide use may increase toxicity with propofol (cardiorespiratory instability); may increase cyclosporine levels; and may increase the risk of developing osteomalacia in patients receiving phenytoin or phenobarbital. Concomitant topiramate use may increase the risk of nephrolithiasis and paresthesia; and concomitant salicylates increase acetazolamide serum levels, resulting in CNS toxicity. Acetazolamide increases lithium excretion.

Compatible Diluents/Administration

Reconstituted injectable formulation at 100 mg/mL concentration is stable for 1 week refrigerated. It may be diluted further in D5W or NS for I.V. infusion, with a stability of 5 days at room temperature and 44 days refrigerated.

Osmotic Diuretics

Mannitol

Indication

Mannitol is used to promote diuresis in the treatment of oliguria or anuria caused by acute renal failure. Mannitol is also used to reduce increased intracranial pressure associated with cerebral edema.

Mechanism of Action

Mannitol is an osmotic diuretic that increases the osmotic pressure of the glomerular filtrate, inhibits the tubular reabsorption of water and electrolytes, and increases urinary output.

Dosing
Children:

Test dose (to assess adequate renal function): 200 mg/kg (maximum, 12.5 g) over 3 to 5 minutes to produce a urine flow of at least 1 mL/kg/ h for 1 to 3 hours

Initial: 0.5 to 1 g/kg over 20 minutes as a 20% solution

Maintenance: 0.25 to 0.5 g/kg administered every 4 to 6 hours

Adults:

Test dose: 12.5 g (200 mg/kg) over 3 to 5 minutes to produce a urine flow of at least 30 to 50 mL of urine per hour over the next 2 to 3 hours

Initial: 0.5 to 1 g/kg (50–100 g)

Maintenance: 0.25 to 0.5 g/kg administered every 4 to 6 hours

Pharmacokinetics
The onset of action of mannitol begins within 1 to 3 hours after injection and persists for 3 to 8 hours. The drug remains confined to the extracellular space except in high concentrations or acidosis. The half-life of mannitol is 1.1 to 1.6 hours and it is primarily eliminated in urine by glomerular filtration.

Monitoring parameters: serum electrolytes, renal function, daily inputs and outputs, serum and urine osmolality (maintain serum osmolality 310–320 mOsm/kg for treatment of elevated intracranial pressure)

Contraindications: severe pulmonary edema or congestion, severe renal disease, dehydration, and active intracranial bleeding

Precautions/Adverse Effects
Mannitol should not be administered until adequate renal function and urine flow is established with test doses and cardiovascular status is evaluated. High doses may cause renal dysfunction—use caution in patients taking other nephrotoxic agents, with sepsis, or underlying renal disease. Keep serum osmolality under 320 mOsm/L to minimize adverse renal effects.

Adverse reactions associated with mannitol include circulatory overload, CHF, headache, convulsions, fluid and electrolyte imbalance, dehydration, hypovolemia, plasma hyperosmolality, hyponatremia or hypernatremia, increased osmolar gap, blurred vision, and pulmonary edema.

Poisoning Information
Symptoms of mannitol overdose include acute renal failure, hypotension, pulmonary edema, cardiovascular collapse, polyuria, oliguria, seizures, hyponatremia, and hypokalemia. Replacement of fluid and electrolyte losses may be necessary. Hemodialysis will clear mannitol and reduce osmolality.

Drug-Drug Interactions

Mannitol use increases lithium toxicity.

Compatible Diluents/Administration

Do not administer mannitol with blood. Inspect mannitol for crystals before administration. Use a filter in administration set. Avoid extravasation.

References

1. Puschett, J. (2000). "Diuretics and the therapy of hypertension." *Am J Med Sci* **319**(1): 1–9.
2. Prandota, J. (2001). "Clinical pharmacology of furosemide in children: a supplement." *Am J Ther* **8**(4): 275–289.
3. Govindarajan, G., Q. Bashir, S. Kuppuswamy, and C. Brooks (2005). "Sweet syndrome associated with furosemide." *South Med J* **98**(5): 570–572.
4. Schwartz, J., R. Bloch, J. Imbs, and M. Spach (1986). "[Diuretics]." *Pathol Biol (Paris)* **34**(7): 861–885.
5. Sica, D. (2003). "Metolazone and its role in edema management." *Congest Heart Fail* **9**(2): 100–105.
6. Materson, B. (1983). "Insights into intrarenal sites and mechanisms of action of diuretic agents." *Am Heart J* **106**(1 Pt 2): 188–208.
7. Ritland, J., K. Egge, S. Lydersen, R. Juul, and S. Semb (2004). "Comparison of survival of exfoliative glaucoma patients and primary open-angle glaucoma patients: impact of acetazolamide use." *Acta Ophthalmol Scand* **82**(4): 397–400.
8. Poca, M. and J. Sahuquillo (2005). "Short-term medical management of hydrocephalus." *Expert Opin Pharmacother* **6**(9): 1525–1538.
9. Brilla, C., M. Schencking, C. Scheer and H. Rupp (1997). "[Spironolactone: renaissance of anti-aldosterone therapy in heart failure?]." *Schweiz Rundsch Med Prax.* **86**(14): 566–574.
10. Borges, H., J. Hocks, and C. Kjellstrand (1982). "Mannitol intoxication in patients with renal failure." *Arch Intern Med* **142**(1): 63–66.

6. β-Blockers

Constantinos Chrysostomou and Traci M. Kazmerski

β-blockers have become an essential component of pharmacological therapy for adults with chronic congestive heart failure (CHF). They have been shown to decrease morbidity and mortality in several randomized controlled studies. Nonetheless, one has to take into consideration some of the differences that exist between pediatric and adult heart failure when considering β-blockers. Heart failure in adults is most often a problem caused by left ventricular (LV) systolic dysfunction that occurs with damage from ischemia, hypertension, or older age. Pediatric heart failure can be secondary to primary systolic dysfunction that is either acquired or congenital but most commonly is caused by congenital structural defects. Patients born with single ventricle defects, and especially those with a single right ventricle, seem to be particularly prone to ventricular dysfunction over time. Despite these differences in the etiology of heart failure, there is substantial evidence that infants and children have alterations in their neurohormonal axes that are similar to adults.[1]

β-blocker therapy for heart failure is based on several proposed mechanisms:

1. *Upregulation of β₁-adrenergic receptors and improved signaling.* In advanced heart failure, there is downregulation of β_1-adrenergic receptors, with resulting decreased contractility, ventricular dilation, and apoptosis.[2–5]
2. *Protection from catecholamine myocyte toxicity.* The high level of circulating catecholamines found in severe heart failure is toxic to the myocardium.[6]
3. *Antiarrhythmic effects.* β-blockers suppress ventricular ectopic activity.[7,8]
4. *Bradycardia.* Bradycardia may improve coronary blood flow and decrease myocardial oxygen demand.[9]
5. *Renin-angiotensin inhibition.* When added to previous angiotensin-converting enzyme (ACE) inhibitor therapy, β-blockade by metoprolol lessens circulating renin and angiotensin II levels, thereby increasing inhibition of the renin-angiotensin system.[9]

The following principles apply to the use of all β-blocker agents:

1. Start with a lower dose and titrate up slowly, watching for side effects, and, if necessary, decrease the dose or advance more gradually.
2. Do not start β-blockers if the patient is hemodynamically unstable, and if possible, do not start β-blockers when the patient is in New York Heart Association (NYHA) Class IV or severe Class III heart failure.
3. Add β-blockers only to existing ACE inhibitors, diuretics, and, possibly, digoxin.
4. Use only β-blockers that have been studied in heart failure, i.e., carvedilol, metoprolol, and bisoprolol. Some of the original β-blockers, including propranolol and atenolol, have not been extensively studied in heart failure. The initiation of

β-blockade is a slow process that requires careful supervision and may temporarily worsen the heart failure.

5. An interesting strategy to appraise tolerance and benefits of β-blockers in a particular patient consists in using intravenous (I.V.) continuous esmolol. Esmolol offers the advantage of being easy to titrate and of having a very short half-life, which may be useful in cases of poor tolerance.

Metoprolol

Indication

Metoprolol has been studied most extensively in adults with acute myocardial infarction, in postinfarct protection, and in stable symptomatic Class II and Class III heart failure.[10] In the pediatric population, three studies showed that metoprolol improved ventricular function and decreased the level of natriuretic peptide and norepinephrine.[11–13]

Mechanism of Action

Metoprolol is a second generation, cardioselective inhibitor of β_1-adrenergic receptors with no intrinsic sympathomimetic activity and weak membrane-stabilizing activity.[14] Its β-selectivity is approximately 75-fold β_1/β_2. β_1-receptor blockade causes a fall in blood pressure, but the exact mechanism is not well known. Blocking of reflex sympathetic stimulation in the heart with a fall in cardiac output and a late decrease in peripheral vascular resistance are possible mechanisms.

Dosing

Neonates/infants: no data available

Children/adolescents: there is limited pediatric dosing information available. Initial oral dosing is 0.1 to 0.2 mg/kg/dose twice daily to a target of 0.25 to 1 mg/kg/dose twice daily[12]

Adults:

Oral: initial oral dosing is 12.5 to 25 mg daily to a target of 200 mg/day (slow release metoprolol)

Dosage in renal failure: no dosage adjustment is required with metoprolol in patients with renal failure

Dosage in hepatic insufficiency: dosage adjustments may be required in patients with hepatic insufficiency because metoprolol is extensively metabolized in the liver. However, studies in patients with hepatic insufficiency are lacking

Pharmacokinetics

Onset of action: immediate release metoprolol has an onset of action as an antihypertensive of 15 minutes and full β-blockade of 1 hour

Duration of action: the β-blocking activity after a single immediate release oral dose is 3 to 6 hours, with longer duration observed with higher doses

Metoprolol is almost completely absorbed when administered orally. Bioavailability ranges between 50 to 70%, because of extensive first-pass metabolism. The half-life varies with neonates, exhibiting times of 5 to 10 hours and, in adults, 3 to 7 hours. Continued administration, however, saturates the hepatic process that removes metoprolol from the circulation, and the effective half-life then becomes significantly longer. Hepatic metabolism of metoprolol varies significantly in individual patients based on the existence of the debrisoquine genetic polymorphism. Extensive hydroxylators may require several doses of the drug daily, whereas poor hydroxylators may do well with a single daily dose.[14]

Drug-Drug Interactions

Interaction with amiodarone may cause a theoretical risk of hypotension, bradycardia, and cardiac arrest. Concomitant therapy with dihydropyridine calcium channel blockers (e.g., nifedipine, amlodipine, felodipine, nicardipine) may cause severe hypotension or impair cardiac performance. These effects are most prevalent in patients with impaired LV function, cardiac arrhythmias, or aortic stenosis. Cimetidine may cause bradycardia or hypotension. Therapy with ciprofloxacin may increase metoprolol concentrations and metoprolol dosage adjustment may be required. Abrupt withdrawal of clonidine while taking a β-blocker may exaggerate the rebound hypertension because of unopposed α-stimulation. Diclofenac and nonsteroidal anti-inflammatory drugs (NSAIDs) may cause a decreased antihypertensive effect. When β-blockers and digoxin are to be administered concomitantly, both atrioventricular (AV) block and potential digoxin toxicity are possible. Diltiazem may cause hypotension, bradycardia, and AV conduction disturbances. Metoprolol toxicity (bradycardia, fatigue, bronchospasm) may be seen with diphenhydramine therapy through the inhibition of metoprolol cytochrome P450. Metoprolol toxicity through increased metoprolol bioavailability may be seen with hydralazine. Insulin may cause hypoglycemia, hyperglycemia, or hypertension. Paroxetine may cause an increased risk of metoprolol adverse effects (shortness of breath, bradycardia, hypotension, acute heart failure) through inhibition of cytochrome P450. Phenobarbital causes decreased metoprolol effectiveness. An exaggerated hypotensive response to the first dose of the α-blocker, phenoxybenzamine, can occur. Propafenone may cause metoprolol toxicity through decreased metoprolol metabolism. Quinidine may cause bradycardia, fatigue, and shortness of breath through decreased metoprolol metabolism or clearance. Rifampin may cause decreased metoprolol effectiveness through increased metoprolol metabolism. Verapamil may cause hypotension and bradycardia.

Adverse Effects

Metoprolol is usually well tolerated, however, caution is warranted in this subset of patients of moderate to severe heart failure because metoprolol may worsen the degree of CHF. Adverse reactions that have occurred include drowsiness, insomnia, nightmares, confusion, depression, bradycardia, worsening of AV block, hypotension, chest pain, peripheral edema, CHF, reduced peripheral circulation, Raynaud's phenomenon, bronchospasm, nausea, abdominal pain, diarrhea or constipation, rash, pruritus, and worsening of psoriasis.

Poisoning Information

Overdose may present as asystole, AV block, bradycardia, hypotension, cyanosis, CHF, hyperreflexia, insomnia, night terrors, confusion, respiratory arrest, seizures, wheezing, or metabolic acidosis. These following general measures can be used if overdose or toxicity is suspected:

Elimination of the drug: gastric lavage should be performed within 1 hour of administration

Bradycardia/hypotension: for bradycardia, atropine should be administered. If there is no response, a continuous infusion of isoproterenol may be used. Temporary transvenous pacing may be required. Alternatively, a high-dose dobutamine infusion may be used to overcome the β-blockade. For hypotension, use I.V. fluid resuscitation and vasopressors (e.g., epinephrine, dopamine). Glucagon bolus of 50 to 150 µg/kg I.V. over 1 minute (usually approximately 10 mg in an adult) then a continuous I.V. infusion of 1 to 5 mg/hour in 5% dextrose in water (D5W) may be used as a first-line agent when an I.V. infusion is needed. Glucagon stimulates formation of cyclic adenine monophosphate (AMP) by bypassing the occupied β-receptors. An infusion of a phosphodiesterase inhibitor, such as milrinone or amrinone should also promote the accumulation of cyclic AMP

Bronchospasm: a β_2-stimulating agent and/or a theophylline derivative should be administered

Carvedilol

Indication

Carvedilol is a nonselective β-blocker that has both α-mediated vasodilatory and antioxidant effects. It has been studied as an additional agent to standard therapy (digoxin, diuretics, and ACE inhibitors) in adults with CHF and in postinfarct LV dysfunction.[15] It has been shown to decrease the risk of death and hospitalization, improve New York Heart Association (NYHA) functional class, and reduce clinical progression in patients with mild CHF.[4] In pediatric patients with cardiomyopathy, carvedilol has been shown to improve symptoms and ventricular function.[16,17]

Mechanism of Action

Carvedilol is a nonselective β-receptor and α_1-receptor antagonist with no intrinsic sympathomimetic activity. The blockade of both β- and α_1-receptors in CHF leads to decreased pulmonary capillary wedge pressure, decreased pulmonary artery pressure, decreased heart rate, decreased systemic vascular resistance, increased stroke volume index, decreased renal vascular resistance, and reduced plasma renin activity. In addition, carvedilol has been shown to inhibit the action of oxygen-free radicals and to demonstrate antiproliferative effects on smooth muscle cells.[18]

Dosing

Neonates: no data available
Infants/children:
Initial dose: 0.03 to 0.08 mg/kg/dose by mouth administered twice daily with a maximum initial dose of 3.125 mg administered twice daily
Maintenance dose: increase (usually double) every 2 to 3 weeks as tolerated. Average maintenance dose at approximately 12 weeks is 0.3 to 0.95 mg/kg/dose twice daily with a maximum of 25 mg administered twice daily. *Note*: Because of increased elimination of carvedilol in pediatric patients, three times daily dosing and a higher target dose per kilogram may be needed in children younger than 3.5 years of age[19]
Adults:
Initial: 3.125 mg by mouth twice daily for 2 weeks
Maintenance: increase (usually double) every 2 to 3 weeks as tolerated, to a maximum of 25 mg twice daily in patients lighter than 85 kg, and 50 mg twice daily in patients heavier than 85 kg
Dosing adjustment in renal impairment: none recommended
Note: mean areas under the curves (AUCs) are 40 to 50% higher in patients with moderate-to-severe renal dysfunction, but the ranges of AUCs are similar to patients with normal renal function
Dosing adjustment in hepatic impairment: carvedilol is extensively metabolized in the liver and dose reductions are suggested in patients with hepatic insufficiency. One study suggests that carvedilol therapy be initiated with approximately 20% of the normal dose in patients with

liver cirrhosis.[20] The manufacturer recommends that carvedilol should not be administered to patients with severe liver failure.

Note: patients with cirrhotic liver disease achieved carvedilol serum concentrations four- to seven-fold higher than healthy patients after a single dose

Pharmacokinetics

Carvedilol has an onset of action of α-blockade within 30 minutes and of β-blockade of within 1 hour. Drug absorption is rapid and extensive, but with a large first-pass effect. Because of this first-pass effect, the bioavailability of the drug is 25 to 35%. Bioavailability is greatly increased in patients with liver disease.[21] Carvedilol is metabolized in the liver primarily via cytochrome P450 isoenzymes. It is metabolized predominantly by aromatic ring oxidation and glucuronidation, and oxidative metabolites undergo conjugation via glucuronidation and sulfation. Half-life of the drug is dependent on age; infants and children 6 weeks to 3.5 years, 2.2 hours; children 5.5 to 19 years, 3.6 hours; and adults in general, 7 to 10 hours.[19] Less than 2% of carvedilol is excreted unchanged in urine, and the metabolites are excreted via the bile into the feces.

Drug-Drug Interactions

Interaction with amiodarone may cause a theoretical risk of hypotension, bradycardia, and cardiac arrest. Concomitant therapy with dihydropyridine calcium channel blockers (e.g., nifedipine, amlodipine, felodipine, nicardipine) may cause severe hypotension or impair cardiac performance. These effects are most prevalent in patients with impaired LV function, cardiac arrhythmias, or aortic stenosis. Cimetidine may cause increased adverse effects of carvedilol (dizziness, insomnia, gastrointestinal symptoms, postural hypotension). Abrupt withdrawal of clonidine while taking a β-blocker may exaggerate the rebound hypertension because of unopposed α-stimulation. Diclofenac and NSAIDs may cause decreased antihypertensive effect. When β-blockers and digoxin are to be administered concomitantly, both AV block and potential digoxin toxicity are possible. Diltiazem may cause hypotension, bradycardia, and AV conduction disturbances. Insulin may cause hypoglycemia, hyperglycemia, or hypertension. An exaggerated hypotensive response to the first dose of the α-blocker phenoxybenzamine may occur. Verapamil may cause hypotension and bradycardia.

Adverse Effects

Carvedilol is usually well tolerated, however, caution is warranted in this subset of patients with moderate to severe heart failure because it may worsen the degree of CHF. The following adverse effects have been reported: AV block, bradycardia, palpitations, syncope, peripheral edema, rebound or withdrawal hypertension after abrupt discontinuation of β-blocker therapy, postural hypotension, dizziness, hyperglycemia, hypertriglyceridemia and weight gain, mild hyperkalemia, decreases in hemoglobin and platelet counts, reversible liver dysfunction, myalgia, joint and back pain, fatigue, headache, insomnia, somnolence, microalbuminuria (in hypertensive patients), erectile dysfunction, bronchospasm, rhinitis, pharyngitis, and dyspnea. Abrupt withdrawal of β-blockers from some patients with angina pectoris may markedly increase the severity and frequency of the angina and result in severe cardiovascular problems (myocardial infarction, arrhythmias, and sudden death). β-blocker therapy should be gradually tapered rather than abruptly discontinued.

Poisoning Information

See metoprolol poisoning information.

Propranolol

Indication

Propranolol is a noncardioselective β-blocking agent with equal effects on β_1 cardiac and β_2 receptors. In patients with CHF, propranolol has been shown to reduce mortality, reduce LV mass, increase LV ejection fraction, and, in addition to digoxin/diuretic therapy, improve CHF symptoms in infants with congenital heart disease. In a prospective, open-label pediatric trial (Congestive Heart Failure In Infants Treated With Propranolol, the CHF-PRO-INFANT trial), infants (n = 20; up to 3 months old) with congenital heart disease and severe CHF caused by left-to-right shunts demonstrated a significant improvement in Ross heart failure score, lower renin and aldosterone levels, and lower mean heart rates.[22]

Mechanism of Action

Propranolol is a nonselective β-blocking agent with equal effects on β_1 (cardiac) and β_2 (bronchial, vasculare smooth muscle) receptors. β_1 blockade produces decreased heart rate and myocardial contractility during periods of high sympathetic activity, such as during exercise. Cardiac output is decreased. Blockade of β-receptors in cardiac conduction tissue results in slowing of AV conduction and suppression of automaticity. β_2 blockade is responsible for many of the adverse effects of propranolol, including bronchospasm, hypoglycemia, and peripheral vasoconstriction.

Dosing

> **Neonates:** limited data is available for neonates. Initial, 0.5 mg/kg/dose by mouth twice daily. Increase by 0.25 mg/kg/dose increments every 2 to 4 weeks, as tolerated, to a maximum of 1.5 mg/kg/dose by mouth twice daily
>
> **Infants/children:** initial, 0.5 mg/kg/dose by mouth twice daily. Increase by 0.25 mg/kg/dose every 2 to 4 weeks, as tolerated, to a maximum of 1.5 mg/kg/dose twice daily
>
> **Adults:**
>
> > *Hypertension:* start with 40 mg twice a day, oral; may increase to a maximum dose of 160 mg twice a day
> >
> > *Angina pectoris:* initiate therapy with 20 to 40 mg twice daily, oral; may increase to 160 mg/d
> >
> > *Arrhythmias:* 10 to 30 mg, three or four times daily, oral
> >
> > *Life-threatening arrhythmias:* 1 to 3 mg, slow I.V., administered under careful monitoring
> >
> > *Postmyocardial infarction:* start with a 20-mg daily dose, oral. If no adverse reaction is noted, increase the dose to 40 mg, three times daily. The maximal dose may be increased to 80 mg, three times daily (20% of patients)
> >
> > *Hypertrophic subaortic stenosis:* 20 to 40 mg, three or four times daily, oral
> >
> > *Dosage adjustment in hepatic impairment:* propranolol is almost entirely eliminated by hepatic metabolism and, thus, patients with liver disease may require variable dosage adjustments and more frequent monitoring. However, the basic approach of dosage titration to the desired therapeutic response will not be altered

Pharmacokinetics

Propranolol is almost completely absorbed from the gastrointestinal tract, but is subject to considerable hepatic tissue binding and first-pass metabolism. Peak effect occurs in 1 to 1.5 hours and, for the sustained-release capsule, in approximately 6 hours. The biological half-life is approximately 3 to 6 hours. Propranolol is highly lipid soluble and crosses the blood-brain barrier and the placenta. It is approximately 90% bound to plasma proteins. It is reported not be significantly dialyzable.

Precautions/Warnings

Propranolol can exacerbate CHF. Use with care in patients with reactive airway disease. Use with caution in diabetes mellitus, hypoglycemia, and renal failure. Use caution when discontinuing propranolol to avoid withdrawal symptoms.

Drug Interactions

Phenobarbital, rifampicin, and cimetidine increase propranolol clearance and decrease its activity. Propranolol's absorption is reduced by aluminum-containing antacids. Phenothiazines may cause an additive hypotensive effect.

Adverse Effects

Propranolol is usually well tolerated, however, caution is warranted in this subset of patients with moderate to severe heart failure because propranolol may worsen the degree of CHF. Other adverse effects reported are AV block, bradycardia, palpitations, syncope, peripheral edema, rebound or withdrawal hypertension after abrupt discontinuation of β-blocker therapy, postural hypotension, dizziness, hyperglycemia, hypertriglyceridemia, reversible liver dysfunction, myalgia, joint and back pain, fatigue, headache, insomnia, somnolence, depression, paraesthesias, erectile dysfunction, bronchospasm, rhinitis, pharyngitis, and dyspnea. Abrupt withdrawal of β-blockers in patients with angina pectoris may markedly increase the severity and frequency of the angina and result in severe cardiovascular problems (myocardial infarction, arrhythmias, and sudden death). β-blocker therapy should be gradually tapered, rather than abruptly discontinued in these patients.

Poisoning Information

See metoprolol poisoning information.

Esmolol

Indication

Esmolol is a β-adrenergic blocker used as a Class II antiarrhythmic agent and as an antihypertensive drug. Esmolol is often used in the acute management of children with arrhythmias and/or hypertension; however, pharmacokinetic studies of esmolol in children have been limited.

Please refer to Chapter 7, Antiarrhythmic Medications.

References

1. Ross RD, Daniels SR, Schwartz DC, et al. (1987). Plasma norepinephrine levels in infants and children with congestive heart failure. *Am J Cardiol* **59**(8): 911–914.

2. Saltissi S, Mushahwar S. (1995). The management of acute myocardial infarction. *Postgrad Med J* 71(839): 534–541.

3. Falkner B, Lowenthal D, et al. (1982). The pharmacodynamic effectiveness of metoprolol in adolescent hypertension. *Pediatr Pharmacol (New York)* 2(1): 49–55.

4. Torp-Pedersen C, Poole-Wilson P, et al. (2005). Effects of metoprolol and carvedilol on cause-specific mortality and morbidity in patients with chronic heart failure—COMET. *Am Heart J* 149(2): 370–376.

5. Stroe A, Gheorghiade M. (2004). Carvedilol: beta-blockade and beyond. *Rev Cardiovasc Med* 5(Supp 1): S18–27.

6. Bristow MR. (2000). β1-adrenergic receptor blockade in chronic heart failure. *Circulation* 101(5): 558–569.

7. Lubbe WF, Podzuweit T, Opie LH. (1992). Potential arrhythmogenic role of cyclic adenosine monophosphate (AMP) and cytosolic calcium overload: implications of prophylactic effects of beta-blockers in myocardial infarction and proarrhythmic effect of phosphodiesterase inhibitors. *J Am Coll Cardiol* 19(7): 1622–1633.

8. Pogwizd SM, Schlotthauer K, Li L, Yuan W, Bers DM. (2001). Arrhythmogenesis and contractile dysfunction in heart failure: Roles of sodium-calcium exchange, inward rectifier potassium current, and residual beta-adrenergic responsiveness. *Circ Res* 88: 1159–1167.

9. RESOLVD Investigators. (2000). Effects of Metoprolol CR in patients with ischemic and dilated cardiomyopathy. The randomized evaluation of strategies for left ventricular dysfunction pilot study. *Circulation* 101(4): 378–384.

10. MERIT-HF Study group. (1999). Effect of metoprolol CR/XL in chronic heart failure: Metoprolol CR/XL randomized trial in congestive heart failure (MERIT-HF). *Lancet* 353(9169): 2001–2007.

11. Shaddy RE, Olsen SL, Bristow MR, et al. (1995). Efficacy and safety of metoprolol in the treatment of doxorubicin-induced cardiomyopathy in pediatric patients. *Am Heart J* 129(1): 197–199.

12. Shaddy RE, Tani LY, Gidding SS, et al. (1999). Beta blocker treatment of dilated cardiomyopathy with congestive heart failure in children: a multi-institutional experience. *J Heart Lung Transplant* 18(3): 269–274.

13. Ishikawa Y, Bach JR, Minami R. (1999). Cardioprotection for Duchenne's muscular dystrophy. *Am Heart J* 137(5): 895–902.

14. Lennard MS, Silas JH, Freestone S, et al. (1982) Oxidation phenotype—a major determinant of metoprolol metabolism and response. *N Engl J Med* 307: 1558–1560.

15. CAPRICORN Investigators. Effects of carvedilol on outcome after myocardial infarction in patients with left ventricular dysfunction: the CAPRICORN randomized trial. *Lancet* 357(9266): 1385–1390.

16. Bruns LA, Chrisant MK, Lamour JM, et al. (2001). Carvedilol as therapy in pediatric heart failure: an initial multicenter experience. *J Pediatr* 138(4): 505–511.

17. Blume ED, Canter CE, Spicer R, et al. (2006). Prospective single-arm protocol of carvedilol in children with ventricular dysfunction. *Pediatr Cardiol* 27(3): 336–342.

18. Moser M, Frishman W. (1998). Results of therapy with carvedilol, a beta-blocker vasodilator with antioxidant properties, in hypertensive patients. *Am J Hypertens* **11**(1 Pt 2): 15S–22S.
19. Laer S, Mir T, et al. (2002). Carvedilol therapy in pediatric patients with congestive heart failure: a study investigating clinical and pharmacokinetic parameters. *Am Heart J* **143**(5): 916–922.
20. Neugebauer G, Gabor M, Reiff K. (1988). Pharmacokinetics and bioavailability of carvedilol in patients with liver cirrhosis. *Drugs* **36**(suppl 6):148–154.
21. Morgan, T. (1994). Clinical pharmacokinetics and pharmacodynamics of carvedilol. *Clin Pharmacokinet* **26**(5): 335–346.
22. Buchhorn R, Hulpke-Wette M, Hilgers R, et al. (2001). Propranolol treatment of congestive heart failure in infants with congenital heart disease: The CHF-PRO-INFANT Trial *Int J Cardiol* **79**(2–3):167–173.

7. Antiarrhythmic Medications

Anne M. Dubin

Class I Antiarrhythmics

Class IA Agents

Class IA agents prolong repolarization and have antivagal effects.

Quinidine

Indication   Quinidine is used as prophylaxis after cardioversion of atrial fibrillation or flutter to maintain normal sinus rhythm; and is used to prevent recurrence of supraventricular tachycardia (SVT) and ventricular tachycardia (VT).

Mechanism of Action   Quinidine is a sodium and potassium channel blocker. Sodium channel blockade predominately occurs in the active state. Quinidine also exhibits low levels of α- and muscarinic-receptor blockade.

Dosing   Dosage is expressed in terms of the salt: 267 mg of quinidine gluconate equals 200 mg of quinidine sulfate.

> **Infants/children:** test dose for idiosyncratic reaction, intolerance, syncope, and thrombocytopenia:
> *Oral, intramuscular (I.M.):* 2 mg/kg or 60 mg/m^2
> *Oral (quinidine sulfate):* 30 mg/kg/day or 900 mg/m^2/day administered in five daily doses, or 6 mg/kg every 4 to 6 hours; range, 15 to 60 mg/kg/day in four to five divided doses
> *Intravenous (I.V.) (quinidine gluconate):* 2 to 10 mg/kg/dose every 3 to 6 hours as needed (I.V. not recommended)
> **Adults:** test dose for idiosyncratic reaction, intolerance, syncope, and thrombocytopenia:
> *Oral:* 200 mg administered several hours before full dose
> *Oral (quinidine sulfate):* 100 to 600 mg/dose every 4 to 6 hours
> *Oral (quinidine gluconate):* 324 to 972 mg every 8 to 12 hours
> *I.M.:* 400 mg/dose every 4 to 6 hours
> *I.V.:* 200 to 400 mg/dose diluted and administered at a rate of at most 10 mg/min
> **Dosing adjustment in renal impairment:** creatinine clearance (Cl_{cr}) less than 10 mL/min, administer 75% of normal dose

Pharmacokinetics   Quinidine is extensively protein bound, and is metabolized extensively in the liver. The half-life of quinidine in children is 2.5 to 6.7 hours; the half-life in adults is 6 to 8 hours. The route of elimination of quinidine is renal. Quinidine is slightly dialyzable by hemodialysis; and is not removed by peritoneal dialysis.[1]

Monitoring Parameters   Complete blood cell count (CBC), with differential, liver and renal function tests, and serum quinidine concentrations should be routinely performed with long-term administration of quinidine.

Contraindications   Contraindications for quinidine are complete atrioventricular (AV) block, marked widening of QRS complex, cardiac glycoside-induced AV conduction disorders, and myasthenia gravis.

Precautions/Warnings   Hemolysis may occur in patients with glucose-6-phosphate dehydrogenase (G-6-PD) deficiency.

Drug-Drug Interactions   Diltiazem, verapamil, amiodarone, and cimetidine may increase quinidine serum concentrations.

Phenobarbital, phenytoin, and rifampin may decrease quinidine serum concentrations.

Quinidine may increase plasma concentration of digoxin; digoxin may need to be decreased by one-half when coadministering quinidine.[2] Quinidine may increase bradycardia when administered with β-blockers; quinidine enhances coumarin anticoagulants. Quinidine potentiates nondepolarizing and depolarizing muscle relaxants.

Quinidine has a potential for interaction with ritonavir; therefore, concurrent use is not recommended.

Adverse Effects

Cardiovascular (CV): syncope, hypotension tachycardia, heart block, ventricular arrhythmias,[3] vascular collapse, severe hypotension with rapid I.V. administration

Central nervous system (CNS): fever, headache

Dermatological: angioedema, rash

Gastrointestinal (GI): GI disturbances, nausea, vomiting, and cramps

Hematological: blood dyscrasias and thrombotic thrombocytopenic purpura

Hepatic: quinidine-induced hepatotoxicity, including granulomatous hepatitis, and jaundice

Respiratory: respiratory depression

Miscellaneous: cinchonism (nausea, tinnitus, headache, impaired hearing or vision, vomiting, abdominal pain, vertigo, confusion, delirium, and syncope)

Poisoning Information   Quinidine has a low toxic-to-therapeutic ratio and may easily produce fatal intoxication. Symptoms include sinus bradycardia, arrest, or asystole; PR, QRS, or QT prolongation; torsade de pointes; depressed myocardial contractility; hypotension; pulmonary edema; dry mouth; dilated pupils; delirium;

seizures; coma; and respiratory arrest. Treatment is primarily symptomatic. Sodium bicarbonate may treat QRS prolongation and hypotension.

Diagnostic or therapeutic endoscopy may be required in patients with massive overdose and prolonged elevated quinidine levels.

Compatible Diluents/Administration   The maximum rate of I.V. infusion is 10 mg/min; with a maximum concentration of 16 mg/mL in dextrose; I.V. tubing should be minimized (quinidine is adsorbed to polyvinyl chloride tubing).

For oral use, do not administer with grapefruit juice. Use of extended-release products is not recommended in children. Bezoar formation is reported in pediatric patients.

Procainamide

Indication   Procainamide is indicated for treatment of VT, paroxysmal atrial tachycardia, and atrial fibrillation.[4] It is also used as a first choice agent by some for the treatment of JET, instead of amiodarone.

Mechanism of Action   Procainamide is a potent sodium channel blocker in the active state and a moderate potassium channel blocker. Procainamide delays repolarization and has a greater effect at faster heart rates.

Dosing

Infants/children:
> *Oral:* 15 to 30 mg/kg/day, divided every 3 to 6 hours (maximum, 4 g/day)
> *I.M.:* 20 to 30 mg/kg/day, divided every 4 to 6 hours (maximum, 4 g/day)
> *I.V.:* loading dose of 3 to 6 mg/kg/dose over 5 minutes, not to exceed 100 mg/dose; may repeat every 5 to 10 minutes to a maximum load of 15 mg/kg; do not exceed 500 mg in 30 minutes
> *Maintenance:* continuous I.V. infusion of 20 to 80 μg/kg/min (maximum dose, 2 g/day)

Adults:
> *Oral:*
>> Immediate release: 250 to 500 mg/dose every 3 to 6 hours
>> Sustained release: 500 mg to 1 g every 6 hours
>> Extended release: 1 to 2 g every 12 hours
>> Usual dose: 50 mg/kg/day or 2 to 4 g/day
> *I.V.:* loading dose of 50 to 100 mg/dose repeated every 5 to 10 minutes until the patient is controlled, or load with 15 to 18 mg/kg (maximum load, 1–1.5 g)
> *Maintenance:* continuous I.V. infusion, 3 to 4 mg/min; range, 1 to 6 mg/min

Dosing adjustment in renal dysfunction:
> Cl_{cr} *10 to 50 mL/min:* administer dose every 6 to 12 hours
> Cl_{cr} *less than 10 mL/min:* administer dose every 8 to 24 hours

Pharmacokinetics   Orally, procainamide is well absorbed. Procainamide is metabolized in the liver to produce the active metabolite, *N*-acetyl procainamide

(NAPA).[5] The half-life of procainamide in children is 1.7 hours; and is 2.5 to 4.7 hours in adults. The NAPA half-life is 6 hours in children, and 6 to 8 hours in adults. Procainamide is excreted in the urine (25% as NAPA). Procainamide is moderately dialyzable by hemodialysis, but not dialyzable by peritoneal dialysis.

Monitoring Parameters   Electrocardiogram (ECG), blood pressure, and CBC with differential should be monitored; cardiac and blood pressure monitoring is required during I.V. administration. Blood levels in patients with renal failure should be monitored. Both procainamide and NAPA levels should be followed during treatment.

Contraindications   Contraindications for use of procainamide are complete AV block or second-degree heart block without pacemaker, torsade de pointes, cardiac glycoside intoxication, myasthenia gravis, or systemic lupus erythematosus (SLE).

Precautions/Warnings   Drug may accumulate in patients with renal or hepatic dysfunction. Procainamide may precipitate or exacerbate congestive heart failure (CHF). Procainamide use may increase ventricular response rate in patients with atrial fibrillation or flutter; therefore, AV conduction should be controlled before initiating use. Hypokalemia may worsen toxicity.

Long-term administration of procainamide leads to the development of a positive antinuclear antibody test in 50% of patients, which may lead to a lupus erythematosus-like syndrome (in 20–30% of patients).

Drug-Drug Interactions   Cimetidine, ranitidine, amiodarone, β-blockers, and trimethoprim may increase plasma procainamide and NAPA levels. Procainamide may potentiate skeletal muscle relaxants; anticholinergic drugs may have enhanced effects.

Adverse Effects

CV: hypotension, tachycardia, arrhythmias, AV block, QT prolongation, widening of QRS complex
CNS: confusion, disorientation
GI: nausea, vomiting, GI complaints
Hematological: agranulocytosis, neutropenia
Hepatic: hepatomegaly, increased liver enzymes
Miscellaneous: drug fever, lupus-like syndrome (arthralgia, positive Coombs' test, thrombocytopenia, rash, myalgia, fever, pericarditis, and pleural effusion)

Poisoning Information   Procainamide has a low toxic-to-therapeutic ratio and can easily produce fatal intoxication. Symptoms include sinus bradycardia and arrest; PR, QRS, and QT prolongation; torsade de pointes; depressed myocardial contractility; hypotension; pulmonary edema; seizures; coma; and respiratory arrest. Treatment of poisoning is symptomatic. Sodium bicarbonate may treat QRS prolongation and hypotension.

Compatible Diluents/Administration   Do not administer procainamide faster than 20 to 30 mg/min. Severe hypotension can occur with rapid I.V. push. Administer an I.V. loading dose over 25 to 30 minutes using a concentration of 20 to 30 mg/mL for the loading dose and 2 to 4 mg/mL for the maintenance infusion.

Disopyramide

Indication   Disopyramide is used in the conversion and management of atrial fibrillation, atrial flutter, and SVT.

Mechanism of Action   Disopyramide is a potent sodium and potassium channel blocker. Disopyramide does not have any α-receptor-blocking activity. Disopyramide prolongs the action potential duration in Purkinje tissue more than the effective refractory period.

Dosing

   Infants/children:
      Oral:
         Younger than 1 year: 10 to 30 mg/kg/day in four divided doses
         1 to 4 years old: 10 to 20 mg/kg/day in four divided doses
         4 to 12 years old: 10 to 15 mg/kg/day in four divided doses[6]
         12 to 18 years: 6 to 15 mg/kg/day in four divided doses
   Adults:
      Oral (controlled release):
         If lighter than 50 kg, administer 100 mg every 6 hours, or 200 mg every 12 hours
         If heavier than 50 kg, administer 150 mg every 6 hours, or 300 mg every 12 hours
   Adult dose adjustment in renal dysfunction:
      Cl_{cr} *30 to 40 mL/min:* 100 mg every 8 hours
      Cl_{cr} *15 to 30 mL/min:* 100 mg every 12 hours
      Cl_{cr} *less than 15 mL/min:* every 24 hours

Pharmacokinetics   Disopyramide is generally highly protein bound. The peak serum concentration is 0.5 to 3 hours. Disopyramide has a half-life of 3 to 5 hours in children. Disopyramide is metabolized in the liver; its major metabolite has anticholinergic and antiarrhythmic effects. Disopyramide is eliminated in the urine.

Contraindications   Contraindications for use of disopyramide are cardiogenic shock, preexisting second- or third-degree heart block (without pacemaker), congenital long QT syndrome, and sick sinus syndrome.

Precautions/Warnings   Use with caution in patients with preexisting urinary retention, existing or family history of glaucoma, myasthenia gravis, CHF, sick sinus syndrome, Wolff-Parkinson-White (WPW) syndrome, and widening of QRS or lengthening of QT interval. Decrease dose in patients with renal or hepatic impairment.

Disopyramide may increase the ventricular response rate in patients with atrial fibrillation or flutter; therefore, AV conduction should be controlled before initiating treatment.

Drug-Drug Interactions Hepatic microsomal enzyme-inducing agents (phenytoin, phenobarbital, rifampin) may increase metabolism of disopyramide, and lower serum concentrations. Clarithromycin and erythromycin may increase disopyramide concentrations and should not be used with disopyramide.

Other antiarrhythmics may increase adverse conduction effects. Adverse effects of disopyramide may be additive with amitriptyline, imipramine, haloperidol, thioridazine, dicapride, and other drugs that prolong the QT.

Do not administer disopyramide 48 hours before or 24 hours after verapamil.

Adverse Effects

CV: CHF, edema, chest pain, syncope and hypotension, AV block, widened QRS and prolonged QT interval

CNS: fatigue, headache, malaise, nervousness, acute psychosis, depression, dizziness

Dermatological: rash

Endocrine and metabolic: hypoglycemia, weight gain, elevated cholesterol and triglyceride levels

GI: xerostomia, dry throat, constipation, nausea, vomiting, diarrhea, pain, gas, anorexia

Genitourinary (GU): urinary retention

Hepatic: elevated liver enzymes

Neuromuscular: weakness

Ocular: blurred vision

Respiratory: dyspnea

Poisoning Information Disopyramide has a low toxic-to-therapeutic ratio and may produce fatal intoxication. Symptoms of poisoning include sinus bradycardia, sinus arrest, and asystole; torsade de pointes; PR, QRS, and QT prolongation; depressed myocardial contractility; hypotension; pulmonary edema; dry mouth; dilated pupils; delirium; seizures; coma; and respiratory arrest. Treatment is symptomatic. Sodium bicarbonate may treat QRS prolongation or hypotension.

Administration Administer disopyramide on an empty stomach.

Class IB Agents

Class IB agents block fast sodium channels and shorten action potential duration and repolarization.

Lidocaine

Indication   Lidocaine is used for treatment of ventricular ectopy, tachycardia, and fibrillation; local anesthetic.

Mechanism of Action   Lidocaine treatment blocks the fast sodium channel and shows frequency dependence. It has little or no effect on tissue above the His bundle.

Dosing

   Infants/children:
     I.V., I.O. (inter osseous): loading dose of 1 mg/kg followed by continuous infusion of 20 to 50 µg/kg/min. May repeat bolus with 0.5 to 1 mg/kg. Patients with shock, hepatic disease, or CHF may require one-half of the loading dose and lower infusion rates
     Tracheal tube: 2- to 10-fold times the I.V. bolus dose
   Adults:
     I.V.: loading dose of 1 to 1.5 mg/kg. May repeat doses of 0.5 to 0.75 mg/kg every 5 to 10 minutes, to a total of 3 mg/kg. Continuous infusion, 1 to 4 mg/min. Decrease the initial bolus of 0.5 to 0.75 mg/kg in patients with CHF
     Tracheal tube: 2 to 2.5 times the I.V. bolus dose

Pharmacokinetics   Metabolism of lidocaine diminished in heart failure. The onset of action is 45 to 90 seconds. The half-life is 2 to 3 hours. Therapeutic levels of lidocaine are in the range of 2 to 5 µg/mL. Lidocaine is eliminated in the urine.

Monitoring Parameters   ECG should be continuously monitored. Measure serum concentrations of lidocaine. Monitor the I.V. site, because local thrombophlebitis has been seen with prolonged infusions.

Contraindications   Sinus, AV, or intraventricular block without pacemaker; WPW syndrome.

Precautions/Warnings   Use lidocaine with caution in patients with hepatic disease, heart failure, hypotension or shock; dose may need to be decreased.

Drug-Drug Interactions   Cimetidine or β-blockers may increase lidocaine serum levels. Class I antiarrhythmics and amiodarone may increase adverse effects.

Adverse Effects

   CV: bradycardia, hypotension, heart block, arrhythmias, cardiovascular collapse
   CNS: lethargy, coma, agitation, slurred speech, seizures, anxiety, euphoria, hallucinations
   GI: nausea, vomiting
   Neuromuscular: paresthesias, muscle twitching
   Ocular: blurred vision, diplopia,

Respiratory: respiratory depression or arrest
Miscellaneous: allergic reaction (rare)

Poisoning Information   Lidocaine has a narrow therapeutic index; severe toxicity is seen slightly above the therapeutic range, especially if lidocaine is administered with other antiarrhythmics.[7] Symptoms include sedation, confusion, coma, seizures, respiratory arrest, sinus arrest, AV block, asystole, hypotension, dizziness, paresthesias, tremor, ataxia, and GI disturbances. Treatment is supportive. Sodium bicarbonate may reverse QRS prolongation, bradyarrhythmias, and hypotension.

Compatible Diluents/Administration   Tracheal tube doses should be diluted to 1 to 2 mL with normal saline (NS).
For I.V. push, dilute lidocaine to a maximum concentration of 20 mg/mL and administer over 5 to 10 minutes. The maximum I.V. push rate is 0.35 to 0.7 mg/kg/min.

Mexiletine

Indication   Mexiletine is indicated for management of ventriculararrhythmias.[8]

Mechanism of Action   Mexiletine inhibits the fast sodium channel with greater effects at faster heart rates. Effects are exaggerated in diseased tissue, dependent on potassium concentration. Mexiletine suppresses early after depolarizations.

Dosing   Mexiletine is only available for enteral administration.

Infants/children:
> *Oral:* 1.4 to 5 mg/kg/dose (mean, 3.3 mg/kg/dose) administered every 8 hours. Increase dose according to effect

Adults:
> *Oral:* initial, 200 mg every 8 hours (may load with 400 mg, if necessary). Adjust dose every 2 to 3 days. Usual dose, 200 to 300 mg every 8 hours; maximum dose, 1.2 g/day

Dosing adjustment in renal impairment: children and adults with Cl_{cr} less than 10 mL/min, administer 50 to 75% of normal dose

Pharmacokinetics   Mexiletine is rapidly absorbed and undergoes hepatic metabolism. The half-life of Mexiletine is 10 to 14 hours. Mexiletine is eliminated in the urine.

Monitoring Parameters   Liver enzymes, CBC, ECG, heart rate, and serum concentrations should be monitored.

Contraindications   Cardiogenic shock and second- or third-degree AV block without a pacemaker are contraindications for Mexiletine.

Precautions/Warnings   Use mexiletine with caution in patients with seizure disorders, severe CHF, hypotension, or hepatic dysfunction. Blood dyscrasias have been reported.

Drug-Drug Interactions   Phenobarbital, phenytoin, rifampin, and other hepatic enzyme inducers may lower mexiletine plasma levels.
   Cimetidine may increase levels of mexiletine.
   Antacids, narcotics, or anticholinergics may decrease absorption of mexiletine.
   Metoclopramide may increase absorption of mexiletine.
   Mexiletine may increase concentrations of theophylline and caffeine.

Adverse Effects

   CV: palpitations, bradycardia, chest pain, syncope, hypotension, atrial or ventricular arrhythmias
   CNS: dizziness, confusion, ataxia
   Dermatological: rash
   GI: nausea, vomiting, diarrhea
   Hematological: thrombocytopenia, leucopenia, agranulocytosis
   Hepatic: elevated liver enzymes, hepatitis
   Neuromuscular: paresthesias, tremor
   Ocular: diplopia
   Otic: tinnitus
   Respiratory: dyspnea

Poisoning Information   Mexiletine has a narrow therapeutic index; severe toxicity is seen slightly above the therapeutic range, especially with other antiarrhythmics. Symptoms include sedation, confusion, coma, seizures, respiratory arrest, sinus arrest, AV block, asystole, hypotension, dizziness, paresthesias, tremor, ataxia, and GI disturbances. Treatment is supportive. Sodium bicarbonate may reverse QRS prolongation, bradyarrhythmias, and hypotension.

Phenytoin

Indication   Phenytoin is indicated for ventricular arrhythmias, including those associated with digitalis intoxication and seizures.[9]

Mechanism of Action   Phenytoin binds primarily to sodium channels in the inactivated state. High concentrations of phenytoin can have some calcium channel-blocking effects with decreases in sinus and AV nodal automaticity. Phenytoin depresses Phase 4 depolarization, which makes it useful for treating digoxin-induced arrhythmias.
   Phenytoin decreases sympathetic effects in the ventricle.

Dosing

Infants/children:
I.V.: loading dose, 1.25 mg/kg every 5 minutes, up to a total load of 15 mg/
kg
Oral, I.V.: maintenance dose, 5 to 10 mg/kg/day in two to three divided doses
Adults:
I.V.: loading dose, 1.25 mg/kg every 5 minutes, may repeat up to a total
loading dose of 15 mg/kg
Oral: loading dose, 250 mg four times per day for 1 day, 250 mg twice
daily for 2 days, and then maintenance at 300 to 400 mg/day in divided
doses one to four times per day

Pharmacokinetics   Peak serum levels occur 3 to 12 hours after dose. Phenytoin is metabolized in the liver. The half-life is up to 24 hours in infants. In patients older than 1 year, the half-life is 8 hours. In adults, the half-life is 24 hours. Phenytoin is eliminated in the urine.

Monitoring Parameters   Serum phenytoin concentration, CBC with differential, liver enzymes, and blood pressure with I.V. use should be monitored.

Contraindications   Heart block and sinus bradycardia are contraindications for phenytoin administration.

Drug-Drug Interactions   Phenytoin may decrease the effectiveness of ritonavir, valproic acid, ethosuximide, warfarin, oral contraceptives, corticosteroids, etoposide, doxorubicin, vincristine, methotrexate, cyclosporine, theophylline, chloramphenicol, rifampin, doxycycline, quinidine, mexiletine, disopyramide, dopamine, or nondepolarizing muscle relaxants.
Serum phenytoin levels may be increased by cimetidine, chloramphenicol, felbamate, zidovudine, isoniazid, trimethoprim, or sulfonamide.
Rifampin, zidovudine, cisplatin, vinblastine, bleomycin, antacids, and folic acid may decrease phenytoin levels.

Adverse Effects

CV: hypotension, bradycardia, arrhythmia, cardiovascular collapse
CNS: slurred speech, dizziness, drowsiness, lethargy, coma, ataxia, dyskine-
sias
Ocular: nystagmus, blurred vision, diplopia
Dermatological: hirsutism, coarsening of facial features, Steven-Johnson
syndrome, rash
Endocrine and metabolic: folic acid depletion, hyperglycemia
GI: nausea, vomiting, gingival hyperplasia, gum tenderness
Hematological: blood dyscrasias, lymphoma
Hepatic: hepatitis
Local: thrombophlebitis
Neuromuscular: peripheral neuropathy
Miscellaneous: SLE-like syndrome

Poisoning Information   Symptoms of phenytoin poisoning include unsteady gait, slurred speech, confusion, nausea, hypothermia, fever, hypotension, respiratory depression, and coma. Treatment is supportive.

Compatible Diluents/Administration   Administer phenytoin by slow injection without dilution and flush with saline immediately, or dilute with NS for infusion to a concentration of less than 6 mg/mL. Do not exceed an I.V. infusion rate of 1 to 3 mg/kg/min and a maximum rate of 50 mg/min. Avoid extravasation.

Class IC Agents

Class IC agents are sodium channel blockers with variable effects on repolarization and some frequency-dependent characteristics.

Flecainide

Indication   Flecainide is indicated for treatment of atrial, junctional, and ventricular arrhythmias.[10,11]

Mechanism of Action   Flecainide blocks slow sodium channels in the activated state, with some mild potassium channel-blocking properties. Flecainide has a long time constant and takes longer to dissociate from sodium channels. In specialized conduction tissue, refractory periods are shortened and automaticity is decreased. Ventricular action potential duration and refractory periods are prolonged.

Dosing

> **Children:**
> > *Oral:* initial dose, 1 to 3 mg/kg/day or 50 to 100 mg/m^2/day, in three divided doses. Increase every few days to usual 3 to 6 mg/kg/day or 100 to 150 mg/m^2/day in three divided doses, up to 8 mg/kg/day or 200 mg/m^2/day
> **Adults:**
> > *Oral:* 50 to 100 mg every 12 hours; increase by 100 mg/day every 4 days. Usual dose, at most 300 mg/day; maximum, 400 mg/day

Pharmacokinetics   Flecainide shows complete absorption. Flecainide is metabolized in the liver. The half-life in newborns is 29 hours; infants, 11 to 12 hours; children, 8 hours; and adults, 12 to 27 hours. Flecainide is eliminated in the urine. Flecainide is not dialyzable.

Monitoring Parameters   ECG, serum flecainide concentration, liver enzymes, and CBC should be monitored.

Contraindications   Contraindications for flecainide administration are preexisting second- or third-degree AV block, complete right bundle branch block (RBBB) with left hemiblock or trifascicular block, cardiogenic shock, and myocardial depression.[12]

Precautions/Warnings   Use flecainide with caution in patients with CHF; conduction abnormalities; and myocardial, renal, or hepatic dysfunction. Proarrhythmia is associated with flecainide.[13]

Drug-Drug Interactions   Other antiarrhythmics may increase adverse cardiac effects.

Flecainide may increase plasma digoxin levels.

β-blockers, disopyramide, or verapamil may result in added negative inotropy.

Antacids, carbonic anhydrase inhibitors, or sodium bicarbonate may decrease clearance of flecainide.

Amiodarone or cimetidine may increase the serum concentration of flecainide.

Use of flecainide with ritonavir is not recommended.

Adverse Effects

CV: bradycardia, heart block, ventricular arrhythmias, CHF, palpitations, chest pain, edema, increased PR interval and QRS duration[14]
CNS: dizziness, fatigue, nervousness, headache
Dermatological: rash
GI: nausea
Hematological: blood dyscrasias
Hepatic: hepatic dysfunction
Neuromuscular: paresthesias, tremor
Ocular: blurred vision
Respiratory: dyspnea

Poisoning Information   Flecainide has a narrow therapeutic index and severe toxicity is seen slightly above the therapeutic range, especially if flecainide is combined with other antiarrhythmics. Acute single ingestion of twice the daily dose is life threatening. Signs include increases in PR, QRS, and QR intervals; AV block; bradycardia; hypotension; ventricular arrhythmias; and asystole. Symptoms include dizziness, blurred vision, headache, and GI upset. Treatment is supportive. Sodium bicarbonate may reverse QRS prolongation, bradycardia, and hypotension.

Compatible Diluents/Administration   Dairy products may interfere with the absorption of flecainide. Serum flecainide levels should be monitored when changing dairy intake.

Propafenone

Indication   Propafenone is indicated for treatment of atrial, junctional, and ventricular arrhythmias.[15]

Mechanism of Action   Propafenone blocks sodium channels with a medium-range time constant for recovery. Propafenone has mild β-blocking properties.

Propafenone has effects on the slow inward calcium current and delayed outward potassium current.

Dosing

Infants/children:
Oral: 150 to 200 mg/m^2/day divided every 8 hours. Upper dose range, 600 mg/m^2/day
Adults:
Oral:
Immediate release: 150 mg every 8 hours; increase every 3 to 4 days to 300 mg every 8 hours
Extended release: 225 mg every 12 hours; increase every 5 days to 325 mg every 12 hours, to a maximum of 425 every 12 hours

Pharmacokinetics   Propafenone is well absorbed. Propafenone is metabolized in the liver, with two genetically determined groups described (fast and slow metabolizers).[16] Propafenone has a half-life of 2 to 8 hours (single dose) or 10 to 32 hours (chronic dosing).

Monitoring Parameters   ECG and blood pressure should be monitored.

Contraindications   Contraindications for propafenone use are sinoatrial (SA), AV, or intraventricular conduction disorders without a pacemaker; sinus bradycardia; cardiogenic shock; uncompensated heart failure; hypotension; bronchospasm; uncorrected electrolyte abnormalities; and concurrent use of ritonavir.

Precautions/Warnings   Monitor for proarrhythmia and increasing CHF with propafenone use. Administer propafenone cautiously in those with significant hepatic dysfunction.

Drug-Drug Interactions   Cimetidine, quinidine, ritonavir (contraindicated), fluoxetine, and miconazole may increase propafenone levels.
Phenobarbital and rifampin may decrease propafenone levels.
Propafenone may increase levels of digoxin, metoprolol, propranolol, theophylline, and warfarin. Use propafenone with caution with Class IA and III agents, erythromycin, cisapride, antipsychotics, and tricyclic antidepressants.

Adverse Effects

CV: proarrhythmia, CHF, AV block, syncope, chest pain, hypotension
CNS: dizziness, fatigue, headache, ataxia, insomnia, anxiety, drowsiness
Dermatological: rash
GI: nausea, vomiting, constipation, dyspepsia, diarrhea, anorexia, abdominal pain
Neuromuscular: tremor, weakness, arthralgia
Ocular: blurred vision
Respiratory: dyspnea

Poisoning Information Propafenone has a narrow therapeutic index and severe toxicity is seen slightly above the therapeutic range, especially if propafenone is combined with other antiarrhythmics. Acute single ingestion of twice the daily dose of propafenone is life threatening. Signs include increased PR, QRS, and QR intervals; AV block; bradycardia; hypotension; ventricular arrhythmias; and asystole. Symptoms include dizziness, blurred vision, headache, and GI upset. Treatment is supportive. Sodium bicarbonate may reverse QRS prolongation, bradycardia, and hypotension.

Class II Antiarrhythmics: β-Blockers

Esmolol

Indication
Esmolol is used for treatment of SVT and atrial fibrillation/flutter (rate control), VT, and hypertension in the postoperative setting.[17,18]

Mechanism of Action
Esmolol is an intravenous β-blocker with predominate β1-receptor selectivity. The predominate sites of action are AV and SA nodes.

Dosing

Infants/children:
I.V.: 100 to 500 μg/kg administered over 1 minute, followed by continuous infusion starting at 50 μg/kg/min. Additional boluses can be administered, with an increase in the infusion rate up to 200 μg/kg/min
Adults:
I.V.: loading dose, 500 μg/kg over 1 minute, followed by a 50 μg/kg/min infusion for 4 minutes. May rebolus and increase continuous infusion to 100 μg/kg/min. Repeat until therapeutic dose or a maximum maintenance dose of 200 μg/kg/min is reached

Pharmacokinetics
Esmolol is metabolized in blood by esterases. The half-life of esmolol is 3 to 10 minutes.

Monitoring Parameters
Blood pressure, ECG, heart rate, and I.V. site should be monitored.

Contraindications
Contraindications of esmolol use are sinus bradycardia or heart block, uncompensated heart failure, and cardiogenic shock.

Precautions/Warnings
Use esmolol with care in patients with reactive airway disease. Use with caution in diabetes mellitus, hypoglycemia, and renal failure. Avoid extravasation. Caution should be exercised when discontinuing esmolol, to avoid withdrawal effects.

Drug-Drug Interactions
Morphine may increase esmolol concentrations.
>Theophylline or caffeine may decrease the effects of esmolol.
>Esmolol may increase digoxin or theophylline serum concentrations.

Adverse Effects
>**CV:** hypotension, bradycardia
>**CNS:** dizziness, somnolence, confusion, lethargy, depression, headache
>**GI:** nausea, vomiting
>**Local:** phlebitis
>**Respiratory:** bronchoconstriction
>**Miscellaneous:** sweating

Poisoning Information
Poisoning signs include hypotension, bradycardia, bronchospasm, CHF, and heart block. Fluid administration is a useful therapy for hypotension. Sympathomimetics can be used to treat bradycardia and hypotension.

Compatible Diluents/Administration
Esmolol must be diluted to a final concentration of 10 mg/mL. Concentrations greater than 10 mg/mL can cause thrombophlebitis.

Propranolol

Indication
Propranolol is used to treat atrial and ventricular tachyarrhythmias and hypertension.[19]

Mechanism of Action
Propranolol is a nonselective β-blocker with membrane effects on the sodium channel. Propranolol has no intrinsic sympathomimetic properties.

Dosing
>**Infants/children:**
>>*I.V.:*
>>>Neonates: 0.01 mg/kg slow I.V. push over 10 minutes; may repeat every 6 to 8 hours as needed, increase slowly to maximum of 0.15 mg/kg/ dose every 6 to 8 hours

Infants/children: 0.01 to 0.1 mg/kg slow I.V. over 10 minutes, maximum dose of 1 mg in infants and 3 mg in children

Oral:

Neonates: 0.25 mg/kg/dose every 6 to 8 hours; increase to maximum of 5 mg/kg/day

Children: 0.5 to 1 mg/kg/day in divided doses every 6 to 8 hours; titrate over 3 to 5 days to usual dose of 2 to 4 mg/kg/day. Do not exceed 16 mg/kg/day or 60 mg/day

Adults:

I.V.: 1 mg/dose slow I.V. push; repeat every 5 minutes up to 5 mg total

Oral: 10 to 20 mg/dose every 6 to 8 hours; increase gradually to a range of 40 to 320 mg/day

Pharmacokinetics

Propranolol has extensive hepatic metabolism and clearance. The half-life of propranolol in infants is 3 to 4 hours; in children and adults, it is 6 hours. Propranolol is excreted in the urine. Propranolol is not dialyzable.

Monitoring Parameters

Monitor ECG and blood pressure with I.V. propranolol administration; monitor heart rate and blood pressure with oral propranolol administration.

Contraindications

Propranolol is contraindicated with uncompensated CHF, cardiogenic shock, bradycardia or heart block, asthma, and chronic obstructive lung disease.

Precautions/Warnings

Use propranolol with care in patients with heart failure, because propranolol can exacerbate CHF. Use with care in patients with reactive airway disease. Use with caution in diabetes mellitus, hypoglycemia, and renal failure. Avoid extravasation. Caution should be exercised when discontinuing propranolol to avoid potential withdrawal.

Drug-Drug Interactions

Phenobarbital and rifampin may increase propranolol clearance and decrease its activity.

Cimetidine may reduce clearance and increase its effects.

Aluminum-containing antacids may reduce absorption.

Additive hypotensive activity can be seen with phenothiazines.

Adverse Effects

CV: hypotension, impaired myocardial contractility, CHF, bradycardia, AV block

CNS: lightheadedness, insomnia, vivid dreams, weakness, lethargy and depression
Endocrine and metabolic: hypoglycemia (especially infants and children), hyperglycemia
GI: nausea, vomiting, diarrhea
Hematological: agranulocytosis
Respiratory: bronchospasm

Poisoning Information
Symptoms include hypotension, bradycardia, bronchospasm, CHF, and heart block. Sympathomimetics can be used to treat bradycardia and hypotension.

Compatible Diluents/Administration
Propranolol is incompatible with bicarbonate; protect from exposure to light.

Atenolol
Indication
Atenolol is used to treat atrial and ventricular tachyarrhythmias and hypertension.[20,21]

Mechanism of Action
Atenolol is a selective β-blocker that primarily affects β1 receptors. Atenolol has no intrinsic sympathomimetic or membrane properties. Atenolol does not cross the blood brain barrier.

Dosing

Infants/children:
   Oral: initial, 0.8 to 1 mg/kg/dose given one daily; maximum dose, 2 mg/ kg/day. Do not exceed the adult maximum dose of 100 mg/day
Adults:
   Oral: initial, 25 to 50 mg/dose administered daily; usual dose, 50 to 100 mg/dose administered daily. Maximum dose, 100 mg/day
Dosing adjustment in renal impairment: If Cl_{cr} 15 to 35 mL/min, use a maximum dose of 50 mg or 1 mg/kg/dose daily. If Cl_{cr} less than 15 mL/ min, use a maximum dose of 50 mg or a 1 mg/kg/dose every other day

Pharmacokinetics
Atenolol reaches a peak concentration 2 to 3 hours after an oral dose; and has a half-life of up to 9 to 10 hours. Atenolol has little hepatic transformation; no

active metabolites; and is eliminated in urine and feces. Atenolol is moderately dialyzable.[22]

Contraindications

Bradycardia, heart block, uncompensated CHF, cardiogenic shock, and pulmonary edema are contraindications for atenolol use.

Precautions/Warnings

Use atenolol with care in patients with renal impairment. Use atenolol with care in patients with reactive airway disease. Use with caution in diabetes mellitus, hypoglycemia, and CHF. Avoid extravasation. Caution should be exercised when discontinuing atenolol to avoid withdrawal.

Drug-Drug Interactions

Atenolol has additive effects with other antihypertensive agents.

Atenolol may reverse the therapeutic effects of theophylline.

Adverse Effects

CV: bradycardia, hypotension, second- or third-degree heart block
CNS: dizziness, fatigue, lethargy headache, nightmares
GI: constipation, nausea, diarrhea
Respiratory: bronchospasm

Poisoning Information

Symptoms include hypotension, bradycardia, cardiogenic shock, and asystole. CNS effects include coma, convulsions, and respiratory arrest. Treatment is symptomatic. Bradycardia may respond to atropine, isoproterenol, or glucagon.

Metoprolol

Indication

Metoprolol is used to treat atrial and ventricular tachyarrhythmias and hypertension. It reduces mortality in adults with CHF.[23]

Mechanism of Action

Metoprolol is a selective β1 blocker. Metoprolol has no intrinsic sympathomimetic activity.

Dosing

Infants/children:
Oral: No pediatric studies are available. For adolescents, limited information suggests 50 to 100 mg twice daily for control of hypertension

Adults:

I.V.: 1.25 to 5 mg every 6 to 12 hours; titrate initial dose to response. Maximum dose, 15 mg every 3 to 6 hours

Oral: initial dosing, 100 mg/day, in one to two doses a day. Increase at weekly intervals. Usual dosage, 100 to 450 mg/day

Pharmacokinetics

Metoprolol undergoes extensive first-pass hepatic transformation. Metoprolol has a half-life of 3 to 8 hours; has no active metabolites; and is excreted in the urine.

Monitoring Parameters

Monitor ECG and blood pressure with I.V. use of metoprolol. Monitor heart rate and blood pressure with oral use.

Contraindications

Sinus bradycardia, second- or third-degree heart block (in patients without a pacemaker), cardiogenic shock, and uncompensated CHF are contraindications for Metoprolol use.

Precautions/Warnings

Use metoprolol with care in patients with heart failure, because metoprolol can exacerbate CHF. Use metoprolol with care in patients with reactive airway disease. Use with caution in diabetes mellitus, hypoglycemia, and renal failure. Avoid extravasation. Caution should be exercised when discontinuing metoprolol to avoid withdrawal.

Drug-Drug Interactions

Reserpine and monoamine oxidase (MAO) inhibitors may have additive effects of hypotension and bradycardia. Antihypertensive agents, diuretics, digoxin, amiodarone, calcium channel blockers, and general anesthetics may have additive effects.

Verapamil may increase the oral bioavailability of metoprolol.

Ciprofloxacin, hydralazine, oral contraceptives, and quinidine may increase metoprolol serum concentrations.

Abrupt withdrawal of clonidine may result in hypertensive crisis.

Nonsteroidal anti-inflammatory drugs (NSAIDs) may decrease antihypertensive effects.

Barbiturate and rifampin may increase the metabolism of metoprolol.

Metoprolol may increase lidocaine serum concentrations.

Adverse Effects

CV: bradycardia, palpitations, CHF, hypotension, peripheral edema, heart block

CNS: dizziness, tiredness, depression, mental confusion, insomnia
Dermatological: rash, pruritus
GI: diarrhea, nausea, abdominal pain, constipation, vomiting
Hematological: agranulocytosis, thrombocytopenia
Hepatic: hepatitis, jaundice
Respiratory: bronchospasm, dyspnea

Poisoning Information

Symptoms include hypotension, bradycardia, cardiogenic shock, and asystole. CNS effects include coma, convulsions, and respiratory arrest. Treatment is symptomatic. Bradycardia may respond to atropine, isoproterenol, or glucagon.

Nadolol

Indication

Nadolol is used to treat atrial and ventricular tachyarrhythmias and hypertension.[24]

Mechanism of Action

Nadolol is a nonselective β-blocker. Nadolol has no intrinsic sympathomimetic or membrane properties.

Dosing

> **Infants/children:**
> > *Oral:* limited information is available. Initial dose, 0.5 to 1 mg/kg, once daily. Gradually increase dose to a maximum dose of 2.5 mg/kg/day
> **Adults:**
> > *Oral:* initial dose, 40 mg once daily. Increase gradually to usual dose of 40 to 80 mg/day, but may need up to 240 to 320 mg/day
> **Dose adjustment in renal impairment (adults):** If Cl_{cr} 10 to 50 mL/min, administer 50% of normal dose. If Cl_{cr} less than 10 mL/min, administer 25% of normal dose

Pharmacokinetics

Nadolol is poorly absorbed, with peak plasma levels 3 to 4 hours after administration. Nadolol has a half-life in infants of 3 to 4 hours, in children, of 7 to 15 hours, and, in adults, of 10 to 24 hours. Nadolol has an increased half-life with decreased renal function. Nadolol is moderately dialyzable.[25]

Monitoring Parameters

Monitor blood pressure and heart rate with nadolol use.

Contraindications

Uncompensated CHF, cardiogenic shock, asthma, and bradycardia or heart block are contraindications for nadolol administration.

Precautions/Warnings

Use nadolol with care in patients with heart failure, because nadolol can exacerbate CHF. Use with care in patients with reactive airway disease. Use with caution in diabetes mellitus, hypoglycemia, and renal failure. Caution should be exercised when discontinuing nadolol to avoid withdrawal.

Drug-Drug Interactions

Diuretic and phenothiazines may increase antihypertensive effects.
Nadolol may enhance the action of neuromuscular blocking agents.
Abrupt withdrawal of clonidine may result in hypertensive crisis.

Adverse Effects

CV: bradycardia, orthostatic hypotension, CHF, edema
CNS: fatigue, dizziness, depression
Dermatological: rash
GI: abdominal discomfort, diarrhea, constipation
Endocrine and metabolic: impotence
Respiratory: bronchospasm

Poisoning Information

Symptoms include hypotension, bradycardia, AV block, cardiogenic shock, and asystole. CNS effects include convulsions, coma, and respiratory arrest. Treatment is symptomatic. Bradycardia and hypotension may respond to atropine, isoproterenol, or pacing.

Class III Antiarrhythmics

Amiodarone

Indication

Amiodarone is used in a wide range of ventricular and atrial tachyarrhythmias that are unresponsive to conventional therapy with less-toxic agents.[26–30] Amiodarone is frequently used to treat postoperative junctional ectopic tachycardia.

Mechanism of Action

Amiodarone inhibits adrenergic stimulation; prolongs the action potential and refractory period of both atrial and ventricular myocardium; and decreases AV and sinus nodal function.

Dosing

Infants/children:

I.V.: 5 mg/kg administered rapid bolus for pulseless VT/ventricular fibrillation (VF); or over 20 to 60 minutes for perfusing tachycardias. May repeat for a total load of 20 mg/kg in 5 mg/kg increments. Maintenance infusion, 5 μg/kg/min, this may be increased to as high as 15 μg/kg/min

Oral: for children younger than 1 year, use body surface area to calculate dose. Loading dose, 10 to 15 mg/kg/day, or 600 to 800 mg/1.73 m²/day in two divided doses for 4 to 14 days. Dosage is then decreased to 5 mg/kg/day or 200 to 400 mg/1.73 m²/day for several weeks. Keep decreasing the dose to the lowest effective dosage possible, usually 1 to 2.5 mg/kg/day

Adults:

I.V.: for pulseless VT/VF, use 300 mg diluted in 20 to 30 mL of 5% dextrose in water (D5W) or NS administered rapid I.V. push. Supplemental bolus doses of 150 mg by rapid I.V. infusion for recurrent pulseless VT/VF may be used. Maximum total dose, 2.2 g/24 hours

Perfusing tachycardias: loading dose, 1000 mg over 24 hours as follows: 150 mg administered over 10 minutes (15 mg/min), followed by 360 mg over 6 hours (at a rate of 1 mg/min), followed with a maintenance dose of 540 mg over 18 hours (0.5 mg/min). After the first 24 hours, the maintenance dose is continued at 0.5 mg/min. Additional supplemental boluses of 150 mg over 10 to 20 minutes may be administered for breakthrough arrhythmia. Maximum daily dose, 2 g

Oral: 800 to 1600 mg/day in one to two doses for 1 to 3 weeks, then 600 to 800 mg/day in one to two doses for 1 month, gradually lower to 100 to 200 mg/day

Pharmacokinetics

Amiodarone is metabolized in the liver. The half-life in adults after an oral dose is 40 to 55 days, and after a single I.V. dose is 20 to 47 days. The half-life is shorter in children. Amiodarone is excreted in the feces and urine. Amiodarone is not dialyzable.

Monitoring Parameters

ECG, blood pressure, chest x-ray, pulmonary function tests, thyroid function tests, serum glucose, serum triglyceride, liver enzymes, and ophthalmological exams should be monitored with amiodarone use.

Contraindications

Severe sinus node dysfunction and second- or third-degree AV block (without a pacemaker) are contraindications for amiodarone use.

Precautions/Warnings

In the United States, amiodarone may not be considered as a first-line antiarrhythmic in some institutions because of its high incidence of toxicity. However, in other countries, the experience with amiodarone is more extensive and it may be considered as a first-line agent to treat various types of tachyarrhythmias. Approximately 75% of patients may experience adverse effects with large doses. Pulmonary and hepatic toxicities may be fatal. Amiodarone may cause hypothyroidism or hyperthyroidism. It may be proarrhythmic. Hypotension with rapid I.V. administration has occurred. Patients should be hospitalized for initiation of therapy and loading dose administration. Some I.V. amiodarone preparations contain benzyl alcohol, which has been associated with the potentially fatal "gasping" syndrome in neonates (metabolic acidosis, respiratory distress, gasping respirations, CNS dysfunction, hypotension, and cardiovascular collapse).

Drug-Drug Interactions

Amiodarone increases plasma concentrations of digoxin, cyclosporine, flecainide, lidocaine, methotrexate, theophylline, procainamide, quinidine, warfarin, and phenytoin. Dosing reduction and monitoring of serum levels are recommended (50% dosage reduction for digoxin, 30% reduction for flecainide, and 30–50% dosage reduction for warfarin).

Combined use with β-blockers, digoxin, or calcium channel blockers may result in bradycardia, sinus arrest, and heart block.

Amiodarone use with Class I antiarrhythmics may cause ventricular arrhythmias.

Amiodarone use with general anesthetics may result in hypotension, bradycardia, and heart block.

Combined amiodarone use with lovastatin or simvastatin may result in an increased risk of myopathy or rhabdomyolysis.

Amiodarone may inhibit the metabolism of dextromethorphan.

St. John's wort may decrease the concentration of amiodarone and is not recommended for concurrent use.

Adverse Effects

CV: proarrhythmia (including torsade de pointes), bradycardia, heart block, sinus arrest, hypotension, heart failure, and myocardial depression. Hypotension may be potentially fatal with I.V. use; in adults, I.V. daily doses greater than 2100 mg have been associated with greater risk of hypotension

Respiratory: interstitial pneumonitis, hypersensitivity pneumonitis, pulmonary fibrosis, and acute respiratory distress syndrome. Use of lower doses may be associated with lower incidence of pulmonary toxicity

CNS: lack of coordination, fatigue, malaise, dizziness, headache, insomnia, nightmares, ataxia, behavioral changes, fever

Dermatological: skin discoloration, photosensitivity, rash, pruritus

Endocrine and metabolic: hypothyroidism or hyperthyroidism, hyperglycemia, elevated triglycerides, syndrome of inappropriate antidiuretic hormone secretion

GI: nausea, vomiting, anorexia, constipation

Hepatic: elevated liver enzymes, bilirubin, serum ammonia, and severe hepatic toxicity. Hepatocellular necrosis, hepatic coma, acute renal failure, and death have been associated with I.V. loading doses of higher concentration and faster rates of infusion than recommended

Neuromuscular and skeletal: paresthesias, tremor, muscle weakness, rhabdomyolysis

GU: sterile epididymitis

Hematological: coagulation abnormalities, thrombocytopenia, neutropenia, pancytopenia, aplastic anemia, hemolytic anemia

Ocular: corneal microdeposits, halos or blurred vision, photophobia, optic neuropathy, optic neuritis

Poisoning Information

Symptoms include sinus bradycardia and/or heart block, hypotension, and QT prolongation. ECG monitoring is necessary for several days. Bradycardia may be atropine resistant.

Compatible Diluents/Administration

I.V.: maximum concentration for peripheral administration is 2 mg/mL; for central administration it is 6 mg/mL. Amiodarone is stable in polypropylene syringes at concentrations of 1 mg/mL and 2.5 mg/mL for up to 26 hours at room temperature without protection from light

Oral: do not administer with grapefruit juice

Sotalol

Indication

Sotalol is used to treat both ventricular and atrial tacharrhythmias.[30]

Mechanism of Action

Sotalol is a nonselective β-blocking agent with Class III effects (prolongation of repolarization); sotalol decreases heart rate and AV nodal conduction. Sotalol increases AV nodal refractoriness. It prolongs atrial and ventricular action potentials, and prolongs the effective refractory period of atrial and ventricular muscle. Sotalol has more Class III effect with higher doses.

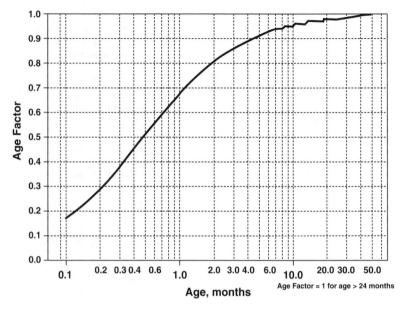

Figure 7-1. Age factor versus age in months for sotalol dosing in children younger than 2 years of age.

Dosing

Infants/children: dosing should be initiated and adjusted in the hospital secondary to possible proarrhythmia

Oral:

For those at least 2 years old, 90 mg/m²/day in three divided doses; dose may be incrementally increased to 180 mg/m²/day divided in three doses. Dose should be gradually increased

For those younger than 2 years, dose should be reduced by the age-related factor obtained from the graph in Figure 7-1. Because younger patients require more time to achieve the steady state, a greater time interval between dose adjustments is necessary

Adults: dosing should be initiated and adjusted in the hospital secondary to possible proarrhythmia

Oral: 80 mg twice a day; dose should be increased gradually to 240 to 320 mg/day. Allow 3 days between dosing increments. Usual range, 160 to 320 mg/day

Dosing in renal impairment (adults): impaired renal function can increase half-life

For treatment of ventricular tachyarrhythmias:

Cl_{cr} *greater than 60 mL/min:* administer every 12 hours

Cl_{cr} *30 to 60 mL/min:* administer every 24 hours

Cl_{cr} *10 to 30 mL/min:* administer every 36 to 48 hours

Cl_{cr} *less than 10 mL/min:* individualize dose

For treatment of atrial arrhythmias:
   Cl_{cr} *greater than 60 mL/min:* administer every 12 hours
   Cl_{cr} *40 to 60 mL/min:* administer every 24 hours
   Cl_{cr} *less than 40 mL/min:* use is contraindicated

Pharmacokinetics

Sotalol is not metabolized. The half-life in neonates is 8.4 hours; in infants/children younger than 2 years old, it is 7.4 hours; in children between 2 to 7 years old, it is 9.1 hours; in children 7 to 12 years old, it is 9.2 hours; and in adults, it is 12 hours. The time to peak concentration in children is 2 to 3 hours and, in adults, it is 2 to 4 hours. Sotalol is excreted in the urine.

Monitoring Parameters

Serum magnesium, potassium, ECG, and renal function tests should be monitored.

Contraindications

Sinus bradycardia, second- or third-degree heart block (without a pacemaker), congenital or acquired long QT syndrome, uncontrolled CHF, asthma, baseline QTc greater than 450 milliseconds, or significantly reduced renal function.

Precautions/Warnings

Initiation of sotalol in a hospital setting with continuous monitoring is required. Dosing should be adjusted gradually, and QT interval monitored. Administer cautiously in heart failure. Use caution when administering with β-blockers or calcium channel blockers. Use sotalol with caution in patients with diabetes mellitus.

Drug-Drug Interactions

Do not use sotalol with drugs that prolong the QT interval (Class I and II antiarrhythmics, phenothiazine, tricyclic antidepressants), because these increase cardiovascular effects.

Class I and II antiarrhythmics should be held for at least three half-lives before initiating sotalol use. Concomitant use of magnesium- and aluminum-containing antacids will decrease absorption of sotalol (administer antacids 2 h after sotalol).

Adverse Effects

CV: proarrhythmia, bradycardia, chest pain, palpitations, CHF, QT prolongation, torsade de pointes, hypotension, syncope[31]
CNS: fatigue, dizziness lightheadedness, confusion, insomnia, depression, mood change, anxiety, headache

Dermatological: rash
GI: diarrhea, nausea, vomiting
Endocrine and metabolic: sexual dysfunction, hyperglycemia in diabetic patients
Hematological: bleeding
Neuromuscular: weakness, paresthesias
Ocular: visual problems
Respiratory: dyspnea, asthma
Miscellaneous: cool extremities, sweating

Poisoning Information

Symptoms of sotalol poisoning include cardiac arrhythmias, CNS toxicity, bronchospasm, hypoglycemia, and hyperkalemia. Most common cardiac symptoms include hypotension and bradycardia. CNS effects include convulsions, coma, and respiratory arrest. Treatment is symptomatic.

Bretylium

Indication

Bretylium has limited applicability in pediatrics. Bretylium is indicated for resuscitation of polymorphic or monomorphic VT or VF that is resistant to standard therapy.[32]

Mechanism of Action

Bretylium causes an initial release of norepinephrine stores in sympathetic ganglia, but prevents further norepinephrine release and reuptake.

Dosing

Infants/children:
I.V.: 5 mg/kg rapid push during VF followed by electrical defibrillation; repeat with 10 mg/kg if VF persists at 15- to 30-minute intervals, to a total of 30 mg/kg. Continuous infusion at 15 to 30 µg/kg/min may be used

Adults:
I.V.: 5 mg/kg over 1 minute; if arrhythmia persists, administer 10 mg/kg over 1 minute and repeat as necessary over 15- to 30-minute intervals to a total dose of 30 to 35 mg/kg

Dosing adjustment in renal impairment: if Cl_{cr} is 10 to 50 mL/min, administer 25 to 50% of the normal dose. If Cl_{cr} is less than 10 mL/min, administer 25% of normal dose or use alternative agent

Pharmacokinetics

The onset of action of bretylium is 6 to 20 minutes, with a peak effect at 6 to 9 hours. The half-life of bretylium is 7 to 11 hours. Bretylium is eliminated in the urine.

Monitoring Parameters
ECG and blood pressure should be monitored with bretylium use.

Contraindications
Severe aortic stenosis or pulmonary hypertension are contraindications for bretylium use.

Precautions/Warnings
Hypotension secondary to decrease in peripheral resistance, which can be severe in patients with fixed cardiac output (severe aortic stenosis or pulmonary hypertension) can occur with bretylium use.

Drug-Drug Interactions
Bretylium has an increased toxicity when used with inotropic agents and digoxin. Other antiarrhythmics may potentiate or antagonize cardiac effects of bretylium.

Adverse Effects

CV: hypotension, bradycardia, flushing
GI: nausea, vomiting
CNS: vertigo, dizziness, syncope

Poisoning Information
Bretylium poisoning is indicated by significant hypertension followed by severe hypotension. Treat with supportive therapy.

Compatible Diluents/Administration
Administer bretylium as an undiluted I.V. push for life-threatening situations. Dilute bretylium to 10 mg/mL for non-life-threatening situations and push over 9 minutes. For I.V. infusion, dilute bretylium to a maximum concentration of 10 mg/mL and administer at a rate of 10 to 20 µg/kg/min. Extravasation may cause tissue necrosis.

Ibutilide

Indication
No data regarding ibutilide is available for children. Ibutilide is used in adult patients for termination of atrial fibrillation and flutter.[33]

Mechanism of Action
The mechanism of action of ibutilide is prolongation of action potential by an unknown mechanism. Ibutilide causes prolonged refractoriness in both atrial and ventricular myocardium.

Dosing

Infants/children: Unknown
Adults:
  I.V.: for patients less than 60 kg, 0.01 mg/kg over 10 minutes. For those greater than 60 kg, 1 mg over 10 minutes. If no results at end of first infusion, may repeat

Pharmacokinetics

Ibutilide has an extensive hepatic metabolism with a half-life of 6 hours. Ibutilide is eliminated in the urine and feces.

Monitoring Parameters

Continuous ECG monitoring should occur for at least 4 hours after infusion or until QTc has returned to baseline. Skilled personnel and proper equipment should be available during ibutilide administration and subsequent monitoring.

Contraindications

Prolonged QTc interval of longer than 440 milliseconds is a contraindications for ibutilide use.

Precautions/Warnings

Potentially fatal arrhythmias can occur with ibutilide administration, usually torsade de pointes. No dosing adjustment is necessary in patients with renal or hepatic dysfunction. Correct hyperkalemia and hypomagnesemia before use. Monitor for heart block.

Drug-Drug Interactions

Ibutilide should not be administered with other Class III antiarrhythmics or Class IA antiarrhythmics secondary to a potential to prolong refractoriness. Avoid other drugs that prolong the QTc (tricyclic antidepressants, phenothiazines, and erythromycin).

Adverse Effects

  CV: 8% of patients experience torsade de pointes, nonsustained VT, hypotension, complete heart block, bradycardia, hypertension, and palpitations
  CNS: headache
  GI: nausea

Poisoning Information

Symptoms of ibutilide poisoning include CNS depression, gasping breath, convulsions, and arrhythmias. Treatment is supportive.

Compatible Diluents/Administration

Ibutilide may be administered undiluted or diluted in 50 mL of diluent (0.9% NS or D5W). Infuse over 10 minutes.

Class IV Antiarrhythmics: Calcium Channel Blockers

Verapamil

Indication

Verapamil is used to treat atrial tachyarrhythmias (SVT, atrial fibrillation, and atrial flutter).

Mechanism of Action

Verapamil blocks calcium channels in vascular smooth muscle and myocardium during depolarization. Verapamil has the greatest influence on cells in the SA and AV nodes. Calcium channel blockade becomes more apparent at faster rates. Verapamil is effective in depressing enhanced automaticity.

Dosing

Infants/children:
Verapamil is not recommended for those younger than 1 year of age. Administer verapamil with continuous ECG monitoring and I.V. calcium at bedside
I.V.: 0.1 to 0.2 mg/kg per dose. May repeat in 30 minutes if no response
For children older than 1 year, 0.1 to 0.3 mg/kg/dose, maximum dose of 5 mg. May repeat in 30 minutes, if necessary
Oral: 4 to 8 mg/kg/day divided every 8 hours
Adults:
I.V.: 5 to 10 mg per dose. May repeat with 10 mg 15 to 30 minutes later, if necessary
Oral: 240 to 480 mg/24 h divided every 8 hours. For sustained release, dose every 12 hours, and, for extended release, dose every 24 hours
Dosing adjustment in renal impairment: children and adults, Cl_{cr} less than 10 mL/min, administer 50 to 75% of normal dose

Pharmacokinetics

Peak effect: oral (immediate release), 1 to 2 hours; I.V., 1 to 5 minutes
Duration: oral (immediate release), 6 to 8 hours; I.V., 10 to 20 minutes
Verapamil is metabolized in the liver with extensive first-pass effect. Verapamil has a half-life in infants of 4 to 7 hours, and, in adults, of 4 to 12 hours. Verapamil is eliminated in the urine.

Monitoring Parameters

ECG and blood pressure should be monitored with verapamil use. Measure hepatic enzymes with long-term verapamil use.

Contraindications

Sinus bradycardia, heart block, VT, severe left ventricular dysfunction, hypotension, and WPW are contraindications for verapamil use.

Precautions/Warnings

Avoid I.V. use in neonates and young infants because of the risk of cardiovascular collapse.[34] Have I.V. calcium chloride 10 mg/kg available at the beside to treat hypotension. Use verapamil with caution in patients with severe left ventricle dysfunction, sick sinus syndrome, hepatic or renal impairment, and hypertrophic cardiomyopathy. Verapamil administration may worsen myasthenia gravis and may decrease neuromuscular transmission in patients with Duchenne's muscular dystrophy.

Drug-Drug Interactions

Verapamil has increased CV effects with β-blocking agents, digoxin, quinidine, and disopyramide. Verapamil may increase serum concentrations of digoxin, quinidine cyclosporine, and carbamazepine. Phenobarbital and rifampin may decrease verapamil serum concentrations. Erythromycin may increase verapamil serum concentration. Concomitant aspirin use may prolong bleeding times. Verapamil may prolong recovery from vecuronium.

Adverse Effects

CV: severe hypotension resulting in asystole and cardiovascular collapse has been reported in infants with I.V. use. Verapamil may also may cause bradycardia, heart block, and worsening of CHF

CNS: dizziness, fatigue, seizures, headache

GI: gingival hyperplasia, constipation, nausea

Hepatic: increase in hepatic enzymes

Respiratory: may precipitate insufficiency of respiratory muscle function in Duchenne's muscular dystrophy

Poisoning Information

Symptoms of verapamil poisoning include hypotension and bradycardia. Intraventricular conduction is usually not affected. Confusion, stupor, nausea, vomiting, metabolic acidosis, and hyperglycemia may also be observed.

Impaired cardiac contractility should be treated with calcium. Glucagon and epinephrine may be used to treat hypotension.

Compatible Diluents/Administration

For I.V. push, dilute with D5W to a maximum concentration of 2.5 mg/mL and administer over 2 to 4 minutes, depending on blood pressure.

For I.V. continuous infusion, use a concentration of 0.4 mg/mL.

Diltiazem

Indication

Diltiazem is used to treat AV nodal blockade in atrial fibrillation and flutter and paroxysmal SVT.[35]

Mechanism of Action

Diltiazem blocks inward calcium channels, with effects on the SA and AV nodes.

Dosing

Infants/children:

I.V.: bolus, 0.15 to 0.45 mg/kg. Continuous infusion, 2 µg/kg/min (0.125 mg/kg/h)

Oral: 1.5 to 2 mg/kg/day divided into three to four doses; maximum, 3.5 mg/kg/day

Adults:

I.V.: initial bolus, 0.35 mg/kg over 2 minutes (average dose, 20 mg); repeat bolus after 15 minutes of 0.35 mg/kg (average dose, 25 mg). Continuous infusion, initiate infusion of 10 mg/h and increase by 5 mg/h to 15 mg/h. When increasing the infusion dose, administer for less than 24 hours at a rate of less than 15 mg/h

Conversion from I.V. to oral dosing: start oral 3 hours after bolus dose. The oral dose (mg/day) is equal to [(I.V. rate in mg/h × 3) + 3] × 10

Oral dose:

Extended release: 180 to 240 mg every day, to 180 to 420 mg/day

Sustained release: 60 to 120 mg every 12 hours, up to 240 to 360 mg/day

Pharmacokinetics

Diltiazem has an extensive first-pass effect. Diltiazem is metabolized in the liver. Diltiazem has a half-life of 3 to 4.5 hours. It is not dialyzable.

Monitoring Parameters

Liver function tests, blood pressure, and ECG should be monitored with diltiazem use.

Contraindications

Severe hypotension, second- or third-degree heart block or sinus node dysfunction, and acute myocardial infarction with pulmonary congestion are contraindications for diltiazem use.

Precautions/Warnings

Use of diltiazem with β-blockers or digoxin can result in conduction abnormalities. Use diltiazem with caution in left ventricular dysfunction. Use with caution in hepatic and renal dysfunction.

Drug-Drug Interactions

Cimetidine use may increase diltiazem serum concentrations.

The risk of bradycardia or heart block is increased with β-blocker or digoxin use.

Diltiazem may decrease metabolism of cyclosporine, carbamazepine, digoxin, lovastatin, midazolam, and quinidine.

Diltiazem use may increase the effect of digoxin and fentanyl.

Rifampin may decrease diltiazem serum concentration.

Cardiac effects of anesthetics may be potentiated by diltiazem.

Adverse Effects

CV: arrhythmia, bradycardia, hypotension, AV block, tachycardia, flushing, and peripheral edema
CNS: dizziness, headache
Dermatological: rash
GI: nausea, constipation, dyspepsia
Hepatic: elevations in liver function tests

Poisoning Information

Symptoms include hypotension (secondary to peripheral vasodilation, myocardial depression, and bradycardia) and bradycardia (secondary to sinus bradycardia, sinus arrest, or second- or third-degree heart block). Usually the QRS duration is normal.

Noncardiac symptoms include confusion, stupor, nausea, vomiting, metabolic acidosis, and hyperglycemia. Calcium may reverse depressed cardiac contractility. Glucagon and epinephrine may treat hypotension and heart rate.

Compatible Diluents/Administration

The final concentration for infusion of diltiazem should be 1 mg/mL.

Miscellaneous Drugs

Adenosine

Indication

Adenosine is indicated for termination of paroxysmal SVT (specifically AV nodal or AV reentrant tachycardia). Adenosine is useful for diagnosing atrial flutter.[36]

Mechanism of Action

Adenosine is an endogenous purinergic agent. Adenosine blocks conduction through the AV node by increasing potassium channel conductance and depressing slow inward calcium current. Adenosine also causes peripheral vasodilation.

Dosing

Infants/children:
> *I.V.:* 0.05 to 0.1 mg/kg per dose. If not effective, increase dose by 0.1 mg/kg increments to total dose of 0.3 mg/kg. ADENOSINE MUST BE ADMINISTERED RAPID I.V. PUSH

Adults:
> *I.V.:* initial dose of 6 mg. If not effective, may double to 12 mg. ADENOSINE MUST BE ADMINISTERED RAPID I.V. PUSH

Pharmacokinetics

Adenosine is metabolized by erythrocytes (cellular uptake) with a half-life of less than 10 seconds.

Monitoring Parameters

Continuous ECG, blood pressure, and respiratory rate should be monitored with adenosine use.

Contraindications

Second- or third-degree heart block or sinus node dysfunction, unless a pacemaker is in place, are contraindications for adenosine use.

Precautions/Warnings

Bronchospasm may occur with adenosine use in asthmatics. Use adenosine with caution in patients with underling SA or AV nodal dysfunction or obstructive lung disease. The initial dose of adenosine should be decreased in patients receiving dipyridamole.

Drug-Drug Interactions

Dipyridamole potentiates the effect of adenosine. Theophylline and caffeine antagonize the effect of adenosine. Carbamazepine increases heart block.

Adverse Effects

CV: flushing, arrhythmias (including atrial fibrillation, bradycardia and heart block), hypotension

CNS: lightheadedness, headache, apprehension, blurred vision

GI: nausea
Respiratory: dyspnea, bronchospasm

Poisoning Information
Adverse events are self-limited because of the short half-life of adenosine.

Compatible Diluents/Administration
Adenosine should be administered by rapid I.V. push followed immediately by a NS bolus.

Atropine

Indications
Atropine is used to treat bradycardia or asystole.[37]

Mechanism of Action
Atropine is an anticholinergic and antispasmodic. Atropine blocks acetylcholine receptors at parasympathetic sites in smooth muscle, secretory glands, and the CNS. It increases cardiac output and antagonizes histamine and serotonin.

Dosing

Infants/children:
I.V., I.O.: 0.02 mg/kg per dose, with a minimum dose of 0.1 mg. Maximum single dose, 0.5 mg in children and 1 mg in adolescents. May repeat in 5 minutes. Total dose of 1 mg for children and 2 mg for adolescents
Tracheal tube: 0.02 mg/kg per dose, with a minimum dose of 0.1 mg. Maximum single dose of 0.5 mg in children and 1 mg in adolescents. May repeat in 5 minutes. Total dose of 1 mg for children and 2 mg for adolescents. Atropine must be diluted if administered via tracheal tube; mix with NS to a total volume of 3 to 5 mL

Adults:
I.V.: 1 mg per dose. May repeat in 3 to 5 minutes. Total dose, 0.04 mg/kg
Tracheal tube: 2 to 2.5 times the usual I.V. dose. Dilute in 10 mL of NS

Pharmacokinetics
Atropine has complete absorption with a wide distribution. Atropine is metabolized in the liver. Atropine has a half-life in children younger than 2 years of 7 hours; in children older than 2 years, of 2.5 hours; and in adults, of 3 hours. Atropine is eliminated in the urine.

Monitoring Parameters

ECG, blood pressure, and mental status should be monitored with atropine use.

Contraindications

Glaucoma, thyrotoxicosis, obstructive disease of the GI or GU tract, and asthma are contraindications for atropine use.

Precautions/Warnings

Psychosis can occur with atropine use in sensitive individuals. Use atropine with caution in hyperthyroidism, CHF, tachyarrhythmias, and hypertension. Use with caution in children with spastic paralysis.

Drug-Drug Interactions

Atropine has additive effects when administered with other anticholinergic drugs. Atropine may interfere with β-blockers.

Adverse Effects

CV: arrhythmias, tachycardia, flushing
CNS: fatigue, delirium, restlessness, tremor, headache, ataxia
Dermatological: dry, hot skin, dry mucous membranes
Ocular: blurred vision, photophobia, dry eyes
GI: impaired GI motility, abdominal distension
GU: urinary retention, impotence

Poisoning Information

Indications of atropine poisoning are dilated and unreactive pupils, blurred vision, dry, hot skin and dry mucous membranes, difficulty swallowing, decreased bowel sounds, urinary retention, tachycardia, hyperthermia, and hypertension. For atropine overdose with severe life-threatening symptoms, physostigmine (0.02 mg/kg; adult dose, 1–2 mg) subcutaneously or slow I.V. may reverse effects.

Compatible Diluents/Administration

Atropine is administered undiluted by I.V. push over 1 to 2 minutes.

Magnesium Sulfate

Indications

Magnesium sulfate is used to treat torsade de pointes in acquired or congenital long QT syndrome[38] and to treat and prevent ventricular tachyarrhythmias, particularly in the postoperative course of cardiac disease.

Mechanism of Action

Magnesium sulfate suppresses early after-depolarizations that can trigger torsade de pointes.

Dosing

Infants/children:
I.V.: 25 to 50 mg/kg per dose, not to exceed 2 g/dose. Infusion rate, 0.5 to 1 mg/kg/h
Adults:
I.V.: 2 g bolus over 10 to 20 minutes. Second bolus may be administered within 5 to 15 minutes. Infusion rate, 0.5 g/h
Dosing in renal impairment: patients with severe renal failure should not receive magnesium

Pharmacokinetics

Magnesium sulfate has an immediate onset of action when administered I.V. The duration of action is 30 minutes.

Monitoring Parameters

Blood pressure and ECG should be monitored with magnesium sulfate use.

Contraindications

Heart block, serious renal impairment, and coma are contraindications for magnesium sulfate use.

Precautions/Warnings

Use magnesium sulfate with caution in patients with renal dysfunction and those receiving digoxin. Monitor serum magnesium levels. Use extreme caution in patients with myasthenia gravis.

Drug-Drug Interactions

Aminoglycosides can potentiate neuromuscular blockade. CNS depressants will increase central depressant effects.
    Use magnesium sulfate with caution with neuromuscular blocking agents.

Adverse Effects

CV: hypotension and asystole with rapid administration, flushing, complete heart block

CNS: somnolence, CNS depression
GI: diarrhea
Neuromuscular: decreased neuromuscular transmission and deep tendon reflexes
Respiratory: respiratory depression

Poisoning Information

Symptoms of magnesium sulfate poisoning usually occur with serum magnesium levels greater than 4 mEq/L. See Adverse Effects. Levels greater than 12 mEq/L may be fatal.

I.V. calcium can reverse respiratory depression or heart block.

Compatible Diluents/Administration

Magnesium sulfate is incompatible when mixed with fat emulsions, calcium gluceptate, clindamycin, dobutamine, hydrocortisone, polymyxin B, procaine hydrochloride, nafcillin, tetracyclines, and thiopental.

References

1. Kim SY, Benowitz NL. Poisoning due to class IA antiarrhythmic drugs. Quinidine, procainamide and disopyramide. Drug Saf 1990;5(6):393–420.
2. Marcus FI. Pharmacokinetic interactions between digoxin and other drugs. J Am Coll Cardiol 1985;5(5 Suppl A):82A–90A.
3. Webb CL, Dick M 2nd, Rocchini AP, et al. Quinidine syncope in children. J Am Coll Cardiol 1987;9(5):1031–1037.
4. Benson DW Jr, Dunnigan A, Green TP, Benditt DG, Schneider SP. Periodic procainamide for paroxysmal tachycardia. Circulation 1985;72(1):147–152.
5. Woosley RL, Drayer DE, Reidenberg MM, Nies AS, Carr K, Oates JA. Effect of acetylator phenotype on the rate at which procainamide induces antinuclear antibodies and the lupus syndrome. N Engl J Med 1978;298(21):1157–1159.
6. Holt DW, Walsh AC, Curry PV, Tynan M. Paediatric use of mexiletine and disopyramide. Br Med J 1979;2(6203):1476–1477.
7. Rosen MR, Hoffman BF, Wit AL. Electrophysiology and pharmacology of cardiac arrhythmias. V. Cardiac antiarrhythmic effects of lidocaine. Am Heart J 1975;89(4):526–536.
8. Moak JP, Smith RT, Garson A Jr. Mexiletine: an effective antiarrhythmic drug for treatment of ventricular arrhythmias in congenital heart disease. J Am Coll Cardiol 1987;10(4):824–829.
9. Garson A Jr, Kugler JD, Gillette PC, Simonelli A, McNamara DG. Control of late postoperative ventricular arrhythmias with phenytoin in young patients. Am J Cardiol 1980;46(2):290–294.
10. Perry JC, McQuinn RL, Smith RT Jr, Gothing C, Fredell P, Garson A Jr Flecainide acetate for resistant arrhythmias in the young: efficacy and pharmacokinetics. J Am Coll Cardiol 1989;14(1):185–191; discussion 92–93.

11. Wren C, Campbell RW. The response of paediatric arrhythmias to intravenous and oral flecainide. Br Heart J 1987;57(2):171–175.

12. Preliminary report: effect of encainide and flecainide on mortality in a randomized trial of arrhythmia suppression after myocardial infarction. The Cardiac Arrhythmia Suppression Trial (CAST) Investigators. N Engl J Med 1989;321(6):406–412.

13. Fish FA, Gillette PC, Benson DW Jr. Proarrhythmia, cardiac arrest and death in young patients receiving encainide and flecainide. The Pediatric Electrophysiology Group. J Am Coll Cardiol 1991;18(2):356–365.

14. Russell GA, Martin RP. Flecainide toxicity. Arch Dis Child 1989;64(6):860–862.

15. Janousek J, Paul T, Reimer A, Kallfelz HC. Usefulness of propafenone for supraventricular arrhythmias in infants and children. Am J Cardiol 1993;72(3):294–300.

16. Kates RE, Yee YG, Winkle RA. Metabolite cumulation during chronic propafenone dosing in arrhythmia. Clin Pharmacol Ther 1985;37(6):610–614.

17. Intravenous esmolol for the treatment of supraventricular tachyarrhythmia: results of a multicenter, baseline-controlled safety and efficacy study in 160 patients. The Esmolol Research Group. Am Heart J 1986;112(3):498–505.

18. Trippel DL, Wiest DB, Gillette PC. Cardiovascular and antiarrhythmic effects of esmolol in children. J Pediatr 1991;119(1 Pt 1):142–147.

19. Pickoff AS, Zies L, Ferrer PL, et al. High-dose propranolol therapy in the management of supraventricular tachycardia. J Pediatr 1979;94(1):144–146.

20. Trippel DL, Gillette PC. Atenolol in children with ventricular arrhythmias. Am Heart J 1990;119(6):1312–1316.

21. Trippel DL, Gillette PC. Atenolol in children with supraventricular tachycardia. Am J Cardiol 1989;64(3):233–236.

22. Buck ML, Wiest D, Gillette PC, Trippel D, Krull J, O'Neal W. Pharmacokinetics and pharmacodynamics of atenolol in children. Clin Pharmacol Ther 1989;46(6):629–633.

23. Frick MH, Luurila O. Double-blind titrated-dose comparison of metoprolol and propranolol in the treatment of angina pectoris. Ann Clin Res 1976;8(6):385–392.

24. Mehta AV, Chidambaram B. Efficacy and safety of intravenous and oral nadolol for supraventricular tachycardia in children. J Am Coll Cardiol 1992;19(3):630–635.

25. Mehta AV, Chidambaram B, Rice PJ. Pharmacokinetics of nadolol in children with supraventricular tachycardia. J Clin Pharmacol 1992;32(11):1023–1027.

26. Perry JC, Knilans TK, Marlow D, Denfield SW, Fenrich AL, Friedman RA. Intravenous amiodarone for life-threatening tachyarrhythmias in children and young adults. J Am Coll Cardiol 1993;22(1):95–98.

27. Coumel P, Fidelle J. Amiodarone in the treatment of cardiac arrhythmias in children: one hundred thirty-five cases. Am Heart J 1980;100(6 Pt 2):1063–1069.

28. Figa FH, Gow RM, Hamilton RM, Freedom RM. Clinical efficacy and safety of intravenous Amiodarone in infants and children. Am J Cardiol 1994;74(6):573–577.

29. Perry JC, Fenrich AL, Hulse JE, Triedman JK, Friedman RA, Lamberti JJ. Pediatric use of intravenous amiodarone: efficacy and safety in critically ill patients from a multicenter protocol. J Am Coll Cardiol 1996;27(5):1246–1250.

30. Maragnes P, Tipple M, Fournier A. Effectiveness of oral sotalol for treatment of pediatric arrhythmias. Am J Cardiol 1992;69(8):751–754.

31. Pfammatter JP, Paul T, Lehmann C, Kallfelz HC. Efficacy and proarrhythmia of oral sotalol in pediatric patients. J Am Coll Cardiol 1995;26(4):1002–1007.

32. Heissenbuttel RH, Bigger JT Jr. Bretylium tosylate: a newly available antiarrhythmic drug for ventricular arrhythmias. Ann Intern Med 1979;91(2):229–238.

33. Ellenbogen KA, Clemo HF, Stambler BS, Wood MA, VanderLugt JT. Efficacy of ibutilide for termination of atrial fibrillation and flutter. Am J Cardiol 1996;78(8A):42–45.

34. Epstein ML, Kiel EA, Victorica BE. Cardiac decompensation following verapamil therapy in infants with supraventricular tachycardia. Pediatrics 1985;75(4):737–740.

35. Dougherty AH, Jackman WM, Naccarelli GV, Friday KJ, Dias VC. Acute conversion of paroxysmal supraventricular tachycardia with intravenous diltiazem. IV Diltiazem Study Group. Am J Cardiol 1992;70(6):587–592.

36. Overholt ED, Rheuban KS, Gutgesell HP, Lerman BB, DiMarco JP. Usefulness of adenosine for arrhythmias in infants and children. Am J Cardiol 1988;61(4):336–340.

37. Stueven HA, Tonsfeldt DJ, Thompson BM, Whitcomb J, Kastenson E, Aprahamian C. Atropine in asystole: human studies. Ann Emerg Med 1984;13(9 Pt 2):815–817.

38. Hoshino K, Ogawa K, Hishitani T, Isobe T, Etoh Y. Successful uses of magnesium sulfate for torsades de pointes in children with long QT syndrome. Pediatr Int 2006;48(2):112–117.

8. Immunosuppressive Agents in Pediatric Heart Transplantation

Indira A. Khimji, Traci M. Kazmerski, and Steven A. Webber

All pediatric heart transplantation programs currently use a calcineurin inhibitor (CNI), either cyclosporine or tacrolimus, as a primary immunosuppressant. Although these drugs have much toxicity, there is insufficient data to show that CNI-free immunosuppression is safe or feasible from the time of transplantation. Most centers also use an additional adjunctive agent, either in the form of an antimetabolite (azathioprine [AZA] or mycophenolate mofetil) or, less commonly, a mammalian target of rapamycin (mTOR) inhibitor. The addition of these agents reduces early acute rejection events and may improve long-term graft and patient outcomes. The most controversial issue is whether corticosteroids should be routinely added to form a "triple therapy." Many pediatric transplant centers have successfully used complete steroid avoidance or early steroid withdrawal. Finally, there is no agreement on whether intravenous antibody induction therapy should be routinely used. If used, there is also no agreement regarding whether it should be in the form of a monoclonal (OKT3) or polyclonal T-cell-depleting antibody (e.g., Thymoglobulin®) or an interleukin (IL)-2 receptor (IL2R) antagonist (e.g., basiliximab or daclizumab). A summary of the options for induction and maintenance therapy is shown in Table 8-1. It should be noted that there have been no large-scale randomized controlled trials of any immunosuppressive therapy in pediatric thoracic transplantation.

Corticosteroids (Methylprednisolone and Prednisone)

Indication

Corticosteroids have broad immunosuppressive and anti-inflammatory effects. Many pediatric heart transplant centers are using steroid-avoidance regimens or early steroid withdrawal to avoid the many side effects and complications associated with long-term steroid use in children. High-dose steroids remain the standard therapy for treatment of acute rejection episodes.

Mechanism of Action

Corticosteroids decrease inflammation through the suppression of the migration of polymorphonuclear leukocytes and the reversal of increased

Table 8-1. Potential combinations of immunosuppressive drugs used in pediatric thoracic transplantation[a]

Number of agents	Potential combinations	Comments
Monotherapy	Tacrolimus or cyclosporine	Monotherapy rarely used with cyclosporine
		Monotherapy not used in lung transplantation
Dual therapy	Tacrolimus or cyclosporine *with* AZA or mycophenolate mofetil or sirolimus/everolimus or corticosteroids	Little experience with the mTOR inhibitors, sirolimus and everolimus, in children
		Steroid avoidance increasingly common in pediatric heart transplantation
Triple therapy	Tacrolimus or cyclosporine *with* corticosteroids *with* AZA or mycophenolate mofetil or sirolimus/everolimus	In triple-therapy regimens, mycophenolate mofetil is being used with increasing frequency in lieu of AZA

[a]All of the above oral maintenance regimens may be used with or without induction therapy with T cell-depleting monoclonal or polyclonal antibody preparations or with the newer IL2R antagonists.
Almost all lung transplant programs use "triple therapy."

capillary permeability. Corticosteroids prevent immune activation by inhibiting antigen presentation, cytokine production, and proliferation of lymphocytes.[1]

Dosing

Acute rejection treatment: high-dose intravenous (I.V.) methylprednisolone is the standard for most episodes of acute rejection; typical dosing is 10 mg/kg once daily for 3 days. Some centers use moderate-dose oral steroids for less severe episodes of acute rejection (e.g., 2 mg/kg).

Maintenance Therapy

Those centers that use long-term maintenance therapy typically use prednisone in doses of 0.5 to 1 mg/kg/day (maximum, 40 mg) orally in single daily dosing for the first 2 weeks after transplantation, with subsequent weaning to long-term maintenance doses of 0.05 to 0.15 mg/kg/day. Some centers continue low-dose prednisone indefinitely, whereas others wean to discontinuation in the first few months if the rejection history is benign. Increasing evidence suggests that complete steroid avoidance beyond the intraoperative period is possible in many children, especially infants.

Pharmacokinetics

The peak and duration are dependent on the route of administration of the drug.

Oral: peak effect occurs within 1 to 2 hours, and the duration is 30 to 36 hours
Intramuscular: peak effect is 4 to 8 days, and the duration is 1 to 4 weeks
Corticosteroids are metabolized in the liver to inactive glucuronide and sulfate metabolites. The half-life is 3 to 3.5 hours, and elimination is via the kidneys.[2]

Precautions/Warning

Acute adrenal insufficiency may occur with abrupt withdrawal after long-term use or with stress; withdrawal or discontinuation of corticosteroids should be performed carefully.

Monitoring Parameters

Blood pressure, weight, height, serum electrolytes, and glucose should be monitored.

Drug-Drug Interactions

Corticosteroids inhibit cytochrome P (CYP)-450 enzymes, CYP2C8 (weak) and CYP3A4 (weak), and are a substrate of CYP3A4 (minor).

Phenytoin, phenobarbital, and rifampin increase clearance of methylprednisolone; potassium-depleting diuretics (furosemide) enhance potassium depletion.

Circulating glucose levels may be increased by corticosteroids.

Permanent diabetes mellitus may be precipitated when corticosteroids are used in combination with cyclosporine or tacrolimus.

Tacrolimus levels may be increased by I.V. bolus doses of methylprednisolone.

Adverse Effects

CV: edema, hypertension
CNS: vertigo, seizures, psychoses, pseudotumor cerebri
Dermatological: Acne, skin atrophy, impaired wound healing, hirsutism
Hematological: transient leukocytosis
Endocrine and metabolic: Cushing's syndrome, pituitary-adrenal axis suppression, growth retardation, glucose intolerance, hypokalemia, alkalosis, weight gain, hyperlipidemia, salt and water retention
Ocular: cataracts, glaucoma
GI: peptic ulcer, nausea, vomiting
Neuromuscular: muscle weakness, osteoporosis, fractures

CNIs (Cyclosporine and Tacrolimus)

Cyclosporine

Indication
Cyclosporine is used in conjunction with other immunosuppressive agents to prevent organ rejection after all forms of solid organ transplantation. Cyclosporine was the most commonly used agent 5 years ago, but, currently, almost half of pediatric heart transplant recipients are receiving tacrolimus. Cyclosporine and tacrolimus have not been compared in large randomized trials in children after transplantation of thoracic organs. One small (26 children), single-center randomized trial in pediatric heart transplantation has been performed but was not powered to identify differences between immunosuppressive regimens.[3]

Mechanism of Action
Cyclosporine is a neutral cyclic polypeptide consisting of 11 amino acids. It is the major metabolic product of the fungus *Tolypocladium inflatum.*

Cyclosporine is a potent immunosuppressant that interferes with IL2 gene transcription that is essential for activation and proliferation of cytotoxic T cells. Cyclosporine crosses the T-cell membrane and binds to cyclophilin. In the presence of intracellular calcium and calmodulin, the cyclosporine-cyclophilin complex binds to an active site on calcineurin. This binding to calcineurin makes calcineurin unable to dephosphorylate nuclear factor of activated T cells (NFAT), thus, inhibiting NFAT from moving into the nucleus and binding to cytokine promoters and, ultimately, impairing cytokine production (IL2 and interferon-γ).[1]

Dosing

The oral dosage for cyclosporine is approximately three times the I.V. dosage.

> **I.V.:** initial, 3 to 5 mg/kg/day as 24-hour continuous infusion or in two divided doses; adjust dose based on serum levels; patients should be switched to oral cyclosporine as soon as possible; reduce the dose by at least 50% if any azole antifungal agent (e.g., fluconazole/itraconazole) is used concomitantly
>
> **Oral:** initial, 10 to 15 mg/kg daily usually divided in two daily doses dosing should be based on serum levels

Pharmacokinetics

Cyclosporine has incomplete and erratic oral absorption. The low absorption of cyclosporine may be caused by metabolism of cyclosporine by CYP450 enzymes in the gastrointestinal tract. The bioavailability of Sandimmune® capsules and the oral solution are equivalent, and the bioavailability of the oral solution is approximately 30% of the I.V. solution. Currently, almost all children receive microemulsion formulations, which have more predictable bioavailability. The bioavailability of Neoral® capsules and the oral solution are equivalent, 43% in children, ranging from 30 to 68%. Cyclosporine is extensively metabolized in the liver by the CYP3A4 enzyme system to at least 25 metabolites. Cyclosporine is metabolized to a lesser extent by the gastrointestinal tract and kidneys, and clearance is affected by age. Pediatric patients clear cyclosporine more rapidly than adults. The half-life of cyclosporine is 7 to 19 hours in children and 19 to 40 hours in adults. Metabolites are excreted primarily through the bile into feces; approximately 6% of cyclosporine is eliminated in the urine, with 0.1% as unchanged drug and the remainder eliminated as metabolites.[2]

Administration

Do not administer liquid cyclosporine from a plastic or Styrofoam cup. Neoral® oral solution may be diluted with orange juice or apple juice. Sandimmune® oral solution may be diluted with milk, chocolate milk, or orange juice. Avoid changing diluents frequently. Mix thoroughly and drink at once. Use the syringe provided to measure the dose. Mix cyclosporine in a glass container and rinse the container with more diluent to ensure that the total dose is taken. Do not rinse the syringe before or after use (rinsing may cause dose variation).[2]

For I.V. use, administer over 2 to 6 hours. However, many transplant centers administer cyclosporine as divided doses (2–3 doses/day) or as a 24-hour continuous infusion. Patients should be under continuous observation for at least the first 30 minutes of the infusion, and should be monitored frequently thereafter.[2]

Monitoring Parameters

Blood/serum drug concentration (trough), renal and hepatic function, serum electrolytes, lipid profile, blood pressure, and heart rate should be monitored.

Reference Range

The reference range of target serum trough concentrations depends on the time after transplantation. Typically, it is 300 ng/mL in the first few weeks, 200 ng/mL over subsequent months, and 100 to 150 ng/mL during long-term follow-up. Trough levels should be obtained 12 hours after oral dose (chronic usage), 12 hours after intermittent I.V. dose, or immediately before the next dose.[2]

When cyclosporine is administered through a single-lumen, silicone central venous catheter and blood samples for therapeutic drug monitoring are drawn through the same catheter, cyclosporine concentrations may be artificially elevated despite appropriate flushing. When central venous administration is used, peripheral venipuncture, capillary pin prick, or a double-lumen catheter should be used to draw blood samples for therapeutic drug monitoring.

Drug-Drug Interactions

Acyclovir, aminoglycosides, diclofenac, amphotericin B, erythromycin, and metoclopramide increase cyclosporine absorption.

Ketoconazole, fluconazole, erythromycin, diltiazem, verapamil, and methylprednisolone increase cyclosporine concentration by inhibiting hepatic metabolism.

Lovastatin, simvastatin, and cimetidine may increase cyclosporine concentration.

Grapefruit and grapefruit juice increase cyclosporine blood concentrations.

Phenytoin and octreotide decrease cyclosporine bioavailability.

Phenytoin, phenobarbital, carbamazepine, primidone, rifampin, trimethoprim, and nafcillin decrease cyclosporine concentration by increasing hepatic metabolism.

St. John's Wort may significantly decrease cyclosporine concentration.

Potassium-sparing diuretics may increase the risk of hyperkalemia.

Sirolimus may aggravate cyclosporine-induced renal dysfunction.

Nonsteroidal anti-inflammatory drugs (NSAIDs) may cause renal dysfunction and add to nephrotoxicity when coadministered with cyclosporine.

Prednisolone, digoxin, and lovastatin may undergo reduced clearance when used with cyclosporine.

Adverse Effects

The principal adverse reactions to cyclosporine therapy are renal dysfunction, hypertension, hyperkalemia, tremor, hyperlipidemia, and gingival hyperplasia. Nephrotoxicity occurs in the majority of patients treated long term.

CV: hypertension, tachycardia, flushing
CNS: headaches, seizure, tremor, paresthesias, insomnia
Endocrine and metabolic: hyperkalemia, hypomagnesemia, hyperuricemia
GI: abdominal discomfort, nausea, diarrhea
Miscellaneous: hepatotoxicity, hirsutism

Poisoning Information

Acute poisoning with cyclosporine is characterized by symptoms such as nausea, headaches, acute sensitivity of the skin, flushing, gum pain and bleeding, and a sensation of increased stomach size. Hypertension, nephrotoxicity, and hepatotoxicity may also occur. Forced emesis may be beneficial if performed within 2 hours of ingestion of oral cyclosporine. Treatment is symptom directed and supportive. Cyclosporine is not dialyzable.

Compatible Diluent/Administration

I.V. cyclosporine diluted in 5% dextrose in water (D5W) to a final concentration of 2 mg/mL is stable for 24 hours in polyvinyl chloride (PVC) containers; I.V. cyclosporine may bind to the plastic tubing in I.V. administration sets.

Tacrolimus

Indication

Tacrolimus is used as an alternative primary immunosuppressant to cyclosporine in all forms of solid organ transplantation in children. Tacrolimus seems to be somewhat more potent in preventing acute rejection than cyclosporine. A recent three-arm randomized trial of tacrolimus versus cyclosporine (along with corticosteroids and either sirolimus or mycophenolate mofetil as adjunctive therapy) in adult heart transplantation showed lower acute rejection rates in patients treated with tacrolimus.[4] To date, there is no definitive evidence that either tacrolimus or cyclosporine is associated with less chronic rejection, less graft loss, or improved survival in thoracic transplantation. Renal toxicity seems comparable between tacrolimus and cyclosporine in pediatric heart transplantation.[5]

Mechanism of Action

Tacrolimus is a macrolide antibiotic produced from *Streptomyces tsukubaensis*. Similar to cyclosporine, tacrolimus inhibits T-cell activation by inhibiting calcineurin. Tacrolimus binds to an intracellular protein, FK-506 binding protein (FKBP)-12, an immunophilin structurally related to cyclophilin, and a complex forms, which inhibits phosphatase activity and prevents dephosphorylation and nuclear translocation of NFAT, inhibiting T-cell activation.

Dosing

Children:

Initial, I.V. continuous infusion: 0.02 to 0.05 mg/kg/day may be used until oral intake is tolerated.[6] However, tacrolimus is now rarely used I.V., and I.V. use may lead to decreased urine output after cardiopulmonary bypass. When renal function is impaired, induction therapy with T-cell-depleting antibodies is generally used with delayed introduction of tacrolimus orally.

Oral: usually three to four times the I.V. dose, or 0.2 mg/kg/day in divided does every 12 hours

Adults:

Initial, I.V. continuous infusion: 0.01 to 0.02 mg/kg/day

Oral: 0.1 to 0.2 mg/kg/day divided every 12 hours

Pharmacokinetics

The oral bioavailability of tacrolimus ranges from 5 to 67%, with an average of 30%. Administration with meals reduces absorption by an average of 33%. Tacrolimus is metabolized in the liver by the CYP450 system (CYP3A) to eight possible metabolites. Plasma protein binding ranges from 75 to 99%. Tacrolimus has an average half-life of 8.7 hours, ranging from 4 to 40 hours. Pediatric patients clear the drug twice as rapidly as adults, and require higher doses on a milligram per kilogram basis to achieve similar blood concentrations. Tacrolimus is primarily eliminated in bile, with less than 1% excreted as unchanged drug in urine.[2]

Monitoring Parameters

Trough blood tacrolimus concentrations, liver enzymes, blood urea nitrogen (BUN), serum creatinine, glucose, potassium, magnesium, phosphorus, complete blood cell count (CBC) with differential, blood pressure, neurological status, and electrocardiogram should be monitored with tacrolimus administration.

Reference Range

The reference range for trough (whole blood enzyme-linked immunosorbent assay [ELISA]) concentrations is 5 to 15 ng/mL. Typical levels are 10 to 15 ng/mL in first few weeks after transplantation, 7 to 10 ng/mL for remainder of first year, and 5 to 7 ng/mL long after transplantation.

Drug-Drug Interactions

Diltiazem, verapamil, nifedipine, fluconazole, itraconazole, ketoconazole, cimetidine, clarithromycin, erythromycin, methylprednisolone, nefazodone, cisapride, protease inhibitors, and oral clotrimazole increase tacrolimus serum concentrations.

Antacids, cholestyramine, sodium polystyrene, sulfonate, carbamazepine, phenobarbital, primidone, phenytoin, rifabutin, rifampin, and St. John's Wort decrease tacrolimus serum concentrations.

NSAIDS, cisplatin, nephrotoxic antibiotics, amphotericin B, and cyclosporine may cause additive nephrotoxicity when administered with tacrolimus.

Tacrolimus should <u>not</u> be used in combination with cyclosporine.

Adverse Effects

Common: neurotoxicity (tremor, headache, paresthesias), hyperglycemia (glucose intolerance when used with corticosteroids)

GI: diarrhea, nausea, vomiting, constipation, dyspepsia

CV: hypertension, QT interval prolongation

Endocrine: hyperkalemia, negative effect on the pancreatic islet β cell, glucose intolerance, diabetes mellitus

Dermatological: pruritus, rash, alopecia

CNS: headache, agitation, seizures, insomnia, dizziness, hyperesthesia, dysarthria

Miscellaneous: opportunistic infections, posttransplantation lympho-proliferative disorders

Poisoning Information

Symptoms of tacrolimus overdose are extensions of immunosuppressive activity and adverse effects. Symptomatic and supportive treatment are required. Tacrolimus is not removed by hemodialysis.

Compatible Diluent/Administration

Tacrolimus is stable for 24 hours when mixed in D5W or normal saline (NS) in glass, polyolefin containers, or plastic syringes; do not store tacrolimus in PVC containers because the polyoxyl 60 hydrogenated castor oil injectable vehicle may leach phthalates from PVC containers; polyvinyl-containing administration sets adsorb drug and may lead to a lower dose being delivered to the patient; do not refrigerate oral suspensions of tacrolimus.

Antimetabolites (AZA and MMF)

Azathioprine

Indication

AZA is used as an adjunctive immunosuppressive agent for the prevention of rejection in heart transplant patients. AZA is used in combination with other agents, such as corticosteroids and CNIs, allowing for enhanced immunosuppressive efficacy while reducing organ toxicities associated with single agents used in high dosage. Most children receive some form of antimetabolite or antiproliferative agent.

Mechanism of Action

AZA is converted to 6-mercaptopurine (6-MP), which is then metabolized to ribonucleotide thioinosinic acid, which becomes incorporated into nucleic acids, causing chromosome breaks, suppression of guanine and adenine synthesis, and synthesis of fraudulent proteins. The ultimate immunosuppressive effect is inhibition of RNA and DNA synthesis, leading to decreased immune cell proliferation.[1]

Dosing

AZA is available in oral and intravenous dosage forms. AZA dosages must be carefully adjusted and individualized according to patient responses. The dosage of AZA must be adjusted in the presence of renal dysfunction and bone marrow suppression.

Oral, I.V.: initial, 2 to 3 mg/kg/dose once daily
Maintenance: 1 to 2 mg/kg/day

Pharmacokinetics

AZA undergoes extensive metabolism by hepatic xanthine oxidase to 6-MP (active), and has 50% bioavailability; the half-life of the parent is 12 minutes and of 6-MP is 0.7 to 3 hours, with anuria, the half-life of AZA increases to 50 hours. A small amount of AZA is eliminated as unchanged drug; 30% is protein bound; metabolites are eliminated eventually in the urine; and AZA crosses the placenta.[2]

Monitoring Parameters

CBC with differential, platelet count, creatinine, total bilirubin, alkaline phosphatase, and liver function should be monitored.

Drug Interactions

Concomitant therapy with angiotensin-converting enzyme (ACE) inhibitors may induce anemia and severe leukopenia. Xanthine oxidase is important in the conversion of AZA to its inactive metabolites. Because allopurinol inhibits this enzyme, dosage reduction of AZA (to 1/3 to 1/4 of normal dose) is necessary when the patient is concurrently receiving allopurinol.

Aminosalicylates (olsalazine, mesalamine, and sulfasalazine) may inhibit thiopurine methyltransferase (TPMT) metabolite, increasing toxicity/myelosuppression of AZA, therefore, caution should be used.

Effects of warfarin may be decreased by AZA use.

Adverse Effects

Hematological: bone marrow suppression, leukopenia, macrocytic anemia, thrombocytopenia. Hematological effects are dose-related. During severe toxicity, the white blood cell (WBC) count and hemoglobin levels drop first, followed by a decreasing platelet count. The WBC count will usually return to normal when the dose of AZA is decreased

GI: nausea, vomiting, anorexia, and diarrhea may occur in patients who are receiving large doses of AZA. These GI effects may be avoided by giving AZA in divided doses and/or with meals. Other GI manifestations of toxicity include ulceration of the oral mucous membranes, esophagitis, and steatorrhea

Infection: there is an increased risk of infection, as with all immunosuppressants. Fungal, protozoal, viral, and uncommon bacterial infections may occur. The risk is increased during leukopenia. When infection occurs, the dosage of AZA and other immunosuppressive agents should be reduced as much as possible and appropriate therapy for infection instituted

Miscellaneous: drug fever, rash, myopathy, pancreatitis

Poisoning Information

Signs and symptoms of AZA overdose are diarrhea, leukopenia (in 2–3 days), and vomiting. Decontamination is with ipecac within 30 minutes or lavage within 1 hour; administer activated charcoal. AZA is slightly dialyzable (5–20%).

Compatible Diluents/Administration

Reconstituted 10 mg/mL AZA injection is stable for 24 hours at room temperature; AZA is stable in neutral or acid solutions, but is hydrolyzed to mercaptopurine in alkaline solutions.

Mycophenolate Mofetil

Indication

MMF is used as an immunosuppressive agent in conjunction with a CNI with or without corticosteroids. AZA was the most commonly used adjunctive therapy throughout the 1980s and 1990s, however, in the past 5 years, its use has dramatically decreased in favor of mycophenolate mofetil.[7] A Phase III study in adults after cardiac transplantation showed a survival benefit for mycophenolate mofetil over AZA.[8]

Mechanism of Action

MMF is a prodrug that is rapidly hydrolyzed to the active drug, mycophenolic acid (MPA), a selective, noncompetitive, and reversible inhibitor of inosine monophosphate dehydrogenase (IMPDH), a critical rate-limiting enzyme in the *de novo* synthesis of the purine biosynthesis pathway. Inhibition of IMPDH results in a depletion of guanosine triphosphate and deoxyguanosine triphosphate and reduction of T- and B-cell proliferation, cytotoxic T-cell generation, and antibody production.

Dosing

Children: oral, I.V., initial, 600 mg/m^2/dose twice daily. Alternative dose, 30 to 45 mg/kg/day divided every 12 hours (some pediatric patients require every 8-h dosing because of rapid clearance). GI side effects are often less noticeable if dosing is started lower (e.g., 20 mg/kg/day divided every 12 h) and dosing is gradually increased as tolerated

Adults: oral, I.V., initial, 2000 mg/day divided twice daily; dosages as high as 3 to 3.5 g/day were used in clinical trials, but no consistent efficacy advantage could be established with the higher doses, and side effects were more common

Pharmacokinetics

MMF has rapid and extensive absorption, and the bioavailability of the active metabolite, MPA, is 94%. Mycophenolate mofetil is metabolized to MPA after oral or intravenous administration and MPA, in turn, is metabolized to the inactive MPA glucuronide (MPAG). MPAG is converted to MPA via enterohepatic recirculation. Parent drug is cleared from blood within minutes. The half-life of MPA is approximately 16 hours. Most of the drug (87%) is excreted in urine as MPAG.[2]

Monitoring Parameters

CBC with differential and platelet count should be monitored. Use of therapeutic drug monitoring remains controversial.

Drug-Drug Interactions

Antacids containing aluminum or magnesium hydroxide decrease absorption of mycophenolate.

Cholestyramine or other drugs that affect enterohepatic circulation may decrease plasma MPA concentrations via binding free MPA in the intestines.

Acyclovir and ganciclovir compete with MPAG for tubular secretion, possibly resulting in increased concentrations of MPAG and the antiviral agents in the blood.

Drugs that inhibit tubular secretion (e.g., probenecid) increase mycophenolate and MPAG concentrations.

Adverse Effects

Principal adverse effects are gastrointestinal and hematological and include leukopenia, diarrhea, and vomiting.

> **CNS:** fever, headache
> **GI:** constipation, nausea, dyspepsia, diarrhea; a delayed release tablet (Myfortic®) was designed to reduce adverse GI events by slowly delivering drug to the small intestines
> **Hematological:** neutropenia, anemia, thrombocytopenia
> **Miscellaneous:** as with other immunosuppressives, there is a possible increased risk of infection

Poisoning Information

Symptoms of mycophenolate overdose may include nausea, vomiting, diarrhea, increased incidence of infections, and unusual bleeding or bruising with mycophenolate mofetil use. Pursue symptomatic and supportive treatment.

Mammalian Target of Rapamycin

Sirolimus

Indication

Sirolimus is indicated for the prevention of organ rejection in patients receiving a CNI. Calcineurin-free regimens based around the use of high-dose mTOR inhibitors (with mycophenolate mofetil and steroids) are not routinely used in thoracic transplantation, because their ability to prevent rejection is unproven. There is little experience with these agents in the pediatric population, especially after thoracic transplantation. The most interesting aspect of the use of mTOR inhibitors is their possible role in the prevention of posttransplantation coronary artery disease.[9]

Mechanism of Action

Sirolimus inhibits T-lymphocyte activation and proliferation after the activation of IL2 and other T-cell growth factors. The drug's action requires the formation of a complex with the immunophilin, FKBP-12, which will bind to and inhibit the mammalian kinase, mTOR, a key enzyme in cell-cycle progression to the S phase. In this way, sirolimus inhibits acute rejection of allografts and prolongs graft survival.

Dosing

> **Children:** *dosing is poorly defined.* Typical starting dose, 1 mg/m²/day administered daily or as twice daily dosing (especially in infants and

young children). Subsequent dosing is adjusted to maintain sirolimus trough levels between 3 and 7 ng/mL. Doses should be taken consistently either with or without food

Adults: oral, initial dose, 2 to 5 mg/day. Subsequent dosing, adjust dose to maintain sirolimus trough levels between 3 and 7 ng/mL. Higher target levels may be used when there is a clinical indication to maintain CNI dosing at very low levels because of side effects. Data from clinical trials suggest that creatinine levels will be higher when cyclosporine is used with sirolimus than when used with mycophenolate mofetil or AZA. Careful monitoring of renal function is, therefore, required. Because of impaired wound healing, sirolimus should not be started until surgical wounds are completely healed

Pharmacokinetics

Sirolimus is absorbed rapidly and reaches a peak concentration within 1 to 3 hours. Bioavailability is approximately 14% and protein binding is approximately 92%. Sirolimus is hepatically metabolized by CYP3A4 and is transported by P-glycoprotein. Seven major metabolites of sirolimus have been identified in whole blood, as well as in the urine and feces. Some of these metabolites are active; however, sirolimus remains the major component in the immunosuppressive effect. The half-life of sirolimus is less than 24 hours in children and 62 hours in adults. The majority (91%) of sirolimus is eliminated in the feces.[2]

Monitoring Parameters

Whole blood sirolimus trough concentration, serum cholesterol and triglycerides, and serum creatinine, CBC with differential, hemoglobin, platelet count, CNI blood levels, and healing of surgical wounds should be monitored.

Reference Range

A reference range for target trough concentrations of 3 to 7 ng/mL has been used in heart transplantation. Higher levels, up to 15 ng/mL, have been used in calcineurin-sparing or avoidance regimens.

Drug-Drug Interactions

Note: although not documented, drug interactions, qualitatively, are expected to be similar to tacrolimus or cyclosporine. Sirolimus is a substrate of CYP3A4.

Cyclosporine and tacrolimus increase the maximum concentration (C_{max}) and area under the curve (AUC) of sirolimus during concurrent therapy. Clearance of these drugs may be reduced during administration of sirolimus. Inhibitors of CYP3A4 (calcium channel blockers, azole antifungal agents, macrolide antibiotics, and human immunodeficiency virus protease inhibitors) may increase sirolimus concentrations.

Inducers of CYP3A4 (rifampin, phenobarbital, carbamazepine, rifabutin, and phenytoin) are likely to decrease serum concentrations of sirolimus. Grapefruit juice may reduce the metabolism of sirolimus and should not be used during sirolimus therapy.

Adverse Effects

Common: hyperlipidemia, thrombocytopenia, mouth ulcers
CV: hypertension, peripheral edema
Hematological: anemia, neutropenia, thrombocytopenia
Endocrine: hypercholesterolemia, hypertriglyceridemia
CNS: fever, headaches, pain, insomnia, weakness, tremor
Dermatological: acne, rash, pruritus, impaired wound healing
GI: nausea, diarrhea, constipation, mouth ulceration
Renal: increased serum creatinine in combination with CNIs
Hepatic: abnormal liver function
Respiratory: noninfectious pneumonitis

Poisoning Information

Symptoms of sirolimus overdose are not known.

Polyclonal Antibodies

Thymoglobulin and Atgam

Indication

Thymoglobulin® (rabbit antithymocyte globulin) and Atgam® (equine antithymocyte globulin) are used in the treatment of steroid-resistant acute cellular rejection (ACR) in kidney and other solid organ transplant recipients and for the prevention of graft-versus-host disease in bone marrow transplant recipients. Thymoglobulin is also used for induction in the immediate post-transplantation period to prevent acute rejection.

Mechanism of Action

The mechanisms of action of Thymoglobulin® and Atgam® are elimination of T lymphocytes from the peripheral blood or altered T-cell function. The exact mechanisms of action are unknown. Polyclonal antibodies have broad antigen specificity, and bind to various cellular antigens on T lymphocytes in addition to cellular antigens on platelets, erythrocytes, and leukocytes. Complete, or nearly complete, depletion of T lymphocytes from the peripheral circulation generally occurs after two to three doses. There may also be variable depletion of T lymphocytes from peripheral lymphoid tissues.

Dosing

Thymoglobulin

> **Induction:** 1.5 mg/kg/day I.V. once daily for 5 days (range, 3–7 days)
> **Rejection:** 1.5 mg/kg/day once daily for 7 to 14 days

Atgam An intradermal skin test of Atgam is recommended before administration of the initial dose; use 0.1 mL of a 1:1000 dilution in NS; observe the skin test every 15 minutes for 1 hour; a local reaction of at least 10-mm diameter with a wheal or erythema or both should be considered a positive skin test.

> **Cardiac allograft:** 10 mg/kg/day for 7 days or as per protocol
> **Rejection prevention:** various protocols used. 15 mg/kg/day for 7 days; initial dose should be administered within 24 hours of transplantation
> **Rejection treatment:** 10 to 15 mg/kg/day for 7 to 14 days

Atgam® is currently used much less frequently than Thymoglobulin®.
Administer premedications 30 minutes before Thymoglobulin® or Atgam®; acetaminophen (10 mg/kg, orally), diphenhydramine (1 mg/kg, I.V.), and methylprednisolone (1–2 mg/kg, I.V.). With prolonged administration times (>6 h), acetaminophen and diphenhydramine can be repeated. If the first dose is well tolerated, the dose of steroid premedication is often reduced (or even eliminated) for subsequent doses.

Pharmacokinetics

Thymoglobulin peak levels occur 4 to 8 hours after I.V. doses of 1.25 to 1.5 mg/kg, with an average concentration of 22 µg/mL. Peak levels increase to an average of 87 µg/mL after 7 to 10 days of continuous dosing. Serum half-life after the first dose is approximately 44 hours and increases with subsequent doses up to 13 days. Atgam has poor distribution into lymphoid tissues; it binds to circulating lymphocytes, granulocytes, platelets, and bone marrow cells. The plasma half-life is 1.5 to 12 days; 1% of dose excreted in urine.

Monitoring Parameters

CBC with differential and platelet count, lymphocyte profile (T-cell enumeration), vital signs during administration, and renal function should be monitored.

Warnings

Anaphylaxis (symptoms can include hypotension, respiratory distress, pain in the chest, rash, and tachycardia) may occur at any time during therapy. Epinephrine and oxygen should be readily available to treat anaphylaxis.

Drug-Drug Interactions

Other drugs that suppress the immune system may increase the adverse effects of Thymoglobulin.

Adverse Effects

Infusion-related reactions, such as fever, chills, headache, and rash are adverse effects. To prevent or minimize febrile reactions, premedicate with an antipyretic, an antihistamine, and/or a corticosteroid. Some of these effects reflect a cytokine release syndrome. This is generally less severe than that observed with OKT3 (see below).

> **CV:** hypertension, tachycardia, edema
> **CNS:** seizures, fever, headache, chills, pain
> **Dermatological:** rash, pruritus, urticaria
> **GI:** abdominal pain, diarrhea, gastritis, nausea
> **Hematological:** leukopenia, thrombocytopenia, neutropenia
> **ID:** pneumonia, primary or reactivation of cytomegalovirus (CMV) infection
> **Hypersensitivity:** hypersensitivity may reflect anaphylaxis and may be indicated by hypotension and acute respiratory distress. Serum sickness reactions may also be observed

Poisoning Information

Excessive dosing for prolonged periods may increase the risk of opportunistic infection and lymphoproliferative disorders.

Compatible Diluents/Administration

> **Atgam:** dilute in half-normal NaCl or 0.9% NaCl at a maximum concentration of 4 mg/mL
> **Thymoglobulin:** use within 4 hours of reconstitution if stored at room temperature; compatible with D5W or 0.9% NaCl; Dilute dosage of Thymoglobulin in 50 to 500 mL of 0.9% NaCl injection or 5% dextrose injection

Monoclonal Antibodies

Muromonab

Indication

Muromonab is indicated for the treatment of steroid-resistant acute allograft rejection in cardiac and hepatic transplant patients.[10] A small number of centers also use muromonab for induction therapy. Overall use of muromonab has markedly declined in recent years.

Mechanism of Action

Muromonab binds to CD3, a monomorphic component of the T-cell receptor complex involved in antigen recognition, cell signaling, and proliferation. Muromonab binds to the CD3 receptor complex to activate circulating

T cells, resulting in transient cellular activation, release of cytokines, and generally very rapid T-cell depletion from the peripheral circulation. T cells that appear in the circulation are CD3 negative and are incapable of T-cell activation. Muromonab also coats the circulating T cells, subjecting them to opsonization by the reticuloendothelial system. This continued reduction in function can be defined by a lack of IL2 production and great reduction in the production of multiple cytokines. The repeat use of muromonab may be limited by a neutralizing antimouse antibody response. Acute adverse reactions related to T-cell activation and systemic cytokine release are common and have led to a reduction in popularity of this agent in favor of other antibody preparations.[8]

Dosing

Children less than 30 kg: I.V., 2.5 mg/day once daily
Children at least 30 kg and adults: I.V., 5 mg/day once daily

The period of usage is highly variable. Often 5 to 10 doses are administered. In general, muromonab is used for shorter periods for induction therapy compared with treatment of refractory rejection.

Pharmacokinetics

Muromonab reduces the number of circulating CD3-positive T cells within hours after administration. T-cell function usually returns to normal within weeks. The route of metabolism for the drug is unclear; it may be removed by opsonization by the reticuloendothelial system when bound to T lymphocytes or by human antimurine antibody production (approximately 85% of patients treated with muromonab develop these antibodies).[11]

Administration

Note: children and adults, premedication with acetaminophen, diphenhydramine, and methylprednisolone sodium succinate at 2 mg/kg I.V. administered 2 hours before the first muromonab administration is strongly recommended to decrease the incidence of reactions to the first one or two doses; patient temperature should not exceed 37.8°C (100°F) at the time of administration. Before administration, assess the patient's volume status. There should be no clinical evidence of volume overload, uncontrolled hypertension, or uncompensated heart failure.

Monitoring Parameters

Chest x-ray, weight gain, CBC with differential, BUN and creatinine, vital signs (blood pressure, temperature, pulse, respiration), and T-cell counts should be monitored.

Drug-Drug Interactions

Other immunosuppressant drugs may lead to increased immunosuppression when used with muromonab. Consider reducing the dose of other agents. Echinacea administration is not advised during muromonab therapy. Indomethacin may cause encephalopathy and other CNS effects when used with muromonab.

Warnings

Cytokine release syndrome is attributed to the release of cytokines by activated/lysed lymphocytes. This release of cytokines stimulates the production of leukotrienes, prostaglandins, and endoperoxides contributing to fever, decreased cardiac contractility and hypotension, coronary vasospasm, increased pulmonary capillary permeability, and alterations in bronchial and GI smooth muscle control.[1] Clinical manifestations of the cytokine release syndrome (see below) typically appear within 1 hour after the first few doses and may persist for several hours. The severity and frequency of the cytokine release syndrome diminishes with each successive dose. Increasing the amount of muromonab or resuming treatment after a hiatus may result in reappearance of the cytokine release syndrome.

Adverse Effects

A major side effect of anti-CD3 therapy is cytokine release syndrome, which includes the clinical manifestations of high fever, chills/rigor, headache, tremor, nausea and vomiting, diarrhea, abdominal pain, malaise, muscle/joint aches and pains, respiratory distress, pulmonary edema, and generalized weakness.

CV: tachycardia, hypertension, hypotension, peripheral cyanosis, pulmonary edema
Dermatological: pruritus, rash
CNS: aseptic meningitis, headache, seizure, encephalopathy
Renal: increased BUN and creatinine
Respiratory: dyspnea, pulmonary edema, wheezing
Miscellaneous: flu-like symptoms, anaphylactic-type reactions; a high rate of "rebound" rejection has been witnessed after cessation of muromonab treatment[12]

Poisoning Information

Overdose with muromonab is commonly characterized by hyperthermia, myalgia, severe chills, diarrhea, vomiting, edema, oliguria, pulmonary edema, and acute renal failure. Neurotoxicity induced by muromonab is commonly seen through aseptic meningitis, however, some cases have reported the manifestation of a neurological syndrome characterized by akinetic mutism, blepharospasm, anomic aphasia, and delirium.[13]

Alemtuzumab

Indication
Alemtuzumab is primarily used in the treatment of B-cell chronic lymphocytic leukemia. Alemtuzumab is used as induction therapy in a small number of solid organ transplant programs. However, there is minimal use of alemtuzumab in pediatrics at this time.

Mechanism of Action
Alemtuzumab binds to CD52, a nonmodulating antigen present on the surface of B and T lymphocytes as well as a majority of monocytes, macrophages, and natural killer cells. After binding to CD52-positive cells, antibody-dependent lysis occurs.[2]

Dosing
I.V. infusions of 30 mg/dose for one to two doses (before transplantation with or without a second dose on Day 1 after transplantation) have been used in adult solid organ transplantation. No dosing requirements have been established for pediatric usage.

Pharmacokinetics
Clearance decreases with repeated dosing, because of loss of CD52 receptors in the periphery; this results in a seven-fold increase in the AUC. The elimination half-life is initially 11 hours and increases to 6 days after repeat doses.[14]

Monitoring Parameters
Vital signs should be monitored, carefully monitor blood pressure, especially in patients with ischemic heart disease or on antihypertensive medications; CBC and platelets should be monitored weekly; signs and symptoms of infection should be monitored; and T-lymphocyte counts should be monitored after treatment until recovery. Patients should be monitored closely for infusion reactions (including hypotension, rigors, fever, shortness of breath, bronchospasm, chills, and/or rash).

Drug-Drug Interactions
Allergic reactions may be increased in patients who have received diagnostic or therapeutic monoclonal antibodies because of the presence of human antichimeric antibody (HACA).

Administration of live vaccines should be avoided in immunosuppressive therapy.

Adverse Effects

Infusion-related adverse events are common, rigors, hypotension, drug-related fever, nausea, vomiting, rash, fatigue, urticaria, dyspnea, pruritus, headache, and diarrhea. To prevent or ameliorate infusion-related events, antihistamine, acetaminophen, meperidine, corticosteroids, and antiemetics, as well as incremental dose escalation may be used.

CV: hypotension, peripheral edema
CNS: fever, fatigue, headache, dysthesias, dizziness
Dermatological: rash, urticaria, pruritus
GI: nausea, vomiting, anorexia, diarrhea, stomatitis/mucositis, abdominal pain
Hematological: neutropenia, anemia
Neuromuscular and skeletal: rigors, skeletal muscle pain, weakness, myalgia
Respiratory: dyspnea, cough, bronchitis/pneumonitis, pneumonia, pharyngitis
Miscellaneous: infection (incidence may be reduced with prophylactic regimens), diaphoresis, sepsis

Warning

The US Food and Drug Administration (FDA) has posted an "Alert for Health-care Professionals" concerning the use of alemtuzumab. Development of severe (fatal in one case) idiopathic thrombocytopenic purpura (ITP) has occurred in a clinical study of alemtuzumab (Campath®) for multiple sclerosis. The labeling for alemtuzumab contains boxed warnings describing serious hematological toxicities, including autoimmune ITP, pancytopenia, marrow hypoplasia, and autoimmune hemolytic anemia.[14]

Poisoning Information

Overdose symptoms of alemtuzumab are likely to be extensions of adverse events and may include hematological toxicity, respiratory distress, bronchospasm, or anuria. Cumulative doses greater than 90 mg/wk have been associated with pancytopenia and severe (and occasionally fatal) ITP. Treatment is symptom directed and supportive.[2]

Antibodies to IL2R (Basiliximab and Daclizumab)

Basiliximab

Indication

Basiliximab is used for prophylaxis of acute organ rejection. Experience with basiliximab in heart transplantation is limited. In a cohort study in children, two doses of basiliximab were associated with low acute rejection rates despite intentional subtherapeutic dosing of CNIs in the immediate posttransplantation period.[15]

Mechanism of Action

Basiliximab is chimeric (murine/human) monoclonal antibody that blocks the α-chain of the IL2R complex; this specific high-affinity binding to IL2R competitively inhibits IL2-mediated activation of lymphocytes, a critical pathway in the cellular immune response involved in allograft rejection.

Dosing

In pediatric patients weighing less than 35 kg, the recommended regimen is two I.V. doses of 10 mg each. In pediatric patients weighing at least 35 kg, the recommended regimen is two I.V. doses of 20 mg each. The first dose should be administered within 2 hours before transplantation surgery. The recommended second dose should be administered 4 days after transplantation. The second dose should be withheld if complications, such as severe hypersensitivity reactions to basiliximab, occur.

Each dose should be infused over 20 minutes via a peripheral or a central line.

Pharmacokinetics

The pharmacokinetics of basiliximab are: mean duration, 36 days (determined by IL2R α saturation); and elimination half-life in children 1 to 11 years old, 9.5 days; adolescents 12 to 16 years, 9.1 days; and adults, 7.2 days.

Drug Interactions

No dose adjustment is necessary when basiliximab is added to triple-immunosuppression regimens including cyclosporine, corticosteroids, and either AZA or mycophenolate mofetil.

Vaccine (dead organism): basiliximab may decrease the effect of vaccines
Vaccine (live organism): basiliximab may increase the risk of vaccinial infection

Adverse Effects

GI: abdominal pain, vomiting
CV: hypertension, edema
CNS: headache, tremor, insomnia, pain, fever
Hematological: anemia
Renal: dysuria
Respiratory: dyspnea, upper respiratory tract infection
Dermatological: surgical wound complications, acne

Warning

Severe acute hypersensitivity reactions including anaphylaxis have been observed with initial and reexposure doses. These reactions may include hypotension, tachycardia, cardiac failure, dyspnea, wheezing, bronchospasm, pulmonary edema, respiratory failure, urticaria, rash, pruritus, and/or sneezing. If a severe hypersensitivity reaction occurs, therapy with basiliximab should be permanently discontinued. Medications for the treatment of severe hypersensitivity reactions including anaphylaxis should be available for immediate use.[16]

Poisoning Information
Monoclonal antibodies: allergic reactions may be increased in patients who have received diagnostic or therapeutic monoclonal antibodies because of the presence of HACA.[2]

Compatible Diluents/Administration
Basiliximab is diluted in 25 to 50 mL 0.9% NaCl or D5W and infused over 20 to 30 minutes via a peripheral or central line.

Daclizumab

Indication
Daclizumab is used as induction therapy in conjunction with CNIs and other adjunctive agents to prevent rejection in organ transplant recipients. In a large analysis of adult heart transplant recipients (Scientific Registry of Transplant Recipients), daclizumab was shown to decrease acute rejection (compared with no induction) without increased mortality or infectious mortality.[17] In a recent study of pediatric and adult cardiac recipients, daclizumab seemed as efficacious as muromonab as induction therapy (compared with historical controls) but with lower complication rates.[18]

Mechanism of Action
Daclizumab is a humanized IgG_1 monoclonal antibody produced by recombinant DNA technology that binds specifically to the α-subunit of the human high-affinity IL2R (CD25) on the surface of activated lymphocytes. This action inhibits IL2 binding, thereby blocking IL2-mediated activation of lymphocytes involved in allograft rejection.[19]

Dosing

Children and adults: I.V., initial dose, 1 mg/kg/dose administered no more than 24 hours before transplantation, followed by 1 mg/kg/dose administered every 14 days for a total of five doses; maximum dose, 100 mg

Pharmacokinetics

Serum levels of daclizumab have been shown to be somewhat lower in pediatric transplant patients than in adult transplant patients. The half-life of the drug is 20 days for adults and 13 days for children.

Monitoring Parameters

CBC with differential, vital signs, immunological monitoring of T cells, renal function, and serum glucose should be monitored.

Drug-Drug Interactions

Other immunosuppressant drugs may lead to increased immunosuppression when used with daclizumab. Consider reducing the dose of other agents.

Echinacea administration is not advised during daclizumab therapy because it has been found to antagonize the immunosuppressive effect of the drug.

Adverse Effects

CV: hypotension, tachycardia
CNS: headache, fever, chills, tremors
GI: rash, nausea, diarrhea, vomiting, abdominal pain
Dermatological: pruritus
Neuromuscular: arthralgia, myalgia, back pain, diaphoresis
Miscellaneous: increased susceptibility to infection. Increased risk for developing lymphoproliferative disorders has not been established

Poisoning Information

If an overdose is suspected, follow laboratory parameters, including serum creatinine, BUN, serum uric acid tests, and CBC.

Compatible Diluents/Administration

Dilute daclizumab in 50 mL of 0.9% NaCl solution; in fluid-restricted patients, the maximum concentration is 1 mg/mL; administer over 15 minutes in a peripheral or central line.

References

1. Smith SL. Immunosuppressive therapies on organ transplantation. *Organ Transplant* 2002. C 2002 Medscape. http://www.medscape.com/viewarticle/437182.
2. Taketomo CK, Hodding JH, Kraus DM. Pediatric Dosage Handbook, 13th edition. Lexicomp, 2006–2007.

3. Pollock-Barziv SM, Dipchand AI, McCrindle BW, Nalli N, West LJ. Randomized clinical trail of tacrolimus- vs cyclosporine-based immunosuppression in pediatric heart transplantation: preliminary results at 15-month follow-up. *J Heart Lung Transplant* 2005; 24:190–194.

4. Kobashigawa J, Miller LW, Russell SD, et al. Tacrolimus with mycophenolate mofetil (MMF) or sirolimus vs. cyclosporine with MMF in cardiac transplant patients: 1-year report. *Am J Transplant* 2006; 6:1377–1386.

5. English RF, Pophal SA, Bacanu S, Fricker FJ, Boyle GJ, Miller SA, Law Y, Ellis D, Harker K, Sutton R, Pigula F, Webber SA. Long-term comparison of tacrolimus and cyclosporine induced nephrotoxicity in pediatric heart transplant recipients. *Am J Transplant* 2002; 2:769–773.

6. Robinson BV, Boyle GJ, Miller SA, Law Y, Griffith BP, Webber SA. Optimal dosing of intravenous tacrolimus following pediatric heart transplantation. *J Heart Lung Transplant* 1999; 18:786–791.

7. Boucek MM, Edwards LB, Keck BM, Trulock EP, Taylor DO, Hertz MI. Registry of the International Society for Heart and Lung Transplantation: eighth official pediatric report—2005. *J Heart Lung Transplant* 2005; 24:968–982.

8. Eisen HJ, Kobashigawa J, Keogh A, et al. Three-year results of a randomized, double-blind, controlled trial of mycophenolate mofetil versus azathioprine in cardiac transplant recipients. *J Heart Lung Transplant* 2005; 24:517–525.

9. Webber SA, McCurry K, Zeevi A. Heart and lung transplantation in children. *Lancet* 2006; 368: 53–69.

10. Ortho Biotech Products, L.P. Orthoclone OKT3® Package Insert. November 2004.

11. Hooks M, Wade C, Millikan WJ. Muromonab CD-3: a review of its pharmacology, pharmacokinetics, and clinical use in transplantation. *Pharmacotherapy* 1991; 11(1): 26–37.

12. Wilde M, Goa K. Muromonab CD3: a reappraisal of its pharmacology and use as prophylaxis of solid organ transplant rejection. *Drugs* 1996; 51(5): 865–894.

13. Pittock S, Rabinstein A, Edwards B, Wijdicks E. OKT3 neurotoxicity presenting as akinetic mutism. *Transplantation* 2003; 75(7):1058–1060.

14. Genzyme Corporation. Campath® Package Insert. July 2005.

15. Ford KA, Cale CM, Rees PG, Elliott MJ, Burch M. Initial data on basiliximab in critically ill children undergoing heart transplantation. *J Heart Lung Transplant* 2005; 24:1284–1288.

16. Smith J, Nemeth T, McDonald R. Current immunosuppressive agents: efficacy, side effects, and utilization. *Pediatr Clin N Am* 2003; 50:1283–1300.

17. Kobashigawa J, David K, Morris J, et al. Daclizumab is associated with decreased rejection and no increased mortality in cardiac transplant patients receiving MMF, cyclosporine, and corticosteroids. *Transplant Proc* 2005; 37:1333–1339.

18. Chin C, Pittson S, Luikart H, et al. Induction therapy for pediatric and adult heart transplantation: comparison between OKT3 and daclizumab. *Transplantation* 2005; 80:477–481.

19. Hoffman-La Roche Inc. Zenapax® Package Insert. September 2005.

9. Extracorporeal Membrane Oxygenation and Drug Clearance

Peter D. Wearden, Victor O. Morell, and Ricardo Munoz

The prolonged use of extracorporeal membrane oxygenation (ECMO) in the pediatric, and particularly neonatal, population to support patients for days to weeks has become increasingly commonplace over the past two decades. Along with little advancement in the underlying technology, there has been a relative paucity of research into the effects of ECMO on drug metabolism and elimination in children. By its very nature, ECMO is used in the most critically ill children, those who are often already receiving maximal pharmacological support with multiple vasoactive agents to improve their circulation. High doses of sedatives and muscle relaxants are common adjuncts to the management of the child on ECMO. The increased risk of infection requires the use of prophylactic or therapeutic antibiotics, and diuretics are frequently used to maintain fluid balance. Unlike most patients in the intensive care unit (ICU) setting, the successful use of ECMO generally requires full anticoagulation with heparin. This chapter reviews the general ways in which ECMO may affect drug clearance, and summarizes specific information regarding selected drugs that are used frequently in clinical practice.

The half-life of a drug is affected by both its volume of distribution and its clearance. Drug clearance and the volume of distribution can be affected by a number of different mechanisms; these same mechanisms may be fundamentally altered during ECMO support. The volume of distribution relates the total amount of drug in the body to the concentration of the drug in blood or plasma. The volume of distribution is affected by the pKa of the drug, the degree to which the drug binds to plasma or tissue proteins, and how lipophilic or hydrophobic (partition coefficient) the drug is, among other properties. ECMO alters the apparent volume of distribution of drugs in a number of fashions. The most obvious of these is the degree to which the ECMO circuit changes the extracellular volume. With ECMO circuit priming volumes traditionally between 200 and 400 mL, the circulating blood volume of an infant (80–85 mL/kg) can be doubled acutely. The magnitude of this effect exerts a much greater influence on a drug with a small volume of distribution than on a drug with a greater volume of distribution. The dilutional effect of the prime is often exacerbated by the ongoing intravenous (I.V.) fluid requirements of a critically ill child because of hypovolemia from bleeding or the systemic inflammatory response. Bleeding complications often necessitate multiple transfusions of red blood cells, platelets, and plasma. Loss of fluid from the intravascular compartment requires repeated I.V. fluid boluses to maintain adequate levels of circuit flow (Vrancken, 2005).[1] A 30% increase in the body weight of infants with respiratory failure placed on ECMO has been noted. Using the sodium bromide and deuterium oxide technique, the increase was attributed to expansion of the extracellular fluid volume and total body water (Anderson, 1992).[2] The degree to which ECMO itself expands the intracellular and extracellular fluid compartments is debatable, and the increase is more likely related to the underlying disease process than to ECMO per se (Kazzi, 1990).[3] These effects are only exacerbated by the additional increase in volume and loss of existing drug during ECMO circuit changes.

Conversely, the prime and multiple transfusions also dilute plasma proteins, resulting in decreased drug binding, increased free concentration of drug, and an apparent decreased volume of distribution. The increased fraction of free drug is, however, more likely to result in redistribution to the tissues, which may increase the apparent volume of distribution. Additional effects on plasma proteins include binding of protein by heparin and potential denaturation of proteins passing through the membrane oxygenator. More importantly, however, the chemical constructs [polyvinyl chloride (PVC) and silicone] of the pump tubing and oxygenator may also bind the drug, resulting in an increased volume of distribution. This effect may change over time as these binding sites become saturated with proteins. Oxygenators, because of their large surface areas, may in particular affect drug levels and apparent volume of distribution. Silicone oxygenators have been demonstrated to have a higher affinity for more lipophilic drugs (Rosen, 1990).[4] Dagan et al. examined preoxygenator and postoxygenator concentrations of several drugs in an in vitro model. These investigators used both new circuits and circuits that had been used to support patients. When examining drug loss in the new ECMO circuits, a significant decrease in the concentration of drugs was seen after flow through the oxygenator. Phenytoin decreased by 43%, vancomycin and morphine by 36%, phenobarbital by 17%, and gentamicin by 10%. In circuits that had been used in a patient for 5 days, the loss was significantly less; the decreases were morphine, 16%; vancomycin, 11%; and phenobarbital, 6%. These findings suggested saturation of binding sites over several days in circuits used to support patients (Dagan, 1993).[5] In a separate but similar study examining sedatives, even more significant drug loss was observed. Using a circuit with distilled water instead of blood (which would decrease plasma or blood binding and magnify loss to the circuit), diazepam concentrations decreased by 88%, midazolam by 68%, and lorazepam by 40%. Propofol, because of its highly lipophilic nature, decreased by 98%. Pretreatment with albumin magnified the loss of drug to PVC tubing, but significantly reduced uptake by a silicon oxygenator. Only lorazepam was observed at expected concentrations. The presence of the drugs in the tubing and membrane was demonstrated by high-performance liquid chromatography (HPLC), but the authors did not examine the possible liberation of drug back into the patient (Mulla, 2000).[6] These findings suggest that one must also be cognizant of the different effects that can occur when the drug is administered directly into the circuit versus into the patient. When drugs are administered directly to the circuit, different effects may be observed whether the drug is administered before or after the oxygenator, as well as with the type of oxygenator used. The partition coefficient has been demonstrated to be of particular importance in determining the amount of drug lost to the circuit (Mulla, 2000).[6]

There may also be incomplete mixing of drug in the circuit. Silicone venous reservoirs or bladders are often used as a safety measure. When there is inadequate return of blood, such as occurs with kinking of circuit tubing or hypovolemia, an alarm sounds and the pump shuts down to avoid intraining air. The venous reservoir is then subject to low and more laminar flow. It has been demonstrated that dye injected distal to the reservoir in the ECMO circuit mixes completely in 10 minutes. Drug injected proximal to the reservoir did not mix thoroughly. In the same study, flow rates less than 250 mL/min were associated with pooling in the system (Hoie, 1993).[7]

The clearance, or rate of elimination, of a drug is also affected during ECMO. Similar to the volume of distribution, the clearance of a drug can be affected by the degree to which ECMO impacts bound or unbound drug levels. Drugs generally are cleared as a result of processes in the liver and kidneys, but drugs may also be cleared by the lungs and other organs. Clearance is intimately related to the amount of drug presented to these organs, i.e., the blood flow to each organ, the volume of distribution, and the bound and unbound fractions of the drug. ECMO can result in altered end organ perfusion, most prominently by a lack of pulsatility in venoarterial ECMO. The lack of pulsatile flow may result in an increase in systemic vascular resistance, decreased capillary flow, and decreased lymphatic flow (Shevde, 1987[8]; Mavroudis, 1978[9]). The renal response is altered in the absence of pulsatility, resulting in decreased function and activation of the renin-angiotensin system. Decreases in hepatic blood flow may also affect drug metabolism (Hynynen, 1989[10]; Bartlett, 1990[11]). Decreased capillary flow and decreased flow to skeletal muscles, adipose tissue, bone, and skin, as well as the liver and kidneys, will decrease the volume of distribution and clearance and alter the half-life. There also may be alterations in end organ perfusion related to the underlying disease state. If induced hypothermia is used for cerebral protection while on ECMO, there will be even more pronounced alterations in perfusion and enzymatic function. In venoarterial ECMO, only bronchial flow is delivered to the lungs; this profoundly alters drug binding or elimination of drugs that are distributed or metabolized by the lungs (Bentley, 1983).[12] Importantly, the kidneys, liver, and other organs frequently have suffered an insult before the initiation of ECMO, and such an insult may affect their intrinsic ability to clear drug.

Thus, the concentration and half-life of drugs administered to patients on ECMO can be significantly different than when the same drugs are administered to a patient not receiving ECMO support. The following is a discussion of the current, albeit limited, knowledge of these effects for specific drugs.

Heparin

Heparin is likely the most commonly used and monitored (indirectly via activated clotting time [ACT]) drug during ECMO support, as most centers use this agent for the requisite anticoagulation. Despite its nearly universal use and frequent monitoring, bleeding and thrombosis remain frequent and significant complications of ECMO support. Green et al. studied heparin clearance in infants on ECMO and after decannulation. Up to 50% of the heparin administered seemed to be eliminated by the circuit. They further observed that the clearance of heparin was 3.8 ± 1.9 L/kg/min while on ECMO. After decannulation, heparin clearance decreased to 1.6 ± 0.5 m/kg/min. Clearance in an isolated circuit was 2.1 ± 0.8 m/kg/min. When comparing circuits before and after decannulation, more than half of the loss of heparin was related to the circuit itself. The authors speculated that heparin was being bound or destroyed by the circuit or that the prolonged exposure to the circuit resulted in it being bound or destroyed by blood products (Green, 1990).[13]

Gentamicin

Although gentamicin is now less commonly used, the effects of ECMO on its pharmacokinetics have been studied extensively. In 1989, Southgate et al., in the first prospective study, determined that the half-life of gentamicin was roughly doubled with ECMO; they recommended initiating therapy with an 18-hour dosing regimen and determining subsequent dosing by measuring gentamicin levels (Southgate, 1989).[14] Others observed an increased volume of distribution and decreased rate of clearance on ECMO when compared with the same children after the cessation of ECMO (Cohen, 1990[15]; Dodge, 1994[16]). A retrospective study confirmed the findings of an increased volume of distribution and decreased half-life (Bhatt-Metta, 1992[17]). Interestingly, one group was not able to demonstrate any impact of ECMO on the pharmacokinetics of gentamicin (Munzenberger, 1991[18]). Based on the above studies, Buck suggests an empirical regimen of 2.5 to 3 mg/kg every 18 to 24 hours to achieve peak serum concentrations of 5 to 10 mg/mL and trough concentrations of 0.5 to 1.0 mg/mL (Buck, 2003[19]).

Vancomycin

With the increase in multidrug resistant gram-positive organisms, vancomycin use has increased in neonatal and pediatric ICUs and in ECMO patients. Hoie et al. found an increased volume of distribution of vancomycin in patients receiving ECMO, and, although the authors had difficulty identifying appropriate controls, they anticipated a prolonged elimination (Hoie, 1990[20]). Amaker et al. observed an even more pronounced alteration in the volume of distribution and half-life of vancomycin and recommended 24-hour dosing in patients on ECMO (Amaker, 1996[21]). A retrospective study of 15 ECMO patients compared with controls did not find a statistically increased volume of distribution or rate of clearance, although there were trends in that direction. The authors did observe a prolonged half-life and elimination rate constant when compared with controls (Buck, 1998[22]). In an examination of 45 patients on ECMO ranging in age from neonates to adults, Mulla and Pooboni observed a significantly decreased clearance and increased volume of distribution. When compared with critically ill non-ECMO patients of similar age, their findings suggested an altered disposition of vancomycin on ECMO (Mulla, 2005[23]). Based on the above findings, a suggested dosing regimen for infants would be 15 to 20 mg/kg every 18 to 24 hours (Buck, 2003[19]). Trough levels should be monitored during the course of therapy.

Diuretics

Despite the frequent need for diuretics in the ECMO patient, and particularly in preparation for weaning, only a single study has examined the affects of ECMO on diuretics. Wells et al. found an increased volume of distribution, decreased plasma and renal clearance, and increased half-life for bumetanide in 11 neonates on ECMO when compared to term and preterm infants. Interestingly, they also found considerable interpatient variability, and they estimated nonrenal clearance to be 47 to 97% higher than expected. They speculated that this could be related to drug loss in the circuit (Wells, 1992[24]). Similar findings with regard to adsorption by the circuit were observed in for furosemide in in vitro circuits. An analysis of furosemide administered to four ECMO circuits observed a 63 to 87% reduction over a 4-hour period (Scala, 1996[25]).

Ranitidine

Wells also examined the effects of ECMO on ranitidine. Like the other drugs, the volume of distribution was increased, clearance decreased, and the plasma half-life nearly doubled when compared with controls (Wells, 1998[26]).

Nitroglycerin

Nitroglycerin, which is well known to be adsorbed by plastics, has been demonstrated to have significant adsorption in the ECMO circuit (Dasta, 1983[27]).

Amrinone and Milrinone

Twenty percent of an initial Amrinone dose was taken up by the circuit. Milrinone seemed to be less bound, as would be expected, because it is less lipid soluble and protein bound and has a greater volume of distribution (Williams, 1995[28]; Bailey, 1994[29]).

Neuromuscular-Blocking Agents

Neuromuscular blocking agents tend to have small volumes of distribution and are, therefore, subject to a significant decrease in their concentrations at the initiation of ECMO support. They may also, however, be subject to decreased clearance and alterations in distribution (Bogaert WA, 1989[30]; Weekes, 1995[31]).

Morphine

Increased requirements for narcotics on ECMO, particularly morphine and fentanyl, are well described (Caron, 1990[32]; Arnold, 1990[33]; Arnold, 1991[34]; Burda, 1999[35]; Franck, 1998[36]). The reasons for this increased requirement are somewhat unclear. Physiological tolerance and dependence are common in this population because of their length of treatment and need to maintain high levels of sedation. As discussed earlier, it is also known that there is some loss of drug in the circuit. One group observed a 20 to 40% loss of morphine over 6 hours in an in vitro circuit, with the loss being in the PVC tubing (Bhatt-Mehta, 2005[37]). Dagan observed that the clearance of morphine on ECMO was 0.574 ± 0.3 L/kg/h, and that it increased to 1.058 ± 0.727 L/kg/h after the cessation of support. The authors hypothesized that this change was related both to a decrease in hepatic blood flow and a decrease in pulmonary metabolism while on ECMO. This rapid increase in clearance after decannulation may play a role in opioid withdrawal (Dagan, 1994[38]).

Fentanyl

There is even greater sequestration of fentanyl by the ECMO circuit than morphine, with approximately 70% of an I.V. dose lost in the first passage through the circuit. The primary site of sequestration is the membrane oxygenator, and the binding seems to be irreversible (Rosen, 1986[39]; Koren, 1984[40]; Hynynen, 1987[41]). In an in vivo study, Leuschen found no correlation between the plasma levels and the infusion rate of fentanyl or the time spent on ECMO (Leuschen, 1993[42]). Arnold recorded steadily increasing plasma fentanyl concentrations in neonates on ECMO and a 57% rate of neonatal abstinence syndrome (NAS) in these same patients. ECMO duration was the greatest predictor of the development of NAS (Arnold, 1990[33]). The increasing concentrations with time would be observed if circuit _binding sites became saturated. There was, however, no plateau in the need for increasing infusion rates.

Lorazepam

Lorazepam, an agent commonly used for sedation in this patient population, was demonstrated to have 30 to 50% lower concentrations at 3 hours in an in vitro circuit. This loss had a plateau at 3 hours, and based on their study design, the authors of one study speculated that the majority of the loss took place in the PVC tubing (Bhatt-Mehta, 2005[37]).

Midazolam

Rosen suggested that circuit binding of midazolam was so great that it was not possible to sedate a child on ECMO with midazolam (Rosen 1991[43]). Mulla has extensively studied the effects of ECMO on midazolam pharmacokinetics. In 20 ECMO patients, he observed the need for significantly greater dosing when the drug was administered to the circuit rather than directly to the patient. Drug levels were significantly below expected for the first 24 hours, but by 48 hours, they exceeded the expected concentration. A prolonged plasma half-life was also found. His findings suggested an increased volume of distribution and circuit sequestration in the first 24 hours. However, by 48 hours, dosing could be reduced because of an increased half-life, probably because of reversible circuit binding. The authors further suggested that midazolam be administered directly to the patient rather than to the circuit (Mulla, 2003a[44]; Mulla, 2003b[45]).

Propofol

Propofol is highly lipophilic and protein bound. Propofol levels can fall to 45% of their expected level after the initiation of cardiopulmonary bypass, and to 37% after 10 minutes. In an in vitro preparation, 75 to 98% of the drug was bound by the circuit (Hynynen, 1994[46]; Mulla, 2000[6]).

Phenobarbital

Phenobarbital, which is used to treat seizures, has also been studied. A retrospective chart review of 20 neonates found that the doses required to maintain acceptable serum concentrations were twice those needed for neonates not being treated with ECMO (Marx, 1991[47]). The same group examined levels in vitro, and, although they found that up to half of a phenobarbital dose could be adsorbed (47–90%) by the ECMO tubing, this process was very variable. As noted earlier, Dagan observed a 17% loss of phenobarbital in an in vitro circuit (Dagan, 1994[38]). As with many of the other drugs, there is a greater apparent volume of distribution with variable clearance (Elliot, 1999[48]).

Conclusions

ECMO can potentially have a myriad of effects on the clearance of drugs in the pediatric population. Universally, the volume of distribution is increased. The magnitude of this effect depends on the size of the child, the size of the ECMO prime, and the volume of distribution for the drug in a patient not on ECMO. Drugs with small volumes of distribution are more greatly affected than those with large volumes of distribution. Generally, drug clearance seems to be decreased in children receiving ECMO support. This process is most likely multifactorial and related to alterations in end organ function caused by the underlying illness, as well as to changes in organ perfusion associated with ECMO support. The increased volume of distribution and decreased clearance results in prolonged drug half-life. The most variable effect of ECMO on drug action is the degree to which the circuit and oxygenator bind the agent. This seems to be greatest for drugs with a high partition coefficient (i.e., more lipophilic). These alterations in drug pharmacokinetics are clearly most acute when the circuit is new, and they diminish over time. Therefore, increased drug dosing may be necessary earlier in an ECMO run compared with a later time. The binding process may be irreversible or reversible and may contribute to drug tachyphylaxis, dependency, and prolonged action after discontinuation. The clinician should be aware that all of these effects on the volume of distribution and clearance are magnified at initiation and discontinuation of the ECMO run or during circuit changes. Frequent monitoring of drug levels and therapeutic effects are recommended to ensure proper dosing in the child receiving ECMO support.

References

1. Vrancken SL, Heijst, AF, Zegers M, et al. Influence of volume replacement with colloids versus crystalloids in neonates on venoarterial extracorporeal membrane oxygenation on fluid retention, fluid balance, and ECMO runtime. ASAIO J 2005; 51: 808–812.

2. Anderson HL, Coran AG, Drongowski RA, et al. Extracellular fluid and total body water changes in neonates undergoing extracorporeal membrane oxygenation. J Pediatr Surg 1992; 27: 1003–1008.

3. Kazzi NJ, Schwartz CA, Palder SB, et al. Effect of extracorporeal membrane oxygenation on body water content and distribution in lambs. ASAIO Transactions 1990; 36: 817–820.

4. Rosen DA, Rosen KR, Leong P. Uptake of lorazepam and midazolam by the Scimed membrane oxygenator. Anesthesiology 1990; 73: A474.

5. Dagan O, Klein J, Greunwald C, et al. Preliminary studies of the effects of extracorporeal membrane oxygenator on the disposition of common pediatric drugs. Ther Drug Monit 1993; 15: 233–236.

6. Mulla H, Lawson G, von Anrep C, et al. In vitro evaluation of sedative drug losses during extracorporeal membrane oxygenation. Perfusion 2000; 15: 21–26.

7. Hoie EB, Hall MC, Schaff LJ. Effects of injection site and flow rate on the distribution of injected solutions in an extracorporeal membrane oxygenation circuit. Am J Hosp Pharm 1993; 50: 1902–1906.

8. Shevde, K, DuBois WJ. Pro: pulsatile flow is preferable to nonpulsatile flow during cardiopulmonary bypass. J Cardiothorac Anesth 1987; 1: 165–168.

9. Mavroudis C: To pulse or not to pulse. Ann Thorac Surg 1978, 25: 259–271.

10. Hynynen M, Olkkola KT, Naveri E, et al. Thiopentone pharmacokinetics during cardiopulmonary bypass with a nonpulsatile or pulsatile flow. Acta Anaesthesiol Scand 1989; 33:554–560.

11. Bartlett RH. Extracorporeal life support for cardiopulmonary failure. Curr Prob Surg 1990; 27: 621–705.

12. Bentley JB, Conahan TJ III, Cork RC. Fentanyl sequestration in the lungs during cardiopulmonary bypass. Clin Pharmacol Ther 1983; 34: 703–706.

13. Green PT, Isham-Schopf B, Irmiter JR, et al. Inactivation of heparin during extracorporeal circulation in infants. Clin Pharmacol Ther 1990; 48: 148–153.

14. Southgate WM, DiPiro JT, Robertson AF. Pharmacokinetics of gentamicin in neonates on extracorporeal membrane oxygenation. Antimicrob Agents Chemother 1989; 33: 817–819.

15. Cohen P, Collart L, Prober CG, et al. Gentamicin pharmacokinetics in neonates undergoing extracorporeal membrane oxygenation. Pediatr Infect Dis J 1990; 9: 562–566.

16. Dodge WF, Jeliffe RW, Zwichenberger JB, et al. Population pharmacokinetic models: effect of explicit versus assumed constant serum concentration assay error patterns upon parameter values of gentamicin in infants on and off extracorporeal membrane oxygenation. Ther Drug Monit 1994; 16:552–559.

17. Bhatt-Metta V, Johnson CE, Schumacher RE. Gentamicin pharmacokinetics in term neonates receiving extracorporeal membrane oxygenation. Pharmacotherapy 1992; 12: 28–32.

18. Munzenberger PJ, Massoud N. Pharmacokinetics of gentamicin in neonatal patients supported with extracorporeal membrane oxygenation. ASAIO Transactions 1991; 37: 16–18.

19. Buck ML. Pharmacokinetic changes during extracorporeal membrane oxygenation: implications for drug therapy in neonates. Clin Pharmacokinet 2003; 42: 403–417.

20. Hoie EB, Swigart SA, Leuschen MP, et al. Vancomycin pharmacokinetics in patients undergoing extracorporeal membrane oxygenation. Clin Pharm 1990; 9: 711–715.

21. Amaker RD, DiPiro JT, Bhatia J. Pharmacokinetics in critically ill infants undergoing extracorporeal membrane oxygenation. Antimicrob Agents Chemother 1996; 40: 1139–1142.

22. Buck ML. Vancomycin pharmacokinetics in neonates receiving extracorporeal membrane oxygenation. Pharmacotherapy 1998; 18: 1082–1086.

23. Mulla H, Pooboni S. Population pharmacokinetics of vancomycin in patients receiving extracorporeal membrane oxygenation. Br J Clin Pharmacol 2005; 60: 265–275.

24. Wells TG, Fasules JW, Taylor BJ, et al. Pharmacokinetics and pharmacodynamics of bumetanide in neonates treated with extracorporeal membrane oxygenation. J Pediatr 1992; 121: 974–980.

25. Scala JL, Jew RK, Poon CY, et al. In vitro analysis of furosemide disposition during extracorporeal membrane oxygenation (ECMO) [abstract]. Pediatr Res 1996; 39: 78A.

26. Wells TG, Heulitt M, Taylor BJ, et al. Pharmacokinetics and pharmacodynamics of ranitidine in neonates treated with extracorporeal membrane oxygenation. J Clin Pharmacol 1998; 38: 402–407.

27. Dasta JF, Jacobi J, Wu LS, et al. Loss of nitroglycerin in the cardiopulmonary bypass apparatus. Crit Care Med 1983; 11: 50–52.

28. Williams GD, Sorensen GK, Oakes R, et al. Amrinone loading during cardiopulmonary bypass in neonates, infants and children. J Cardiothorac Vasc Anesth 1995; 9: 278–282.

29. Bailey JM, Levy JH, Kikura M, et al. Pharmacokinetics of intravenous milrinone in patients undergoing cardiac surgery. Anesthesiology 1994; 81: 616–622.

30. Bogaert WA, Herregods LL, Mortierr EP. Cardiopulmonary bypass and pharmacokinetics of drugs. Clin Pharmacokinet 1989; 17: 10–26.

31. Weekes LM, Keneally JP, Goonetillek PH, Ramzan IM. Pharmacokinetics of alcuronium in children with acyanotic and cyanotic cardiac disease undergoing cardiopulmonary bypass surgery. Paediatr Anaesth 1995; 5: 369–374.

32. Caron E, Maguire DP. Current management of pain, sedation and narcotic physical dependency of the infant on ECMO. J Perinat Neonatal Nurs 1990; 4: 63–74.

33. Arnold JH, Truog RD, Orav EJ, et al. Tolerance and dependence in neonates sedated with fentanyl during extracorporeal membrane oxygenation. Anesthesiology 1990; 73: 1136–1140.

34. Arnold JH, Truog RD, Scavone JM, et al. Changes in pharmacodynamic response to fentanyl in neonates during continuous infusion. J Pediatr 1991; 119: 639–643.

35. Burda G, Trittenwein G. Issues of pharmacology in pediatric cardiac extracorporeal membrane oxygenation with special reference to analgesia and sedation. Artif Organs 1999; 23: 1015–1019.

36. Franck LS, Vilardi J, Durand D, et al. Opioid withdrawal in neonates after continuous infusions of morphine or fentanyl during extracorporeal membrane oxygenation. Am J Crit Care 1998; 7: 364–369.

37. Bhatt-Mehta V, Annich G. Sedative clearance during extracorporeal membrane oxygenation. Perfusion, 2005; 20: 309–315.

38. Dagan O, Klein J, Bohn D, et al. Effects of extracorporeal membrane oxygenation on morphine pharmacokinetics in infants. Crit Care Med 1994; 22: 1099–1101.

39. Rosen DA, Rosen KR. A comparison of fentanyl uptake by three different membrane oxygenators. Anesthesiology 1986; 65: A128.

40. Koren G, Crean P, Klein J, et al. Sequestration of fentanyl by the cardiopulmonary bypass. Eur J Clin Pharmacol 1984; 27: 51–56.

41. Hynynen M. Binding of fentanyl and alfentanil to the extracorporeal circuit. Acta Anaesthesiol Scand 1987; 31: 706–710.

42. Leuschen MP, Willett LD, Hoie EB, et al. Plasma fentanyl levels in infants undergoing extracorporeal membrane oxygenation. J Thorac Cardiovasc Surg 1993; 105: 885–891.

43. Rosen DA, Rosen KR. Midazolam for sedation in the pediatric intensive care unit. Intens Care Med 1991; 17: S15–19.

44. Mulla H, Lawson G, Peek GJ, et al. Plasma concentrations of midazolam in neonates receiving extracorporeal membrane oxygenation. ASAIO J 2003; 49: 41–47.

45. Mulla H, McCormack P, Lawson G, et al. Pharmacokinetics of midazolam in neonates undergoing extracorporeal membrane oxygenation. Anesthesiology 2003; 99: 275–282.

46. Hynynen M, Hammaren E, Rosenberg PH. Propofol sequestration within the extracorporeal circuit. Can J Anaesth 1994; 41: 583–588.

47. Marx C, et al. Investigation of increased phenobarbital dose requirement for newborn infants on ECMO. In vitro adsorption in ECMO circuit. Pharmacotherapy 1991; 11: 270.

48. Elliot ES, Buck ML. Phenobarbital dosing and pharmacokinetics in a neonate receiving extracorporeal membrane oxygenation. Ann Pharmacother, 1999; 33: 419–422.

10. Pharmacological Treatment of Pulmonary Hypertension

Mary P. Mullen and David L. Wessel

Pathophysiology of Pulmonary Hypertension

Elevated pulmonary arterial pressure arises from three well-characterized vascular changes: vasoconstriction, thrombus formation, or proliferation of smooth muscle and/or endothelial cells in the pulmonary vessels.[1] Thus, pulmonary hypertension is associated with conditions causing chronic vasoconstriction, thrombosis, or abnormalities of vessel function.

Recent advances in molecular biology have allowed for the identification of several key mediators of vascular function in the pulmonary vasculature. This, in turn, has enabled development of specific pharmacological therapies for the disease.

Arachidonic acid metabolites, such as prostacyclin and thromboxane A_2, are active in the pulmonary vessels, associated with vasodilation and vasoconstriction, respectively. In addition, prostacyclin is a platelet inhibitor and is capable of inhibiting endothelial cell proliferation, whereas thromboxane A_2 is a platelet activator. Endothelin-1 is a vasoconstrictor that causes smooth-muscle proliferation in pulmonary vessels.[2] Nitric oxide (NO), produced by endothelial cells, induces vasodilation through a cyclic guanosine monophosphate (cGMP)-dependent pathway[3,4] and additionally inhibits platelet function and smooth vessel proliferation.

Clinical studies of adults and children with idiopathic pulmonary arterial hypertension (PAH) suggest imbalances in these potent vasoactive factors, as well as in other vasoactive compounds, such as vascular endothelial cell growth factor, adrenomedullin, serotonin, and vasoactive peptides, in patients with pulmonary hypertension. With great consistency, patients with pulmonary hypertension have been found to have altered homeostatic balances of these factors, tending toward prothrombotic, vasoconstrictive physiology. These clinical findings suggest that acquired alterations in normal vascular physiology contribute to the onset of pulmonary hypertension.

Other conditions that contribute to chronic changes in the pulmonary vasculature include hypoxemia and small vessel thrombosis. Chronic hypoxemia contributes to pulmonary vasoconstriction. Thrombotic events in the microvasculature contribute to hypoxia and also release acute mediators that contribute to vasoconstriction.

The pathological vascular changes associated with pulmonary hypertension and congenital heart disease (CHD) were described by Heath and Edwards in patients with pulmonary hypertension secondary to septal defects.[5] Classic initial changes (Heath and Edwards Grade 1 and 2) include medial hypertrophy, smooth muscle extension into nonmuscular arteries, and intimal cell proliferation from smooth muscle thickening. Progressive changes include intimal fibrosis, and eventual thinning of the media with dilation of the vessels (Grade 3 and 4). Eventually, medial fibrosis and necrotizing arteritis (Grade 5 and 6) changes arise in the pulmonary vessels.

Children with many forms of CHD are prone to develop pulmonary hypertension over time. Some of the important factors that contribute to elevation in pulmonary vascular resistance (PVR) in CHD include pulmonary artery pressure and flow, left atrial pressure, length of exposure to these adverse hemodynamic forces associated with increased shear and stress, and the extent of pulmonary vascular and especially endothelial damage. Longstanding exposures to high flow and pressure in the pulmonary circulation are associated with gradual reduction in endothelial function.[6] The ensuing microvascular and ultrastructural changes bear striking similarities to idiopathic forms of PAH.[7] Overproduction of vasoconstrictors and mitogens and reduced levels of local vasodilators are associated with pulmonary vascular pathology in CHD, just as they are with adult forms of PAH.[8-10] Undoubtedly, genetic predisposition affects the vulnerability of a patient with any given heart disease over another patient with the same disease to develop refractory pulmonary hypertension.[11]

These observations suggest that the pathophysiology of pulmonary hypertension is governed by alterations in the normal function of vascular tone, hemostatic activity, and vascular cell biology. Imbalances between vasodilators/vasoconstrictors, platelet activation/inhibition, and endothelial and smooth muscle cell proliferation/inhibition conspire to cause chronic pathological changes in pulmonary vessels and worsening clinical symptoms (Figure 10-1). Importantly, these contributing factors to the pathophysiology of pulmonary hypertension also serve as emerging targets for treatment. Strategies that reverse these underlying contributors to pulmonary hypertension seem able to improve clinical function in patients. We will review drug therapies for treatment of acute pulmonary hypertension, usually associated with CHD and conclude with available therapies for chronic idiopathic PAH.

Drug Therapy for Inpatient Treatment of Acute Pulmonary Hypertension in CHD

Perioperative elevation in PVR may complicate the postoperative course, when transient myocardial dysfunction requires optimal control of right ventricular afterload.[12] Assessment and treatment of pulmonary hypertension among patients with heart disease can be life saving (Tables 10-1 and 10-2). Historically, the incidence of true postoperative pulmonary hypertensive crises in patients who were judged preoperatively to be at risk for these events was high, probably greater than 50%.[13] The challenge to improve care and treatment of these patients at that time was highlighted by the postmortem observation in these patients that the microscopic findings in the lung vasculature

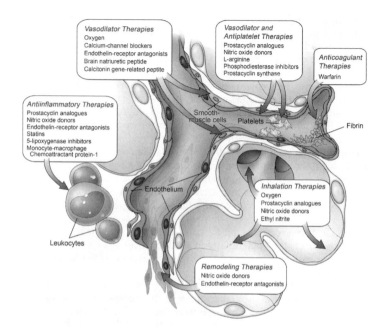

Figure 10-1. Pathophysiological factors and therapeutic targets in pulmonary hypertension. (*Source:* adapted from Farber and Loscalzo, 2004.)

Table 10-1. Vasodilators by class

Drug class	Advantages	Disadvantages
Nitrates	Easily titratable, rapid onset and offset	1. Nonspecific 2. Tachycardia 3. Tachyphylaxis 4. Cyanide toxicity
α antagonists	Powerful, dense blockade, blocks sympathetic vasolability	1. Nonspecific 2. Very long duration of action 3. Serious systemic hypotension
ACE inhibitors	Orally active, facilitates myocardial remodeling	1. Little effect on pulmonary circulation
Calcium channel blockers	Orally active, best defined role in patients with idiopathic pulmonary hypertension who respond to acute testing	1. Myocardial depression 2. Raises end diastolic pressure 3. Bradycardia 4. Sudden death 5. Hypotension in infants
Prostaglandins	Good afterload reduction, increase cardiac output, some pulmonary selectivity, titratable, long-term benefit	1. Intravenous forms produce systemic hypotension 2. Increases intrapulmonary shunt 3. Value in acute illness unproven

Table 10-1. (continued)

Drug class	Advantages	Disadvantages
	for remodeling, antiplatelet and cytoprotective effect. Aerosolized forms are selective and potent and efficacious in adult PAH	4. Long-term administration 5. Requires central vascular access 6. Expensive for long-term intravenous use 7. Aerosolized delivery systems not well established, with frequent administration required
Endothelin receptor blockers	Effective for disease states with high endothelin levels, may be tailored to have some pulmonary specificity	1. Oral agents improve status of adults with idiopathic PAH 2. Minimal experience in critically ill patients on mechanical ventilation 3. Slow onset of effect 4. Potential for hepatic toxicity 5. Intravenous forms more suitable for postoperative setting but not yet approved for use in humans
β agonists	Increases cardiac output, titratable	1. Nonspecific 2. Tachycardia 3. Increases myocardial oxygen demand 4. Maldistribution of cardiac output 5. Arrhythmogenic
Phosphodiesterase inhibitors type III	Increases contractile function, reduces afterload, lowers filling pressures, acts synergistically with catecholamines, not arrhythmogenic	1. Nonspecific 2. Hypotension at high doses for refractory pulmonary hypertension 3. Slightly long duration of action (1–3 h)
Phosphodiesterase inhibitors type V	Orally active, act synergistically with inhaled NO to raise cGMP, attenuate withdrawal response to NO, may have use as single-agent pulmonary vasodilator, may have additive effects with prostacyclin analogs	1. Improves status of adults with idiopathic PAH 2. May be a nonspecific vasodilator 3. Longer-acting oral forms under development 4. Concomitant nitrate therapy contraindicated (hypotension) 5. No intravenous preparation approved
Inhaled NO	Selective potent pulmonary vasodilator, rapid onset, improves intrapulmonary shunt, no myocardial depression, may have benefit from selected long-term applications	1. Methemoglobin 2. Nitrogen dioxide 3. Complex delivery compared with oral medication 4. Rebound effects 5. Short acting 6. Expensive

Table 10-2. Common therapeutic agents for pediatric patients with pulmonary hypertension

Agent	Mechanism of action	Dose/therapeutic range	Side effects
Oxygen	Vasodilator	Titrate to provide symptom relief, reduce hypoxemia	
Warfarin	Anticoagulant	Standard prophylaxis: INR 1.5 to 2	Bleeding
		Patients prone to trauma, such as toddlers: INR < 1.5	
		Patients with known hypercoagulable state: INR 2.5 to 3.5	
Digoxin	Positive inotrope; antiarrhythmic	8 to 10 μg/kg daily or divided twice daily, depending on age for management of right heart failure	Dysrhythmia
Diuretics	Through diuretic action, heart size, filling pressure, and lung water are reduced	Titrate to manage volume status in patients with right heart failure	Hypotension; electrolyte disturbance
Nifedipine	Calcium channel blocker acts as vasodilator	Titrated dose based on decrease in pulmonary pressures with maintenance of cardiac output and pulmonary wedge pressure	Hypotension, hemodynamic compromise
Inhaled NO	Increases CCOPM in smooth muscle	Titrated to effect 5–20 ppm, may do short-term testing at 80 ppm	Rebound hypertension with cessation of prolonged therapy; methemoglobinemia; nitrogen dioxide
Sildenafil	Phosphodiesterase V inhibitor	0.35–0.5 mg/kg thrice daily	Headache, flushing, nasal congestion
Bosentan	Endothelin receptor antagonist	1–2 mg/kg twice daily oral dose for 4 wk then 2–4 mg/kg twice daily	Transaminase elevations/hepatic toxicity, flushing, syncope, teratogen, anemia
Prostacyclin	Vasodilator via cAMP and inhibitor of platelet aggregation	Intravenous, epoprostenol or treprostinil 1–2 ng/kg/min, and increase as tolerated Inhaled iloprost, 2.5 μg over 10 minutes through mouthpiece 6–8 times/d	Headache, diarrhea, jaw pain, leg pain, rash, nausea, flushing, syncope, catheter complications (intravenous)

were rarely indicative of irreversible disease. Treatment has advanced considerably since that era. Improvements in cardiopulmonary bypass (CPB) and the inflammatory response to surgery, combined with earlier age at operation and development of focused postoperative therapies have all served to markedly reduce the incidence of postoperative pulmonary hypertension and mortality associated with this condition. Lindberg et al. estimated that, between 1994 to 1998, 2% of children operated on for CHD had severe postoperative pulmonary hypertension; this was higher (14%) after correction of atrioventricular septal defect repair.[14] Even in the recent era, morbidity associated with postoperative elevation in PVR occurs frequently and prompts us to further refine our treatments.[15]

Inhaled NO

Mechanism of Action

In 1980, Furchgott and Zawadski[16] reported the obligatory role of the endothelium in acetylcholine-induced vasodilation and proposed the existence of an endothelium-derived relaxing factor, now accepted to be NO.[3,17] NO formed from L-arginine and molecular oxygen in a reaction catalyzed by NO synthase induces vasodilation through a cGMP-dependent pathway.[18] Because NO exists as a gas, it can be delivered by inhalation to the alveoli to the blood vessels that lie in close proximity to ventilated lung.

Because of its short half-life and rapid inactivation by hemoglobin, inhaled NO achieves selective pulmonary vasodilation when pulmonary vasoconstriction exists,[19–23] whether secondary to endothelial dysfunction or as a result of abundance of vasoconstricting influences. Inhalational NO may achieve better oxygenation when administered in the presence of ventilation perfusion mismatch.[24–28] It has advantages over intravenously administered vasodilators, which cause systemic hypotension and increase intrapulmonary shunting.

The effectiveness of inhaled NO as a pulmonary vasodilator, together with the diminished response to the endothelium-dependent vasodilator acetylcholine, in patients in whom endothelial injury is associated with the disease state[20,22,24] raises the question whether a deficiency of endogenously released NO is responsible for the elevation in pulmonary vascular tone. NO is thought to be released continuously under basal conditions and inhibition of basal release may lead to an increase in systemic vascular resistance.[29] The perfusion of isolated human lungs with methylene blue, an inhibitor of NO-mediated vessel relaxation, leads to an increase in PVR.[30] Thus, endothelial damage with a reduction in endogenous NO could account for pulmonary vasoconstriction. Inhaled NO has been used as a probe to test the effect of CPB on pulmonary endothelial function.[22] CPB may result in damage to the pulmonary endothelium,[31,32] and the degree of pulmonary hypertension is correlated to the extent of such damage.[33] Moreover, measurement of exhaled NO suggests transient reduction in endogenous production of NO as a result of CPB.[34] Inhaled NO can, therefore, be used to selectively manipulate the pulmonary vasculature after endothelial injury[35] and represents an important advance in pharmacological strategies aimed at treatment of the diseased or abnormally reactive pulmonary circulation.

Relaxation at both precapillary and postcapillary levels by inhaled NO has been demonstrated in animal models of pulmonary hypertension.[36–39] Rimar and Gillis demonstrated that inhaled NO affected primarily arterial vessels but, under extreme venous constriction, could dilate at the postcapillary level as well.[40] In adults with acute lung injury, Benzing has shown that NO has a predominant vasodilating effect on the pulmonary venous vasculature.[41] The increased responsiveness seen in pediatric patients with pulmonary venous hypertension to NO may result from pulmonary vasorelaxation at a combination of precapillary and postcapillary vessels.[20] It does seem that inhaled NO, unlike intravenous NO donors, is limited in action to small resistance arteries and veins, and is unable to dilate larger capacity vessels, likely as a factor of rapid inactivation by hemoglobin.[37]

Pulmonary vascular endothelial dysfunction contributes to post-CPB pulmonary hypertension.[22] Pulmonary hypertensive crises are dramatic events that threaten the life of an infant despite a good surgical repair.[13,42,43] In such situations, the pulmonary artery pressure rises to systemic or suprasystemic levels, the systemic blood pressure falls, and the transcutaneously monitored arterial oxygen saturation decreases. In an early report of a series from one large center, half of the postoperative cardiac children who had pulmonary hypertensive crises died during their hospitalization.[13] Journois et al. have shown dramatic response to inhaled NO among patients demonstrating severe pulmonary hypertensive crises.[44] In more recent work, they have reasoned that use of inhaled NO is an independent predictor of improved survival in postoperative patients with atrioventricular defects who were at risk for having serious postoperative pulmonary hypertension.[45] Others concur that inhaled NO improves outcomes of the postoperative child with CHD.[46] Many single-center trials support this contention, but it has been difficult to design and execute placebo-controlled multicenter trials to test efficacy in CHD given the unusual manner in which inhaled NO became standard-of-care treatment for postoperative pulmonary hypertension. Inhaled NO selectively lowers pulmonary artery pressure after CPB compared with controls, reduces time on mechanical ventilation in a randomized trial of patients at risk for developing postoperative pulmonary hypertension, and also reduces need for extracorporeal membrane oxygenation (ECMO) in pivotal placebo-controlled, blinded trials in newborns with persistent pulmonary hypertension. Clinicians and investigators are reluctant to join a placebo-controlled trial for this drug. Consequently, there is a paucity of randomized controlled trials to demonstrate efficacy of the drug and establish evidence-based practice for its use.[47]

Dosage of Inhaled NO

Measurements of NO and NO_2 currently are made at or near the airway. The alveolar concentration of NO or NO_2 after therapeutic inhalation is unknown. NO uptake by bronchial epithelium and lung fluid may affect final alveolar concentrations and may vary with disease. Because these effects are still not clarified, establishment of lowest effective dosage therapy is indeed more important to minimize possible toxicities.

Animal work using experimental models of pulmonary hypertension and preliminary adult human investigations yield conflicting results with greatly varying conclusions regarding the dose of NO required to produced either a threshold response or 50% of maximal reduction in pulmonary artery pressure.[19,27,28,48–52] Both animal and human studies have begun to suggest that there is a dose-response relationship regarding maximal pulmonary vasodilation up to doses of 80 ppm or more.[23,48,53–55] Optimal dosing of inhaled NO that will maximize pulmonary vascular relaxation without incurring toxic side effects, systemic hypotension, or deleterious effects on venous admixture is unclear.

Maximal pulmonary vasodilator response to inhaled NO may occur at higher doses than that which produce optimal ventilation perfusion matching in patients with elevated pulmonary artery pressure and severe pulmonary parenchymal disease.[56] By redistributing pulmonary blood flow away from underventilated alveoli toward normally ventilated areas of lung, inhaled NO in very low concentrations (<1 ppm) may improve intrapulmonary shunt fraction and raise PaO_2. It has been suggested that this effect may be optimized at doses of inhaled NO that are low (1–10 ppm) even though maximal pulmonary vasodilation occurred in the same patients at higher NO doses (10–100 ppm) among 12 adult patients with acute respiratory distress syndrome (ARDS).[50] Improved oxygenation was lost at the higher NO doses in these patients, where pulmonary vasodilation was maximized. Presumably, this occurred from a "spillover" effect of NO into poorly ventilated lung, with loss of preferential delivery to and vasodilation of better-ventilated areas. No data are available for childhood diseases comparing the NO-induced dose-response changes in oxygenation simultaneously with changes in PVR. This is especially important in the critically ill population of children with acute severe pulmonary parenchymal disease that complicates their pulmonary hypertensive CHD, in whom, dose response may be quite variable.[52,57] Day recently reported no difference between outcome variables in pediatric patients with severe lung disease between 11 and 60 ppm. Although we have seen a continued dose-response relationship in pulmonary artery pressure up to 80 ppm on NO among patients with CHD, Demirakca et al. studied 17 neonatal and pediatric patients with ARDS and determined that the best effective dose was 10 ppm in pediatric patients and 20 ppm in neonatal patients with ARDS plus persistent pulmonary hypertension of the neonate (PPHN).[58] Thus, the desirable dose may depend in part on the severity of the pulmonary artery hypertension versus the severity of intrapulmonary shunting from lung disease.

Toxicity of Inhaled NO

At the relatively low levels of NO used therapeutically (1–80 ppm), the metabolic fate of inhaled NO is an accumulation of nitrate and nitrite in plasma, a small increase in methemoglobin but little detectable nitrosylhemoglobin.[59] Possible toxicities of inhaled NO include methemoglobinemia caused by the intravascular binding to hemoglobin,[60] cytotoxic effects in the lung caused by either free radical formation, development of excess nitrogen dioxide, peroxynitrite production, or injury to the pulmonary surfactant system.[61] Carcinogenic and teratogenic potentials of inhaled NO exist, as well as effects on glutathione metabolism, unknown effects on immature or immunocompromised lung, potential interaction with other heme-containing proteins, and effects on platelet function and hemostasis.

Caution should be exercised when administering NO to patients with severe left ventricular dysfunction and pulmonary hypertension. In adults with ischemic cardiomyopathy, sudden pulmonary vasodilation may occasionally unload the right ventricle sufficiently to increase pulmonary blood flow and harmfully augment preload in a compromised left ventricle.[62,63] The attendant rise in left atrial pressure may produce pulmonary edema.[64] This is not likely to arise from any negative inotropic effect of NO[65] and may be ameliorated with vasodilators or diuretics.

Abrupt withdrawal effects of NO or even rebound pulmonary hypertension are important issues. Appreciation of the transient characteristics of withdrawal of NO may facilitate weaning from NO and has important implications for patients with persistent pulmonary hypertensive disorders when interruption of NO is necessary.[66,67] If the underlying pulmonary hypertensive process has not resolved, then the tendency for an abrupt increase in pulmonary artery pressure may be hazardous when NO therapy is withdrawn or interrupted.[37,68,69] If withdrawal of NO is necessary before resolution of the pathological process, hemodynamic instability may be expected. If a labile patient with pulmonary hypertension is stabilized with NO before transfer to a specialized center for further management, NO should be available during patient transport. If withdrawal of NO is necessary before resolution of the pathological process, hemodynamic instability may be expected. We have previously suggested that the withdrawal response to inhaled NO can be attenuated by pretreatment with the type V phosphodiesterase inhibitor, sildenafil.[70]

Intravenous Vasodilators

Many intravenous vasodilators have been used with variable success in patients with pulmonary hypertensive disorders and CHD. Older style vasodilators, such as tolazoline, phenoxybenzamine, nitroprusside, or isoproterenol had little biological basis for selectivity or enhanced activity in the pulmonary vascular bed. Moreover, they seldom targeted the pathophysiology, which is now better understood. However, if myocardial function is depressed and the afterload reducing effect on the left ventricle is beneficial to myocardial function and cardiac output, then there may be considerable value to these drugs. Phenoxybenzamine is still proclaimed to reduce sympathetic vasolability in postoperative patients and has its devotees among cardiac surgeons.[71,72] When resources are severely limited, some have recently suggested that phenoxybenzamine together with nitroprusside offer a reasonable cost-effective therapy for postoperative pulmonary hypertensions.[73]

Prostacyclin

Prostacyclin therapy has been widely studied in treatment of pulmonary hypertension. Because of its potent vasodilatory activity in the pulmonary vasculature, it is a useful drug for such patients, although the precise mechanism of action is not known. Prostacyclin therapy has been shown to improve hemodynamic function, exercise tolerance, quality of life, and survival for patients with pulmonary hypertension (Barst et al., 1996). Prostacyclin (epoprostenol) is most commonly administered as a continuous intravenous infusion through a central venous catheter. The initial dose is 1 to 2 ng/kg/min, which is carefully titrated over time, based on patient tolerability and response. Epoprostenol can be effective regardless of clinical response to acute pulmonary vasodilator testing. Because epoprostenol requires continuous intravenous access, patients are subject to a variety of complications, including catheter sepsis and significant hemodynamic changes if treatment is interrupted inadvertently. Children can thrive on epoprostenol over long periods. The mechanisms of resistance or tolerance to prostacyclin therapy are not well characterized. Because of the usefulness of epoprostenol, a variety of prostacyclin formulations have been developed that allow oral (beraprost), inhaled (iloprost), or subcutaneous (treprostinil) administration.

Prostacyclin seems to have somewhat more selectivity for the pulmonary circulation, but, at high doses, can precipitate a hypotensive crisis in unstable postoperative patients with refractory pulmonary hypertension. Similarly, iloprost, the longer-acting analog of prostacyclin, produces significant systemic hypotension in children with CHD and may have more use when administered in aerosolized form.[74] Chronic administration of prostacyclin has the potential to facilitate reversal of vascular remodeling through its antiplatelet effects, antimitogenic activity, or other indirect effects of raising intracellular cAMP (see chronic therapy below). Administration of aerosolized iloprost requires multiple doses during 24 hours in critically ill patients. The pharmacokinetics, when iloprost is administered by this route, are not well worked out for adults or children.

Other Vasodilators for Acute Pulmonary Hypertension and Comparison with Inhaled NO

Concurrent with studies exploring the therapeutic uses of inhaled NO in disorders with pulmonary vasoconstriction have been studies of other vasodilators both in comparison with and in addition to inhaled NO. In a group of six adults with primary pulmonary hypertension, oxygen and inhaled NO seemed to have less potent selective pulmonary vasodilation compared with aerosolized prostacyclin and iloprost.[75] However, animal model comparisons of inhaled NO, inhaled prostacyclin, and intravenous prostacyclin show similar selective pulmonary vasodilation for the inhaled agents, and improvement to a lesser extent with intravenous prostacyclin.[76] In an experimental model of hypoxic vasoconstriction inhaled prostacyclin reduced PVR to only 65% of the effect of inhaled NO, and only with NO did right ventricular ejection fraction increase.[77] A prospective randomized cross-over trial involving 13 children with pulmonary hypertension after cardiac repair showed both more effective and more selective pulmonary vasodilation with NO at 20 ppm compared with intravenous prostacyclin at 20 ng/kg/min.[78] Carroll et al.[79] have suggested that inhaled prostacyclin may be useful in postoperative children who had an incomplete response to inhaled NO.[79] However, circuit malfunctions on ventilators incorporating aerosolized prostacyclin, when added to the vagaries of dose delivery necessary to achieve pulmonary vasodilation but avoid systemic hypotension, have been obstacles to widespread adoption of this form of therapy. Promising therapy is offered by inhaling the more stable and longer-acting analog of prostacyclin, iloprost.[80–82] Although approved for use in the treatment of adult PAH, it may also have potential application in children with CHD. Rimensberger et al.[83] showed efficacy and selectivity of aerosolized iloprost in a small group of preoperative and postoperative children with CHD. The effect was comparable to inhaled NO during short-term administration. Application of the US Food and Drug Administration-approved adult outpatient disc-dose inhaler to critically ill children on mechanical ventilation is feasible, but little experience has, to date, been generated outside of selected European centers. It is noteworthy that adults with PAH whose clinical condition deteriorates with aerosolized iloprost respond to intravenous iloprost.[84] Unfortunately, intravenous iloprost is associated with hypotension in children with CHD.[74] Synergistic use of NO with aerosolized iloprost or intravenous prostacyclin,[85,86] atrial natriuretic peptide,[87] dipyridamole,[88,89] or specific type V phosphodiesterase inhibitors[90] holds considerable promise for more effective control of pulmonary hypertension in the postoperative setting. In addition to its vasodilator effect, inhaled NO indirectly improves right ventricular failure in pulmonary hypertensive situations, such as CHD or lung transplantation, and in cardiomyopathy.[91] Inhaled NO has been shown to assist the management of patients with right heart failure in those already on left ventricular assist device, thereby obviating the need for ECMO.[92]

Sildenafil inhibits the inactivation of cGMP within the vascular smooth muscle cell and has the potential to augment the effects of endogenous or exogenously administered NO to effect vascular smooth muscle relaxation. Sildenafil has been thought beneficial to children with pulmonary hypertensive disease, including structural heart disease.[93] This may suggest an important therapeutic application of a suitable preparation in postoperative congenital heart surgery. The intravenous form, as with all vasodilators, runs the risk of increasing any intrapulmonary shunt and inducing systemic vasodilation. However, there is much to recommend the oral form for use in weaning patients from inhaled NO.[94–96] NO inhalation in combination with sildenafil may offer superior drug therapy for postoperative pulmonary hypertension and facilitate weaning from inhaled NO. Sildenafil has crept into common practice as adjunctive therapy in the intensive care unit without benefit of properly controlled clinical trials.

Undoubtedly, because the cause of pulmonary hypertension in the intensive care setting is frequently multifactorial, our "best" therapy will be multiply targeted. Adding phosphodiesterase inhibitors to prostacyclin infusion or inhalation, endothelin blockers, thromboxane inhibitors, inhaled NO, and sildenafil may all have individual and combined merit with synergism enhancing efficacy. The combined approach to treatment has been recently reviewed.[97]

Drugs for Outpatient Treatment of Chronic and Idiopathic PAH

The true incidence of idiopathic PAH is not known. Estimates suggest one to two cases per 1 million people in the population. There is a predominance of cases in girls/women, with a female-to-male ratio of 1.7 or 1.8 to 1. As recently as the 1980s, pulmonary hypertension carried a grave prognosis in children, with a median life expectancy of less than 1 year.[98] Recent advances in diagnosis and treatment have radically altered the natural history of pulmonary hypertension in pediatric patients. Indeed, recent data suggest median survival well in excess of 5 years in patients with access to vasodilator therapy, such as prostacyclin and calcium channel blocker treatment.[99] Prolonged survival is particularly observed among patients with response to vasodilator treatment. This finding places a premium on the correct classification of patients as responders/nonresponders to acute vasodilator testing.

There are several unique challenges when interpreting the treatment literature for pulmonary hypertension. First, pulmonary hypertension is a heterogeneous disorder, arising from many different etiological factors, not all of which are known. This diversity complicates the understanding of the treatment and expected outcomes for patients. Second, pulmonary hypertension, particularly in the pediatric population, is a relatively rare disorder. Thus, treatment principles for children are often derived from observations in adults, without large clinical experiences in younger people to confirm independently the same observations. There are reasons why data from adults may not be easily extrapolated to children, including the different natural life expectancy, different etiologies for pulmonary hypertension, different intrinsic pulmonary vascular reactivity, and the historically worse natural history of the disease in children. Third, the critical end points for clinical trials are widely debated. Many trials have reported on mean changes in 6-minute walking distance or changes in hemodynamic function. Both of these may be challenging in younger pediatric populations. Beyond these technical challenges, relatively few studies have reported on long-term clinical outcomes, such as survival, or on quality of life or functional status, which may be crucial measures for children and their families. For all of these reasons, treatment of pediatric patients with pulmonary hypertension remains individualized. Although many algorithms have been promulgated to guide treatment choices, the exact sequence, duration, combination, and timing of treatments have not been characterized.

The therapeutic approach to the pediatric patient with pulmonary hypertension begins with a thorough identification of underlying causes and with first treatments directed at these factors.[100] These may include such measures as supplemental oxygen for patients with parenchymal lung disease, anti-inflammatory therapies for patients with collagen-vascular disease, continuous positive airway pressure therapy and/or tonsillectomy for patients with obstructive sleep apnea, and anticoagulation and potential thromboendarterectomy for chronic thromboembolic disease.

Anticoagulation

In adults with primary pulmonary hypertension, warfarin therapy is associated with improved survival.[101] The benefits of anticoagulation include treatment of chronic thromboembolism. Because microvessel thrombosis may contribute to the ongoing pathogenesis of pulmonary hypertension, anticoagulation may help minimize damage to the vasculature even in the absence of overt hypercoagulable states or proven thromboembolism. The optimal dosing of warfarin for pediatric patients is not well characterized. In clinical practice, a target international normalized ratio (INR) of 1.5 to 2.0 is sought. For toddlers or patients at risk for bleeding, lower INR levels, less than 1.5, are appropriate. Patients with documented thromboembolism or hypercoagulable states, such as positive cardiolipin or lupus anticoagulant tests, or known inherited thrombotic disorders, merit higher levels of anticoagulation.

Oxygen

Supplemental oxygen therapy can be valuable in certain patients with pulmonary hypertension to alleviate chronic hypoxemia. Such patients include those with sleep apnea or other hypoventilation syndromes, patients with intrinsic lung disease or acute respiratory infection, and patients with exercise-induced hypoxia. Patients with advanced right heart failure and resting oxygen desaturation may also benefit from oxygen therapy.

Drugs for Treatment of Right Heart Failure

Patients with pulmonary hypertension and right heart failure may benefit from cardiac glycosides, such as digoxin, and from diuretic therapy. Because pulmonary hypertension patients are vulnerable to reductions in cardiac preload, the initiation of diuretic therapy needs to be performed cautiously to avoid excessive volume depletion and hypotension. The use of angiotensin-converting enzyme (ACE) inhibitors and β-blockers for right heart failure associated with pulmonary hypertension has not been adequately studied in children.

Calcium Channel Blockers

Historic experience with use of calcium channel blockers as vasodilator therapy suggested that these drugs can prolong survival in patients with response to therapy.[102] To date, there are no randomized clinical trials involving calcium channel blockers for pulmonary hypertension. Because of the potential for severe hemodynamic collapse during initial challenge with calcium channel blockers, these drugs are not appropriate as first-line treatment during diagnostic challenge. Instead, acute vasodilator testing is performed with oxygen, NO, or prostacyclins.[49] Patients with response to such therapies are candidates for initiation of calcium channel blocker treatment, performed with close hemodynamic monitoring. Patients who tolerate initiation of calcium channel blockers and who have sustained hemodynamic benefit are continued on standing oral therapy. Patients without sustained benefit during initiation of therapy should have treatment with calcium channel blockers discontinued. The literature regarding treatment of adults with pulmonary hypertension suggests that fewer than 20% have clinical response to calcium channel blocker treatment; in children, a greater proportion—nearly 40%—seem to respond to such therapy.[103,104] The dose of therapy is cautiously titrated to optimize cardiac output and minimize pulmonary hypertension.

Endothelin Receptor Antagonists

Endothelin-1, a potent vasoconstrictor, mediates its activity through two types of endothelin receptors, ET_A and ET_B. Newer treatments for pulmonary hypertension include the dual-receptor antagonist, bosentan, and the ET_A selective receptor antagonist, sitaxsentan. Bosentan has been shown in randomized clinical trials to improve functional capacity and hemodynamics in adults with pulmonary hypertension.[105] A two-center study examined the pharmacokinetics, safety, and response to Bosentan in pediatric patients and found the results to be similar to those observed in adults.[106] Bosentan has been associated with reversible elevation of liver function tests and anemia. Careful monitoring of transaminases and hemoglobin levels is warranted in patients receiving treatment. In addition, Bosentan is a potential teratogen. Young patients need to be counseled regarding these effects and use effective forms of contraception.

Type 5 Phosphodiesterase Inhibitors

Sildenafil inhibits the inactivation of cGMP within the vascular smooth muscle cell and has the potential to augment the effects of endogenous or exogenously administered NO to effect vascular smooth muscle relaxation. Sildenafil is most readily available in oral forms and has been shown to have somewhat selective pulmonary vasodilating capacity while lowering the left atrial pressure and providing a modest degree of afterload reduction. Chronic oral administration of sildenafil to adults with primary pulmonary hypertension improves the exercise capacity and reduces pulmonary artery pressure.[107-110] It also is beneficial to children with pulmonary hypertensive disease, including structural heart disease.[93] Sildenafil is also being studied in combination with prostacyclin analogs as well as with endothelin receptor blockers. However, the optimal use of sildenafil is still under study.

References

1. Farber HW, Loscalzo J. Pulmonary arterial hypertension. *New England Journal of Medicine* 351(16):1655–1665, 2004.
2. Hassoun PM, Thappa V, Landman MJ, Fanburg BL. Endothelin 1: mitogenic activity on pulmonary artery smooth muscle cells and release from hypoxic endothelial cells. *Proceedings of the Society for Experimental Biology & Medicine* 1992;165–170.
3. Palmer RM, Ferrige AG, Moncada S. Nitric oxide release accounts for the biological activity of endothelium-derived relaxing factor. *Nature* 1987; 327:524–526.
4. Ignarro LJ, Buga GM, Wood KS, Byrns RE, Chaudhuri G. Endothelium-derived relaxing factor produced and released from artery and vein is nitric oxide. *Proc Natl Acad Sci U S A* 1987; 84:9265–9269.
5. Heath D, Edwards JE. The pathology of hypertensive pulmonary vascular disease: a description of six grades of structural changes in the pulmonary arteries with special attention to congenital cardiac septal defects. *Circulation* 1958; 18:533–547.
6. Celermajer DS, Cullen S, Deanfield JE. Impairment of endothelium-dependent pulmonary artery relaxation in children with congenital heart disease and abnormal pulmonary hemodynamics. *Circulation* 1993; 87:440–446.
7. Haworth SG. Normal pulmonary vascular development and its disturbance in congenital heart disease. 1981.
8. Adatia I, Barrow SE, Stratton PD, Miall-Allen VM, Ritter JM, Phil D, et al. Thromboxane A2 and prostacyclin biosynthesis in children and adolescents with pulmonary vascular disease. *Circulation* 1993; 88[part 1]:2117–2122.
9. Adatia I, Haworth SG. Circulating endothelin in children with congenital heart disease. *Br Heart J* 1993; 69:233–236.
10. Adatia I, Barrow SE, Stratton PD, Ritter JM, Haworth SG. Effect of intracardiac repair on thromboxane A2 and prostaglandin biosynthesis in children with left to right shunt. *Br Heart J* 1994; 72:452–456.
11. Canter J, Summar ML, Smith HB, et al. Genetic variation in the mitochondrial enzyme carbamyl-phosphate synthetase I predisposes children to increased pulmonary artery pressure following surgical repair of congenital heart defects: A validated genetic association study. *Mitochondrion* 2007; 7(3):204–210.
12. Wessel DL. Current and future strategies in the treatment of childhood pulmonary hypertension. *Prog Ped Cardiol* 2001; 12:289.

13. Hopkins RA, Bull C, Haworth SG, De Leval MR, Stark J. Pulmonary hypertensive crises following surgery for congenital heart defects in young children. *European Journal of Cardio-Thoracic Surgery* 1991; 5(12):628–634.

14. Lindberg L, Olsson AK, Jogi P, Jonmarker C. How common is severe pulmonary hypertension after pediatric cardiac surgery? *The Journal Of Thoracic And Cardiovascular Surgery* 2002; 123:1155–1163.

15. Schulze-Neick I, Li J, Penny DJ, Redington AN. Pulmonary vascular resistance after cardiopulmonary bypass in infants: effect on postoperative recovery. *The Journal Of Thoracic And Cardiovascular Surgery* 2001; 121:1033–1039.

16. Furchgott RF, Zawadzki JV. The obligatory role of endothelial cells in the relaxation of arterial smooth muscle by acetylcholine. *Nature* 1980; 288:373–376.

17. Ignarro LJ, Buga GM, Woods KS, Byrns RE, Chaudhuri G. Endothelium-derived relaxing factor produced and released from artery and vein is nitric oxide. *Proc Natl Acad Sci* 1987; 84:9265–9269.

18. Palmer RMJ, Ashton DS, Moncada S. Vascular endothelial cells synthesize nitric oxide from L-arginine. *Nature* 1988; 333:664–666.

19. Day R, Lynch J, Shaddy R, Orsmond G. Pulmonary vasodilatory effects of 12 and 60 parts per million inhaled nitric oxide in children with ventricular septal defect. *Am J Cardiol* 1995; 75:196–198.

20. Adatia I, Perry S, Landzberg M, Moore P, Thompson JE, Wessel DL. Inhaled nitric oxide and hemodynamic evaluation of patients with pulmonary hypertension before transplantation. *J Am Coll Cardiol* 1995; 25:1656–1664.

21. Atz AM, Adatia I, Jonas RA, Wessel DL. Inhaled nitric oxide in children with pulmonary hypertension and congenital mitral stenosis. *Am J Cardiol* 1996; 77:316–319.

22. Wessel DL, Adatia I, Giglia TM, Thompson JE, Kulik TJ. Use of inhaled nitric oxide and acetylcholine in the evaluation of pulmonary hypertension and endothelial function after cardiopulmonary bypass. *Circulation* 1993; 88:2128–2138.

23. Roberts JD, Jr., Lang P, Bigatello LM, Vlahakes GJ, Zapol WM. Inhaled nitric oxide in congenital heart disease. *Circulation* 1993; 87:447–453.

24. Adatia I, Lillehei C, Arnold JH, Thompson JE, Palazzo R, Fackler JC, et al. Inhaled nitric oxide in the treatment of postoperative graft dysfunction after lung transplantation. *Annals of Thoracic Surgery* 1994; 57(5):1311–1318.

25. Roberts JD, Polaner DM, Lang P, Zapol WM. Inhaled nitric oxide in persistent pulmonary hypertension of the newborn. *Lancet* 1992; 340:818–819.

26. Kinsella JP, Neish SR, Ivy DD, Shaffer E, Abman SH. Clinical responses to prolonged treatment of persistent pulmonary hypertension of the newborn with low doses of inhaled nitric oxide. *J Pediatr* 1993; 123:103–108.

27. Finer NN, Etches PC, Kamstra B, Tierney AJ, Peliowski A, Ryan CA. Inhaled nitric oxide in infants referred for extracorporeal membrane oxygenation: dose response. *J Pediatr* 1994; 124:302–308.

28. Rossaint R, Falke KJ, Lopez F, Slama K, Pison U, Zapol WM. Inhaled nitric oxide for the adult respiratory distress syndrome. *New England Journal of Medicine* 1993; 328:399–405.

29. Vallance P, Collier J, Moncada S. Effects of endothelium-derived nitric oxide on peripheral arteriolar tone in man. *Lancet* 1989; 2:997–1000.

30. Cremona G, Dinh-Xuan AT, Higenbottam TW. Endothelium-derived relaxing factor and the pulmonary circulation. *Lung* 1991; 169:185–202.

31. Turner-Gomes SO, Andrew M, Coles J, Trusler GA, Williams WG, Rabinovitch M. Abnormalities in von Willebrand factor and antithrombin III after cardiopulmonary bypass operations for congenital heart disease. *Journal of Thoracic & Cardiovascular Surgery* 1992; 103(1):87–97.

32. Kirshbom MP, Jacobs TM, Tsui SLSDRL, Schwinn AD, Ungerleider MR, Gaynor WJ. Effects of cardiopulmonary bypass and circulatory arrest on endothelium-dependent vasodilatation in the lung. *J Thorac Cardiovasc Surg* 1996; 111:1248–1256.

33. Koul B, Willen H, Sjöberg T, Wetterberg T, Kugelberg J, Steen S. Pulmonary sequelae of prolonged total venoarterial bypass: Evaluation with a new experimental model. *Ann Thorac Surg* 1991; 51:794–799.

34. Beghetti M, Silkoff PE, Caramori M, Holtby HM, Slutsky AS, Adatia I. Decreased exhaled nitric oxide may be a marker of cardiopulmonary bypass-induced injury. *Ann Thorac Surg* 1998; 66:532–534.

35. Rimar S, Gillis CN. Pulmonary vasodilation by inhaled nitric oxide after endothelial injury. *Journal of Applied Physiology* 1992; 73(5):2179–2183.

36. Hillier SC, Graham JA, Hanger CC, Wagner WW, Jr. Inhaled nitric oxide reverses hypoxic vasoconstriction in <100 micron canine pulmonary microvessels. *Anesth Analg* 1995; 80:S187.

37. Roos CM, Rich GF, Uncles DR, Daugherty MO, Frank DU. Sites of vasodilation by inhaled nitric oxide vs. sodium nitroprusside in endothelin-constricted isolated rat lungs. *Journal of Applied Physiology* 1994; 77(1):51–57.

38. Gao Y, Zhou H, Raj JU. Endothelium-derived nitric oxide plays a larger role in pulmonary veins than in arteries of newborn lambs. *Circ Res* 1995; 76:559–565.

39. Mikiyasu S, Shimouchi A, Kawaguchi AT, Ninomiya I. Inhaled nitric oxide: diameter response patterns in feline small pulmonary arteries and veins. *Am J Physiol* 1996; 270:H974–H980.

40. Rimar S, Gillis CN. Site of pulmonary vasodilation by inhaled nitric oxide in the perfused lung. *Journal of Applied Physiology* 1995; 78(5):1745–1749.

41. Benzing A, Geiger K. Inhaled nitric oxide lowers pulmonary capillary pressure and changes longitudinal distribution of pulmonary vascular resistance in patients with acute lung injury. *Acta Anaesthesiol Scand* 1994; 38:640–645.

42. Wheller J, George BL, Mulder DG, Jarmakani JM. Diagnosis and management of postoperative pulmonary hypertensive crisis. *Circulation* 1979; 60:1640–1644.

43. Del Nido PJ, Williams WG, Villamater J, Benson LN, Coles JG, Bohn D, et al. Changes in pericardial surface pressure during pulmonary hypertensive crises after cardiac surgery. *Circulation* 1987; 76[suppl III]:93.

44. Journois D, Pouard P, Mauriat P, Malhère T, Vouhe P, Safran D. Inhaled nitric oxide as a therapy for pulmonary hypertension after operations for congenital heart defects. *J Thorac Cardiovasc Surg* 1994; 107:1129–1135.

45. Journois D, Baufreton C, Mauriat P, Pouard P, Vouh P, Safran D. Effects of inhaled nitric oxide administration on early postoperative mortality in patients operated for correction of atrioventricular canal defects. *Chest* 2005; 128:3537–3544.

46. Schaffer R, Berdat P, Stolle B, Pfammatter JP, Stocker F, Carrel T. Surgery of the complete atrioventricular canal: relationship between age at operation, mitral regurgitation, size of the ventricular septum defect, additional malformations and early postoperative outcome. *Cardiology* 1999; 91:231–235.

47. Bizzarro M, Gross I. Inhaled nitric oxide for the postoperative management of pulmonary hypertension in infants and children with congenital heart disease. *Cochrane Database Of Systematic Reviews* 2005;CD005055.

48. Dyar O, Young JD, Xiong L, Howell S, Johns E. Dose-response relationship for inhaled nitric oxide in experimental pulmonary hypertension in sheep. *Br J Anaesth* 1993; 71:702–708.

49. Sitbon O, Brenot F, Denjean A, Bergeron A, Parent F, Azarian R, et al. Inhaled nitric oxide as a screening vasodilator agent in primary pulmonary hypertension. A dose-response study and comparison with prostacyclin. *American Journal of Respiratory & Critical Care Medicine* 1995; 151(2 Pt 1):384–389.

50. Gerlach H, Rossaint D, Pappert D, Falke KJ. Time-course and dose-response of nitric oxide inhalation for systemic oxygenation and pulmonary hypertension in patients with adult respiratory distress syndrome. *Euro J Clin Invest* 1993; 23:499–502.

51. Puybasset L, Rouby JJ, Mourgeon E, Stewart TE, Cluzel P, Arthaud M, et al. Inhaled nitric oxide in acute respiratory failure: dose-response curves. *Int Care Med* 1994; 20:319–327.

52. Lonnqvist PA, Jonsson B, Winberg P, Frostell CG. Inhaled nitric oxide in infants with developing or established chronic lung disease. *Acta Paediatr* 1995; 84:1188–1192.

53. DeMarco V, Skimming JW, Ellis TM, Cassin S. Nitric oxide inhalation: effects on the ovine neonatal pulmonary and systemic circulations. *Reproduction, Fertility & Development* 1996; 8:431–438.

54. Rich GF, Roos CM, Anderson SM, Urich DC, Daugherty MO, Johns RA. Inhaled nitric oxide: dose response and the effects of blood in the isolated rat lung. *Journal of Applied Physiology* 1993; 75(3):1278–1284.

55. Berger JI, Gibson RL, Redding GJ, Standaert TA, Clarke WR, Truog WE. Effect of inhaled nitric oxide during group B streptococcal sepsis in piglets. *Am Rev Respir Dis* 1993; 147:1080–1086.

56. Maruyama K, Kobayasi H, Taguchi O, Chikusa H, Muneyuki M. Higher does of inhaled nitric oxide might be less effective in improving oxygenation in a patient with interstitial pulmonary fibrosis. *Anesth Analg* 1995; 81:210–211.

57. Buhrer C, Merker G, Falke K, Versmold H, Obladen M. Dose-response to inhaled nitric oxide in acute hypoxemic respiratory failure of newborn infants: a preliminary report. *Pediatric Pulmonology* 1995; 19:291–298.

58. Demirakca S, Dotsch J, Knothe C, Magsaam J, Reiter HL, Bauer J, et al. Inhaled nitric oxide in neonatal and pediatric acute respiratory distress syndrome: Dose response, prolonged inhalation, and weaning. *Crit Care Med* 1996; 24:1913–1919.

59. Young JD, Sear JW, Valvini EM. Kinetics of methaemoglobin and serum nitrogen oxide production during inhalation of nitric oxide in volunteers. *Br J Anaesth* 1996; 76:652–656.

60. Rimar S, Gillis CN. Selective pulmonary vasodilation by inhaled nitric oxide is due to hemoglobin inactivation. *Circulation* 1993; 88:2884–2887.

61. Hallman M, Bry K, Lappalainen U. A mechanism of nitric oxide-induced surfactant dysfunction. *J Appl Physiol* 1996; 80:2035–2043.

62. Semigran MJ, Cockrill BA, Kacmarek R, Thompson BT, Zapol WM, Dec GW, et al. Hemodynamic effects of inhaled nitric oxide in heart failure. *J Am Coll Cardiol* 1994; 24:982–988.

63. Loh E, Stamler JS, Hare JM, Loscalzo J, Colucci WS. Cardiovascular effects of inhaled nitric oxide in patients with left ventricular dysfunction. *Circulation* 1994; 90:2780–2785.

64. Bocchi EA, Bacal F, Auler Junior JO, Carmone MJ, Bellotti G, Pileggi F. Inhaled nitric oxide leading to pulmonary edema in stable severe heart failure. *Am J Cardiol* 1994; 74:70–72.

65. Hare JM, Shernan SK, Body SC, Graydon E, Colucci WS, Couper GS. Influence of inhaled nitric oxide on systemic flow and ventricular filling pressure in patients receiving mechanical circulatory assistance. *Circulation* 1997; 95:2250–2253.

66. Atz AM, Adatia I, Wessel DL. Rebound pulmonary hypertension after inhalation of nitric oxide. *Ann Thorac Surg* 1996; 62:1759–1764.

67. Francoise M, Gouyon JB, Mercier JC. Hemodynamic and oxygenation changes induced by the discontinuation of low-dose inhalational nitric oxide in newborn infants. *Int Care Med* 1996; 22:477–481.

68. Miller OI, Tang SF, Keech A, Celermajer DS. Rebound pulmonary hypertension on withdrawal from inhaled nitric oxide. *Lancet* 1995; 346:51–52.

69. Lavoie A, Hall JB, Olson DM, Wylam ME. Life-threatening effects of discontinuing inhaled nitric oxide in severe respiratory failure. *Am J Respir Crit Care Med* 1996; 153:1985–1987.

70. Atz AM, Wessel DL. Sildenafil ameliorates effects of inhaled nitric oxide withdrawal. *Anesthesiology* 1999; 91(1):307–310.

71. Tweddell JS, Hoffman GM, Fedderly RT, Berger S, Thomas JP Jr, Ghanayem NS, et al. Phenoxybenzamine improves systemic oxygen delivery after the Norwood procedure. *The Annals of Thoracic Surgery* 1999; 67:161.

72. Bando K, Turrentine MW, Sharp TG, Sekine Y, Aufiero TX, Sun K, et al. Pulmonary hypertension after operations for congenital heart disease: analysis of risk factors and management. *The Journal Of Thoracic And Cardiovascular Surgery* 1996; 112:1600.

73. Kiran U, Makhija N, Das SN, Bhan A, Airan B. Combination of phenoxybenzamine and nitroglycerin: effective control of pulmonary artery pressures in children undergoing cardiac surgery. *Journal of Cardiothoracic and Vascular Anesthesia* 2005; 19:274–275.

74. Hallioglu O, Dilber E, Celiker A. Comparison of acute hemodynamic effects of aerosolized and intravenous iloprost in secondary pulmonary hypertension in children with congenital heart disease. *Am J Cardiol* 2003; 92:1007–1009.

75. Olschewski H, Walmrath D, Schermuly R, Ghofrani HA, Grimminger F, Seeger W. Aerosolized prostacyclin and iloprost in severe pulmonary hypertension. *Ann Intern Med* 1996; 124:820–824.

76. Zobel G, Dacar D, Rodl S, Friehs I. Inhaled nitric oxide versus inhaled prostacyclin and intravenous versus inhaled prostacyclin in acute respiratory failure with pulmonary hypertension in piglets. *Pediatr Res* 1995; 38:198–204.

77. Zwissler B, Welte M, Messmer K. Effects of inhaled prostacyclin as compared with inhaled nitric oxide on right ventricular performance in hypoxic pulmonary vasoconstriction. *Journal Of Cardiothoracic And Vascular Anesthesia* 1995; 9:283–289.

78. Goldman AP, Delius RE, Deanfield JE, Macrae DJ. Nitric oxide is superior to prostacyclin for pulmonary hypertension after cardiac operations. *Annals of Thoracic Surgery* 1995; 60(2):300–305.

79. Carroll CL, Backer CL, Mavroudis C, Cook K, Goodman DM. Inhaled prostacyclin following surgical repair of congenital heart disease—a pilot study. *Journal Of Cardiac Surgery* 2005; 20:436–439.

80. Olschewski H, Simonneau G, Galie N, Higenbottam T, Naeije R, Rubin LJ, et al. Inhaled iloprost for severe pulmonary hypertension. *New England Journal of Medicine* 2002; 347(5):322–329.

81. Max M, Rossaint R. Inhaled prostacyclin in the treatment of pulmonary hypertension. *European Journal of Pediatrics* 1999; 158:S23–S26.

82. Hoeper MM, Schwarze M, Ehlerding S, Adler-Schuermeyer A, Spiekerkoetter E, Niedermeyer J, et al. Long-term treatment of primary pulmonary hypertension with aerosolized iloprost, a prostacyclin analogue. *New England Journal of Medicine* 2000; 342:1866–1870.

83. Rimensberger PC, Spahr-Schopfer I, Berner M, Jaeggi E, Kalangos A, Friedli B, et al. Inhaled nitric oxide versus aerosolized iloprost in secondary pulmonary hypertension in children with congenital heart disease: vasodilator capacity and cellular mechanisms. *Circulation* 2001; 103:544–548.

84. Hoeper MM, Spiekerkoetter E, Westerkamp V, Gatzke R, Fabel H. Intravenous iloprost for treatment failure of aerosolised iloprost in pulmonary arterial hypertension. *The European Respiratory Journal: Official Journal Of The European Society For Clinical Respiratory Physiology* 2002; 20:339–343.

85. Parker TA, Ivy DD, Kinsella JP, Torielli F, Ruyle SZ, Thilo EH, et al. Combined therapy with inhaled nitirc oxide and intravenous prostacyclin in an infant with alveolar-capillary dysplasia. *American Journal Of Respiratory And Critical Care Medicine* 1997; 155:743–746.

86. Schranz D, Huth R, Wippermann CF, Ritzerfeld S, Schmitt FX, Oelert H. Nitric oxide and prostacyclin lower suprasystemic pulmonary hypertension after cardiopulmonary bypass. *European Journal of Pediatrics* 1993; 152:793–796.

87. Ivy DD, Kinsella JP, Wolfe RR, Abman SH. Atrial natriuretic peptide and nitric oxide in children with pulmonary hypertension after surgical repair of congenital heart disease. *Am J Cardiol* 1996; 77:102–105.

88. Kinsella JP, Torielli F, Ziegler JW, Ivy DD, Abman SH. Dipyrimadole augmentation of response to nitric oxide. *Lancet* 1995; 346:647–648.

89. Fullerton DA, Jaggers J, Piedalue F, Grover FL, McIntyre RC. Effective control of refractory pulmonary hypertension after cardiac operations. *J Thorac Cardiovasc Surg* 1997; 113:363–368.

90. Cohen AH, Hanson K, Morris K, Fouty B, McMurtry IF, Clarke W, et al. Inhibition of cyclic 3'-5'-guanosine monophosphate-specific phosphodiesterase selectively vasodilates the pulmonary circulation in chronically hypoxic rats. *J Clin Invest* 1996; 97:172–179.

91. Gatecel C, Mebazaa A, Kong R, Guinard N, Kermarrec N, Mateo J, et al. Inhaled nitric oxide improves hepatic tissue oxygenation in right ventricular failure: value of venous oxygen saturation monitoring. *Anesth* 1995; 82:588–590.

92. Yahagi N, Kumon K, Nakatani T, Matsui J, Sasako Y, Isobe F, et al. Inhaled nitric oxide for the management of acute right ventricular failure in patients with a left ventricular assist system. *Artif Organs* 1995; 19:557–558.

93. Humpl T, Reyes JT, Holtby H, Stephens D, Adatia I. Beneficial effect of oral sildenafil therapy on childhood pulmonary arterial hypertension: twelve-month clinical trial of a single-drug, open-label, pilot study. *Circulation* 2005; 111:3274–3280.

94. Atz AM, Wessel DL. Sildenafil ameliorates effects of inhaled nitric oxide withdrawal. *Anesth* 1999; 91:307–310.

95. Atz AM, Lefler AK, Fairbrother DL, Uber WE, Bradley SM. Sildenafil augments the effect of inhaled nitric oxide for postoperative pulmonary hypertensive crises. *The Journal Of Thoracic And Cardiovascular Surgery* 2002; 124:628–629.

96. Namachivayam P, Theilen U, Butt WW, Cooper SM, Penny DJ, Shekerdemian LS. Sildenafil prevents rebound pulmonary hypertension after withdrawal of nitric oxide in children. *American Journal Of Respiratory And Critical Care Medicine* 2006; 174:1042–1047.

97. Channick RN, Rubin LJ. Combination therapy for pulmonary hypertension: a glimpse into the future? [comment]. *Critical Care Medicine* 2000; 28(3):896–897.

98. D'Alonzo GE, Barst RJ, Ayres SM, Bergofsky EH, Brundage BH, Detre KM, et al. Survival in patients with primary pulmonary hypertension. Results from a national prospective registry. *Annals of Internal Medicine* 1991; 115(5):343–349.

99. Yung D, Widlitz AC, Rosenzweig EB, Kerstein D, Maislin G, Barst RJ. Outcomes in children with idiopathic pulmonary arterial hypertension. *Circulation* 2004; 110(6):660–665.

100. Badesch DB, Abman SH, Ahearn GS, Barst RJ, McCrory DC, Simonneau G, et al. Medical therapy for pulmonary arterial hypertension: ACCP evidence-based clinical practice guidelines. *Chest* 2004; 126(1 Suppl):35S–62S.

101. Fuster V, Steele PM, Edwards WD, Gersh BJ, McGoon MD, Frye RL. Primary pulmonary hypertension: natural history and the importance of thrombosis. *Circulation* 1984; 70(4):580–587.

102. Rich S, Kaufmann E, Levy PS. The effect of high doses of calcium-channel blockers on survival in primary pulmonary hypertension. *New England Journal of Medicine* 1992; 327:76–81.

103. Barst RJ, Maislin G, Fishman AP. Vasodilator therapy for primary pulmonary hypertension in children. *Circulation* 1999; 99:1197–1208.

104. Sandoval J, Bauerle O, Gomez A, Palomar A, Martinez Guerra ML, Furuya ME. Primary pulmonary hypertension in children: clinical characterization and survival. *Journal of the American College of Cardiology* 1995; 25(2):466–474.

105. Channick RN, Simonneau G, Sitbon O, Robbins IM, Frost A, Tapson VF, et al. Effects of the dual endothelin-receptor antagonist bosentan in patients with pulmonary hypertension: a randomised placebo-controlled study. *Lancet* 2001; 358:1119–1123.

106. Barst RJ, Ivy D, Dingemanse J, Widlitz A, Schmitt K, Doran A, et al. Pharmacokinetics, safety, and efficacy of bosentan in pediatric patients with pulmonary arterial hypertension. *Clinical Pharmacology & Therapeutics* 2003; 73(4):372–382.

107. Galie N, Ghofrani HA, Torbicki A, Barst RJ, Rubin LJ, Badesch D, et al. Sildenafil citrate therapy for pulmonary arterial hypertension. *The New England Journal of Medicine* 2005; 353:2148–2157.

108. Humbert M, Sitbon O, Simonneau G. Treatment of pulmonary arterial hypertension. [Review] [97 refs]. *New England Journal of Medicine* 2004; 351(14):1425–1436.

109. Saygili A, Canter B, Iriz E, Kula S, Tunaoğlu FS, Olguntürk R, Ozdoğan ME. Use of sildenafil with inhaled nitric oxide in the management of severe pulmonary hypertension. *J Cardiothorac Vasc Anesth* 2004; 18:775–776.

110. Zhao L, Mason NA, Morrell NW, Kojonazarov B, Sadykov A, Maripov A, et al. Sildenafil inhibits hypoxia-induced pulmonary hypertension. *Circulation* 2001; 104(4):424–428.

11. Anticoagulants, Antithrombotics, and Antiplatelets

Phuong-Tan Nguyen, Jessica Erin Sandy, and Ricardo Munoz

Tests and Monitoring

Alteplase

Indication

Alteplase is used for treatment of acute myocardial infarction (MI), acute ischemic stroke, acute, massive pulmonary embolism, and occluded central venous catheters. Alteplase has also been used in pediatric patients with systemic thrombosis.

Mechanism of Action

Alteplase is a tissue plasminogen activator (TPA) that enhances the conversion of plasminogen to plasmin by binding to fibrin within a thrombus to initiate local fibrinolysis.

Dosing

> **Occluded IV catheters:**
>> dose is listed per lumen; if multiple lumens of a multilumen catheter are occluded, treat one lumen at a time
>
> **"Chest" recommendations:**[1,2]
>> *Central venous catheters:* use a volume equal to the internal volume of the lumen; instill into lumen over 1 to 2 minutes, leave to dwell in catheter for 1 to 2 hours, then aspirate drug out of the catheter after dwell time. DO NOT INFUSE INTO PATIENT. Flush catheter after aspirating with normal saline (NS)
>>
>> Patients weighing at most 10 kg: 0.5 mg diluted in NS
>>
>> Patients weighing more than 10 kg: 1 mg in 1 mL NS; maximum, 2 mg in 2 mL NS
>>
>> *Subcutaneous (S.Q.) port:*
>> Patients weighing at most 10 kg: 0.5 mg diluted with NS to 3 mL
>> Patients weighing more than 10 kg: 2 mg diluted with NS to 3 mL

Manufacturer's Recommendations (Cathflo™ Activase®) for I.V. Catheter Clearance

> **Central venous catheters:** in still the appropriate volume (volume that is equal to 110% of the internal lumen volume of the catheter) into the

occluded catheter and let it dwell in the lumen. Evaluate catheter function after 30 minutes; if the catheter is functional, aspirate 5 mL of blood out of the catheter to remove the drug and residual clot and then flush the catheter with NS. If the catheter is still occluded, leave to dwell in lumen and evaluate again after 120 minutes. If the catheter is functional, aspirate 5 mL of blood and flush with NS. If the catheter remains occluded after 120 minutes, a second dose may be administered by repeating the procedure

Patients weighing at least 10 kg and less than 30 kg: 1 mg/mL concentration; do not exceed 2 mg in 2 mL

Patients weighing at least 30 kg: 2 mg in 2 mL

Systemic thrombosis: initial, 0.1 mg/kg/hour intravenous (I.V.) for 6 hours while monitoring for bleeding and measuring fibrinogen levels. If sufficient response is not reached within 6 hours, increase dose by 0.1 mg/kg/hour at 6-hour intervals, to a maximum of 0.5 mg/kg/hour. Maintain fibrinogen levels greater than 100 mg/dL. Duration of therapy is based on clinical response

Arterial spasm: 0.1 mg/kg followed by an infusion of 0.5 mg/kg/hour for 2 hours followed by a heparin infusion[3]

Venous thrombosis: initial dose of 0.03 mg/kg/hour (0.06 mg/kg/hour in neonates) I.V. and adjust based on clinical response

Pharmacokinetics

For absorption, for coronary thrombolysis, the initial response is seen in 30 minutes, with a peak response in 60 minutes. Therapeutic levels are not clearly established, but the recommended minimal effective plasma concentration is 0.75 μg/mL. For acute MI, the initial response is seen in 20 to 40 minutes, with concentrations ranging from 0.52 to 1.8 μg/mL. The half-life ranges from 4.4 to 7 minutes. The volume of distribution (Vd) is 8.1 mL. Alteplase is metabolized in the liver, with more than 50% of drug cleared within 5 minutes after the infusion has ended and 80% cleared within 10 minutes.

Monitoring Parameters

Signs and symptoms of bleeding, prothrombin time (PT), activated partial thromboplastin time (aPTT), and fibrinogen levels during therapy should be monitored.

Contraindications

Hypersensitivity to alteplase, active internal bleeding, cerebrovascular accident or transient ischemic attack (TIA), intracranial neoplasm, suspected aortic dissection, arteriovenous malformation or aneurysm, bleeding diathesis, severe hepatic or renal disease, hemostatic defects, and severe uncontrolled hypertension are contraindication for alteplase use.

Precautions/Warning

Alteplase may cause bleeding; concurrent use of heparin or oral anticoagulants may increase bleeding; arterial and venous puncture should be minimized; avoid intramuscular (I.M.) injections, recent major surgery, recent trauma, pregnancy, cerebrovascular disease, patients with left heart thrombus (e.g., mitral stenosis with atrial fibrillation), acute pericarditis, subacute bacterial endocarditis, hemostatic defects, significant hepatic or renal dysfunction, hypertension, septic thrombophlebitis or occluded IV cannula at an infected site, advanced age, and known or suspected infection in the catheter that requires clearance. Risks of alteplase therapy may be increased in patients with major early signs of infarct on computed tomographic (CT) scan and in those with severe neurological deficit at presentation.

Drug-Drug Interactions

Anticoagulants and drugs that affect platelet function may increase the risk of bleeding. Safety of the concurrent use of aspirin or heparin with alteplase within the first 24 hours after the onset of symptoms is unknown and should be considered with caution. Defibrotide and lepirudin may increase risk of bleeding. Antifibrinolytic agents may decrease effectiveness. Nitroglycerin may increase the hepatic clearance of alteplase.

Adverse Effects

Adverse effects include gastrointestinal (GI) hemorrhage, genitourinary (GU) hemorrhage, ecchymosis, nausea, vomiting, hypotension, fever, retroperitoneal hemorrhage, epistaxis, gingival hemorrhage, intracranial hemorrhage, and pericardial hemorrhage. Rapid lysis of coronary artery thrombi by thrombolytic agents may be associated with reperfusion-related atrial and/or ventricular arrhythmias.

Poisoning Information

Do not exceed recommended doses. Treatment for alteplase poisoning is symptomatic and supportive. Vital signs, renal and hepatic function, and bleeding should be monitored.

Compatible Diluents/Administration

Alteplase must be used within 8 hours of reconstitution. Administer alteplase I.V. at a concentration of 1 mg/mL in sterile water for injections or dilute further to 0.5 mg/mL with NS or 5% dextrose in water (D5W). Alteplase is **incompatible** with dobutamine, dopamine, heparin, and nitroglycerin infusions; and is physically **compatible** with lidocaine, metoprolol, eptifibatide, and propranolol when administered via a Y site; alteplase is **compatible** with either D5W or NS.

Aminocaproic Acid

Indication
In the United States, aminocaproic acid has been used in the treatment of excessive hemorrhage caused by fibrinolysis and as prophylaxis for intraventricular hemorrhage in neonates supported on extracorporeal membrane oxygenation (ECMO).[4-6]

Mechanism of Action
Aminocaproic acid competitively inhibits activation of plasminogen, resulting in a decreased conversion of plasminogen to plasmin (fibrinolysin).

Dosing

   Children: the I.V. route is the preferred route of administration in the intensive care setting. Oral route of administration is also available
   Oral/I.V.:
       100 to 200 mg/kg/dose as a loading dose, with maintenance dosing of 100 mg/kg/dose every 6 hours (maximum daily dose, 30 g) <u>OR</u>
       100 mg/kg as a one-time loading dose followed by a continuous infusion of 30 mg/kg/hour (daily maximum, 30 g)
   Adults: acute bleeding syndromes caused by elevated fibrinolytic activity:
       Oral: 5 g during the first hour, followed by 1 to 1.25 g/hour for 8 hours or until bleeding stops (maximum daily dose should not exceed 30 g)
       I.V.: 4 to 5 g during first hour followed by continuous infusion at a rate of 1 to 1.25 g/hour, continue for 8 hours or until the bleeding stops
   Dose adjustment for renal impairment: reduce dose to 15 to 25% of normal dose in oliguria or end stage renal disease

Pharmacokinetics
Absorption is rapid with 100% oral bioavailability. Aminocaproic acid widely distributes through intravascular and extravascular compartments. Hepatic metabolism is minimal, and half-life is 2 hours. Forty to 60% of aminocaproic acid is excreted as unchanged drug in the urine within 12 hours.

Monitoring Parameters
Complete blood cell count (CBC) and coagulation panel initially and after treatment, fibrinogen, and fibrin split products; serum potassium, and blood urea nitrogen (BUN) should be monitored. Observe for dyspnea, pulmonary embolism, rhabdomyolysis, and myalgia.

Contraindications
Contraindications to aminocaproic acid use are hypersensitivity to aminocaproic acid, disseminated intravascular coagulation, and evidence of

an intravascular clotting process; risk of thrombus may increase with use of Factor IX concentrate or anti-inhibitor coagulant concentrate.

Precautions/Warnings

Use injection form in premature neonates cautiously because of the presence of benzyl alcohol; use aminocaproic acid cautiously in patients with cardiac, hepatic, or renal insufficiency (drug may accumulate in patients with decreased renal function and may require dosage adjustment); use cautiously in patients with hematuria of upper urinary tract origin or in patients at risk for venoocclusive disease of the liver; a definite diagnosis of primary fibrinolysis must be made before administration.

Drug/Drug Interactions

There is an increased risk of thrombosis with oral contraceptives, estrogens, tretinoin, and Factor IX/anti-inhibitor coagulant complex.

Adverse Effects

Adverse effects of aminocaproic acid include hypotension, bradycardia, arrhythmias, headache, seizures, rash, hyperkalemia, nausea, vomiting, decreased platelet function, agranulocytosis, leukopenia, myopathy, acute rhabdomyolysis, glaucoma, deafness, renal failure, dyspnea, and pulmonary embolism.

Poisoning Information

The therapeutic range of aminocaproic acid is $130\,\mu g/mL$. It is recommended that patients on therapy for longer than 2 weeks and with total doses of greater than 500 g should be monitored carefully for renal, hepatic, or muscle toxicity. Treatment is supportive with no specific antidote. Monitor pulse oximetry and/or arterial blood gases (ABGs), chest x-ray, pulmonary function tests, CBC, urinalysis, and liver and kidney function.

Compatible Diluents/Administration

Rapid I.V. injection (I.V. push) of aminocaproic acid should be avoided because hypotension, bradycardia, and arrhythmia may result; I.V. infusion should be diluted with NS, D5W, or Lactated Ringer's solution (LR) to a final concentration of 20 mg/mL.

Aprotinin

Indication

Aprotinin is used in the United States in adults to prevent hemorrhage after coronary artery bypass graft; it has been used in liver transplantation as a non-US Food and Drug Administration (FDA)-labeled indication. Although not FDA approved for use in pediatrics, aprotinin has been used in the United States and worldwide to reduce or prevent blood loss in patients undergoing cardiac surgery with cardiopulmonary bypass, in those with preexisting coagulopathies, and when a patient's religious beliefs prohibit blood transfusions.

Mechanism of Action

Aprotinin is a serine protease inhibitor; it inhibits plasmin, kallikrein, and platelet activation; and is a weak inhibitor of plasma pseudocholinesterase.

Dosing

A test dose should be administered to all patients at least 10 minutes before administration of the routine dose to assess for allergic reaction.

> **Infants and Children:** data pertaining to dosage recommendations in this population vary, with no conclusive dosing regimen established. Test dose, 0.1 mg/kg I.V. (maximum, 1.4 mg)
> *Body surface area at most 1.16 m²:*
> Loading dose: 240 mg/m² I.V.
> 240 mg/m² into pump prime volume
> 50 mg/m²/hour continuous I.V. infusion during surgery.
> Lower doses of 28 mg/m²/hour I.V. have been used in some institutions, based on a patient's clinical condition
> *Body surface area greater than 1.16 m²:*
> Loading dose: 280 mg/m² I.V.
> 280 mg/m² into pump prime volume
> 70 mg/m²/hour continuous I.V. infusion during surgery
> *Alternative to above dosing:*
> 30,000 Kallikrein inhibitor U (KIU)/kg (4.2 mg/kg) I.V. loading dose
> 30,000 KIU/kg (4.2 mg/kg) into pump prime volume
> 30,000 KIU/kg/hour (4.2 mg/kg/hour) continuous I.V. infusion.
> Lower doses of 1 mg/kg/hour I.V. have been used in some institutions, based on a patient's clinical condition
> **Adults:** loading dose, 1 mL (1.4 mg) I.V.
> *Regimen 1*
> 2 million KIU (280 mg) loading dose, I.V.
> 2 million KIU (280 mg) into pump prime volume
> 500,000 KIU/hour (70 mg/hour) continuous I.V. infusion during surgery
> *Regimen 2*
> 1 million KIU (140 mg) loading dose, I.V.
> 1 million KIU (140 mg) into pump prime volume
> 250,000 KIU/hour (35 mg/hour) continuous I.V. infusion during surgery
> *Note:* in Europe and in Australia, aprotinin is also used in the postoperative period in cases of persistent bleeding, at a dose of 1000 to 4000 KIU/kg/hour

Pharmacokinetics

Aprotinin has a rapid distribution and a slow degradation by lysosomal enzymes, with an elimination half-life of 150 minutes and a terminal elimination of 10 hours. Less than 10% is excreted unchanged in the urine.

Monitoring Parameters

Blood pressure (transient hypotension), CBC, bleeding times, PT, activated clotting time (ACT), platelet count, fibrinogen degradation products, and renal function should be monitored.

Contraindications

Contraindications include hypersensitivity to aprotinin. The FDA has recently issued a contraindication to the use of aprotinin in patients who are suspected to have or have had exposure to aprotinin within a 12-month period because of an increased risk of anaphylactic and potentially fatal reactions. Aprotinin is an ingredient in some fibrin sealant products, and this should also be noted.[7]

Precautions/Warning

Incidence of anaphylactic reaction is increased in patients with a previous exposure to aprotinin, patients with thromboembolic disease on anticoagulant therapy, and patients with renal insufficiency. Consider limiting aprotinin use to patients in whom the benefit of reducing blood loss is essential to management.

The FDA has issued a Public Health Advisory alerting physicians who perform heart bypass surgery and their patients that aprotinin has been linked to higher risk of serious side effects, including nephropathies, MIs, and strokes.

Drug/Drug Interaction

Aprotinin decreases effects of fibrinolytic agents; decreases antihypertensive effects of angiotensin-converting enzyme (ACE) inhibitors; prolongs ACT when used with heparin, and prolonged neuromuscular blockade can be seen in patients on succinylcholine.

Adverse Effects

Adverse effects are anaphylaxis, arrhythmias, MI, heart failure, cerebrovascular events, chest pain, hypotension, pericardial effusion, pulmonary hypertension, fever, seizures, dizziness, hyperglycemia, hypokalemia, acidosis, nausea, vomiting, constipation, diarrhea, GI hemorrhage, hemolysis, anemia, thrombosis, liver damage, phlebitis, arthralgia, renal failure, bronchoconstriction, pulmonary edema, and apnea.

Poisoning Information

Carefully monitor patients for the occurrence of toxicity. Signs and symptoms of aprotinin overdose include possible liver or tubular necrosis (acute) at a dose of 15 million KIU.[8] Treatment of mild to moderate anaphylactic reactions includes an antihistamine with or without β-agonists, corticosteroids, or epinephrine. Severe reactions can necessitate oxygen and airway management.

Compatible Diluents

Aprotinin is incompatible with corticosteroids, amino acid solutions, fat emulsions, heparin, and tetracyclines.

Administration

All patients treated with aprotinin should first receive a 1-mL test dose at least 10 minutes before the loading dose to assess for a potential allergic reaction; patients who have received aprotinin in the past are at increased rate of anaphylactic reactions and should be pretreated with an antihistamine and H2 blocker before administration of the loading dose. Rapid I.V. infusion may cause a transient fall in blood pressure. All doses should be administered via a central line. Administer the loading dose over 20 to 30 minutes with patient in supine position; no other medications should be present in the same line.

Argatroban

Indication

Argatroban is used in the United States for prophylaxis or treatment of thrombosis in adults with heparin-induced thrombocytopenia (HIT) and as an adjunct to percutaneous coronary intervention (PCI) in patients who have or are at risk of coronary artery thrombosis associated with HIT.

Off-label use of argatroban includes treatment of cerebral thrombosis and MI.

Mechanism of Action

Argatroban is a direct, highly selective thrombin inhibitor that reversibly binds to thrombin's active site. Argatroban also inhibits fibrin formation, activation of coagulation Factors V, VIII, and XIII, protein C, and platelet aggregation.

Dosing

Argatroban does not currently have a pediatric indication. Dosing used in this population remains undefined and widely variable. Recommendations on dosing have been extrapolated from the adult literature; however, because of ontogenic differences, such as metabolism, extrapolation may not be accurate. Hursting et al. reported a wide range of doses (0.1–12 μg/kg/min) in pediatric patients for either the prophylaxis or treatment of thrombosis to achieve therapeutic levels of anticoagulation.[9] Children often need higher doses than adults to achieve these therapeutic levels because of increased hepatic metabolism. Neonates and infants, however, may have immature development and function of the liver and require dosing on the more conservative side of the range.[10]

Pharmacokinetics

The onset of action of argatroban is immediate, with a volume of distribution of 174 mL/kg. Protein binding to albumin is 20%, and to α_1-acid glycoprotein is 35%. Metabolism is hepatic via hydroxylation and aromatization. The elimination half-life of argatroban is 39 to 51 minutes and can be as long as 181 minutes in patients with hepatic impairment. The time to steady state is 1 to 3 hours. Excretion is 65% in feces and 22% in the urine.

Monitoring Parameters

Hemoglobin, hematocrit, signs and symptoms of bleeding, liver function tests, and daily international normalized ratio (INR) (if receiving additional warfarin therapy) should be monitored. For HIT, obtain baseline aPTT before start of therapy and check aPTT every 2 hours after initiation of therapy until therapeutic dose has been reached. Adjust the dose, keeping the steady-state aPTT 1.5 to 3 times the initial baseline value (not exceeding 100 s). In PCI, monitor ACT before dosing, 5 to 10 minutes after the bolus dose, and every 5 to 10 minutes thereafter until therapeutic level has been reached. ACT assessments should be made every 20 to 30 minutes during extended procedures.

Contraindications

Contraindications to argatroban are hypersensitivity to argatroban or major bleeding.

Precautions/Warning

Caution should be taken in administering argatroban to patients with increased risk of hemorrhage (e.g., severe hypertension); immediately after lumbar puncture, spinal anesthesia, or major surgery; with congenital or acquired bleeding disorders; or with GI ulcers. Bleeding can occur at any site in the body. Use caution in critically ill patients and patients with hepatic dysfunction.

Drug/Drug Interactions

Drugs that affect platelet function, such as aspirin, nonsteroidal anti-inflammatory drugs (NSAIDs), abciximab, anagrelide, cilostazol, clopidogrel, dipyridamole, eptifibatide, ticlopidine, and tirofiban may potentiate the risk of bleeding. Anticoagulant drugs, such as acenocoumarol, antithrombin III, bivalirudin, dalteparin, danaparoid, drotrecogin alfa, enoxaparin, fondaparinux, heparin, hirudin, lepirudin, nadroparin, tinzaparin, and warfarin can also cause an increased risk of bleeding.

Adverse Effects
Potential adverse effects with argatroban administration are chest pain, hypotension, bleeding, cardiac arrest, ventricular tachycardia, bradycardia, MI, atrial fibrillation, angina, myocardial ischemia, cerebrovascular accident, thrombosis, fever, headache, pain, intracranial bleeding, nausea, diarrhea, vomiting, abdominal pain, urinary tract infection, back pain, abnormal renal function, dyspnea, and cough.

Poisoning Information
A minimum toxic dose of argatroban in humans has not been established. Treatment of possible overdose is symptomatic and supportive, with no specific antidotes available. Monitor for signs of bleeding, vital signs, electrocardiogram, and renal and hepatic function in symptomatic patients. Discontinue or decrease infusion to control excessive anticoagulation with or without bleeding. Reversal of anticoagulant effects may be longer than 4 hours in patients with hepatic impairment. Hemodialysis may remove up to 20% of the drug; however, this is considered clinically insignificant.

Compatible Diluents/Administration
The final concentration for I.V. administration of argatroban is 1 mg/mL. The injectable solution of argatroban may be mixed with NS, D5W, or LR, and may show slight haziness. Do not use if the solution is cloudy. Argatroban is incompatible with other medications.

Aspirin

Indication
In the United States, aspirin is used for the prevention of mortality during suspected acute MI as well as prophylaxis of a recurrent MI; prevention of MI in patients with angina; prevention of recurrent stroke and mortality after a TIA or stroke; adjunctive therapy in coronary artery bypass graft, percutaneous transluminal coronary angioplasty, and carotid endarterectomy; and prevention of thrombosis in patients supported with a ventricular assist device and in patients with endovascular stents. Off-label use of aspirin includes the treatment of Kawasaki Disease and to prevent thrombosis in patients after single ventricle palliation with a shunt, bidirectional Glenn, or Fontan procedure.

Mechanism of Action

Aspirin is a salicylic derivative that inhibits both prostaglandin synthesis and platelet aggregation. Aspirin acts on the hypothalamus heat-regulating center to reduce fever.

Dosing

Children:

Analgesic and antipyretic (oral, rectal): 10 to 15 mg/kg/dose every 4 to 6 hours; maximum dose, 4 grams/day

Anti-inflammatory (oral): initial, 80 to 100 mg/kg/day in divided doses

Kawasaki Disease (oral): 80 to 100 mg/kg/day divided every 6 hours for 2 weeks, then 3 to 5 mg/kg/day once daily for 7 weeks or longer

Antiplatelet effects: adequate pediatric studies have not been performed, therefore, the dose is not well established. Doses ranging from 3 to 10 mg/kg/day administered as a single daily dose have been used; doses are rounded to a convenient amount; maximum, 325 mg/dose

Mechanical heart valves: 6 to 20 mg/kg/day either alone or in combination with dipyridamole

Blalock-Taussig shunt and endovascular stents:[2,11] 1 to 5 mg/kg/day

Fontan procedure: 5 mg/kg/day

Arterial ischemic stroke: 2 to 5 mg/kg/day after discontinuation of anticoagulants

Adults:

Analgesic and antipyretic (oral, rectal): 325 to 1000 mg every 4 to 6 hours (up to 4 grams/day)

Anti-inflammatory (oral): 2.4 to 5.4 grams/day in divided doses; monitor serum concentrations

TIA (oral): 1.3 grams/day in two to four divided doses

Prevention of stroke after ischemic stroke or TIA (oral): 40.5 to 325 mg once daily

Suspected acute MI (oral): initial, 162.5 mg as soon as MI is suspected; then 162.5 mg once daily for 30 days after MI; then consider further aspirin treatment

MI prophylaxis: 81 to 325 mg/day

Pharmacokinetics

Absorption is from the stomach and small intestine. The immediate-release formulation is completely absorbed, whereas the enteric-coated form is erratically absorbed. The drug is widely distributed and is metabolized in the liver. The half-life of the active drug is 6 hours with a time-to-peak serum concentration being 1 to 2 hours (this may be delayed with controlled- or timed-release preparations). Elimination is renal and aspirin is 50 to 100% dialyzable.

Monitoring Parameters
CBC, chemistry profile, blood pressure, fecal occult blood test, liver function at initiation of therapy and every 6 to 12 months thereafter should be monitored. Obtain serum salicylate concentration with chronic use.

Contraindications
Contraindications to aspirin use are hypersensitivity to salicylates or other NSAIDs, bleeding disorders, hepatic failure, and children with chickenpox or flu symptoms because of the risk of Reye's syndrome.[12]

Precautions/Warnings
Use caution in administering aspirin to patients with bleeding disorders, erosive gastritis, peptic ulcer disease, renal failure, and severe hepatic insufficiency. Patients with asthma, rhinitis, or nasal polyps may be more sensitive to the effects of salicylates.

Drug/Drug Interactions
Anticoagulants, such as acenocoumarin, antithrombin III, argatroban, bivalirudin, dalteparin, danaparoid, drotrecogin alfa, enoxaparin, fondaparinux, heparin, hirudin, lepirudin, nadroparin, tinzaparin, and warfarin; other salicylate medications, such as aminosalicylic acid, choline magnesium trisalicylate, salsalate, and sodium salicylate; and NSAIDs, can potentiate bleeding.

Combination therapy of salicylates and carbonic anhydrase inhibitors, such as acetazolamide, brinzolamide, dichlorphenamide, dorzolamide, and methazolamide, has resulted in significant metabolic acidosis in pediatric and adult patients. Salicylates may diminish the antihypertensive effect of ACE inhibitors and may enhance the hypoglycemic effect of sulfonylureas. Aspirin may enhance the adverse GI effects (ulceration or bleeding) of alendronate and systemic corticosteroids, whereas antacids may increase the excretion of salicylates. Nondihydropyridine calcium channel blockers (diltiazem and verapamil) may enhance the anticoagulant effect of salicylates. Salicylates may enhance the adverse/toxic effect of varicella virus-containing vaccines causing Reye's syndrome, and they may increase serum concentration of methotrexate.

Adverse Effects
Adverse effects of aspirin use include rash, urticaria, nausea, vomiting, dyspepsia, epigastric discomfort, occult bleeding, prolongation of bleeding time, leukopenia, thrombocytopenia, hepatotoxicity, bronchospasm, tinnitus, headache, dizziness, confusion, metabolic acidosis, and hyperpyrexia.

Poisoning Information

Salicylate serum concentrations correlate with the pharmacological actions, and adverse effects are observed with serum salicylate levels of approximately 100 mg/dL. Patients with mild-to-moderate intoxication may develop fever, tachypnea, tinnitus, respiratory alkalosis, metabolic acidosis, lethargy, mild dehydration, nausea, and vomiting. Severe intoxication may result in encephalopathy, coma, hypotension, pulmonary edema, seizures, acidemia, coagulopathy, cerebral edema, and dysrhythmias. Treatment of accidental or chronic ingestion is supportive and can include the use of activated charcoal and gastric lavage. Sodium bicarbonate is used to alkalinize the urine and prevent acidosis. Hemodialysis can be considered for patients with high blood salicylate levels (>80 to 100 mg/dL after acute overdose, >50 to 60 mg/dL after chronic overdose).

Compatible Diluents/Administration

For oral administration, administer aspirin with water, food, or milk to decrease GI upset. Do not crush or chew controlled-release, timed-release, or enteric-coated tablets; these are designed to be swallowed whole.

Clopidogrel

Indication

In the United States, clopidogrel has been used in adults with acute coronary syndrome, cerebrovascular accident, MI, PCI, and peripheral arterial occlusive disease. The safety and efficacy in pediatric patients have not yet been established.

Mechanism of Action

Clopidogrel blocks adenosine diphosphate receptors, preventing fibrinogen binding and platelet adhesion and aggregation.

Dosing

Children: Safety and efficacy in pediatric patients are not established; however, clopidogrel has been used in pediatric patients, with data published in infants as young as 6 weeks of age. The dose most commonly used was 1 mg/kg/day (range, 1 to 6 mg/kg/day) by mouth. Clopidogrel was generally well tolerated in the study subjects.[13,14] Soman et al. reported two patients who developed intracranial hemorrhage after receiving both clopidogrel and aspirin for arterial ischemic strokes. Thus, caution should be used in patients with increased risk factors for intracranial hemorrhage and those with intracranial vasculopathies.

Clopidogrel has been used in addition to aspirin therapy in patients with Kawasaki's Disease and giant coronary artery aneurysms. Although there are no published studies in children, doses of 1 mg/kg/day by mouth to a maximum adult dose (75 mg/day) have been used.[15]

Adults:

Recent MI, stroke, or established arterial disease: 75 mg by mouth once daily

Acute coronary syndrome: initial, 300 mg loading dose, followed by 75 mg once daily by mouth (in combination with 75–325 mg aspirin once daily)

PCI: prophylaxis 300 mg before PCI, then 75 mg daily by mouth for 1 month

Dosage adjustment in renal insufficiency: not necessary

Pharmacokinetics

Inhibition of platelet aggregation is detected 2 hours after a 300-mg oral dose is administered. Clopidogrel is well absorbed, with a time-to-peak concentration of 1 hour and at least 50% bioavailability. Clopidogrel is 98% protein bound. It is metabolized extensively through the liver via hydrolysis, with production of an inactive metabolite that is a carboxyl acid derivative. The elimination half-life is 8 hours, with 50% renal excretion and 46% fecal excretion.

Monitoring Parameters

Signs of bleeding, CBC with differential, bleeding time, liver function tests, and periodic hemoglobin and hematocrit should be monitored.

Contraindications

Contraindications to clopidogrel administration are hypersensitivity to clopidogrel and active bleeding (e.g., peptic ulcer disease or intracranial hemorrhage).

Precautions/Warning

Use clopidogrel with caution in patients who may be at risk of increased bleeding. Clopidogrel should be discontinued 5 days before elective surgery. There is an increased risk of bleeding when clopidogrel is used concurrently with other antiplatelet drugs. Use clopidogrel with caution in patients with severe liver disease and renal impairment. Cases of life-threatening thrombotic thrombocytopenic purpura (TTP) have been reported, requiring urgent plasmapheresis.

Drug/Drug Interactions

Anticoagulants or other antiplatelet agents may increase the risk of bleeding. Clopidogrel may increase the antiplatelet effect of aspirin; bleeding time is not prolonged related to clopidogrel alone. Atorvastatin and macrolide antibiotics may attenuate the effects of clopidogrel, and additional monitoring is required. Drotrecogin alfa may increase the risk of bleeding. Concurrent use of NSAIDs may increase GI effects, including GI blood loss. Rifampin may increase the effects of clopidogrel. Thrombolytics may increase the risk of bleeding.

Adverse Effects

With clopidogrel use, bleeding may occur at virtually any site. Other effects include GI side effects, chest pain, edema, hypertension, headache, dizziness, depression, fatigue, general pain, rash, pruritus, hypercholesterolemia, abnormal liver function tests, arthralgia, back pain, dyspnea, rhinitis, bronchitis, cough, flu-like syndrome, atrial fibrillation, cardiac failure, syncope, fever, eczema, gout, hyperuricemia, GI hemorrhage, cystitis, hematoma, anemia, arthritis, leg cramps, neuralgia, paresthesias, weakness, cataracts, and conjunctivitis.

Postmarketing and/or case reports have reported acute liver failure, aplastic anemia, angioedema, erythema multiforme, hepatitis, hypersensitivity, interstitial pneumonitis, lichen planus, pancreatitis, pancytopenia, serum sickness, Stevens-Johnson syndrome, stomatitis, TTP, toxic epidermal necrolysis, and vasculitis.

Poisoning Information

Treatment of clopidogrel overdose is supportive and symptomatic. There is no antidote. However, activated charcoal may be used to help decontaminate. Symptoms of acute toxicity include vomiting, prostration, difficulty breathing, and GI hemorrhage.

Administration

Clopidogrel can be taken with or without food. Take with food if upset stomach occurs.

Dipyridamole

Indication

In the United States, dipyridamole has been used in myocardial imaging and for prophylaxis of prosthetic cardiac valve thrombosis and prosthetic cardiac valve-related embolism. Dipyridamole is also used as a diagnostic agent for coronary artery disease. Off-label indications include maintenance of patency after surgical grafting procedures, including coronary artery bypass and prevention of thromboembolic disorders. Dipyridamole has been used in addition to aspirin therapy for the prevention and treatment of coronary thrombosis in patients with Kawasaki's Disease.

Mechanism of Action

Dipyridamole inhibits the activity of adenosine deaminase and phosphodiesterase, causing an accumulation of adenosine, adenine nucleotides, and cyclic AMP that, together, inhibit platelet aggregation, cause vasodilation, and decrease platelet activation.

Dosing

Children: oral, 3 to 6 mg/kg/day in three divided doses. Doses of 4 to 10 mg/kg/day have been used investigationally to reduce the risk of thromboembolism related to proteinuria in pediatric renal disease

Mechanical prosthetic heart valves: 2 to 5 mg/kg/day (used in combination with an oral anticoagulant in children who have systemic embolism despite adequate oral anticoagulant therapy [INR, 2.5–3.5], and used in combination with low-dose oral anticoagulation [INR, 2–3] plus aspirin in children in whom full-dose oral anticoagulation is contraindicated[2])

Kawasaki Disease: although there are no published studies in children, doses of 2 to 6 mg/kg/day orally in three divided doses have been used[15]

Adults:

Prophylaxis of thromboembolism after cardiac valve replacement (adjunctive use): oral, 75 to 100 mg, four times per day

Dipyridamole stress test (for evaluation of myocardial perfusion): I.V., 0.142 mg/kg/min for a total of 4 minutes (0.57 mg/kg total); maximum dose, 60 mg; inject thallium 201 within 5 minutes after the end of injection of dipyridamole

Pharmacokinetics

Dipyridamole has a slow systemic absorption, with 27 to 66% bioavailability and peak serum concentration within 2 to 2.5 hours. Protein binding is 91 to 99%. Metabolism is hepatic and excretion is biliary. Elimination half-life is 10 to 12 hours.

Monitoring Parameters

Blood pressure, heart rate, electrocardiogram, and vital signs during I.V. infusion; and hepatic function should be monitored.

Contraindications
Hypersensitivity to dipyridamole products is a contraindication to use.

Precautions/Warning
Use caution in administering dipyridamole to patients with hypotension; patients on antiplatelet agents or anticoagulation; or patients with severe coronary artery disease or abnormal cardiac rhythm. Use the I.V. form with caution in patients with Bronchospastie disease or instable angina.

Drug/Drug Interaction
Heparin, warfarin, streptokinase, urokinase, aspirin, alteplase, NSAIDs, cefamandole, cefoperazone, cefotetan, and valproic acid may increase risk of bleeding; decreased coronary artery vasodilation from I.V. dipyridamole may occur in patients receiving theophylline or caffeine.

Adverse Effects
Potential adverse effects of dipyridamole are headache (dose-related), vasodilation, hypotension, flushing, weakness, dizziness, syncope, rash, pruritus, abdominal distress, and diarrhea. Rare but serious effects include angina pectoris, MI, ventricular arrhythmia, and bronchospasm.

Poisoning Information
Use of the I.V. form of dipyridamole has been associated with bronchospasm and chest pain. Use with caution in patients with bronchospastic disease or unstable angina. Bronchodilators should be available in case of bronchospasm with I.V. use. Based on limited experience, signs, and symptoms of oxidose include hypotension, dizziness, headache, weakness, facial flushing, and fainting.

Compatible Diluents/Administration
Dilute I.V. dipyridamole in at least a 1:2 ratio with D5W, NS, or 0.45% NaCl and infuse over 4 minutes.

Enoxaparin

Indication
Enoxaparin is indicated for prophylaxis and treatment of thromboembolic disorders.

Mechanism of Action
Enoxaparin is low molecular weight heparin (LMWH) that inactivates coagulation Factor Xa and Factor IIa (thrombin) activities.

Dosing

Children:
>*Initial S.Q.:*
>>Infants younger than 2 months: prophylaxis, 0.75 mg/kg every 12 hours; treatment, 1.5 mg/kg every 12 hours
>>Infants older than 2 months and children at most 18 years: prophylaxis, 0.5 mg/kg every 12 hours; treatment, 1 mg/kg every 12 hours
>>*Maintenance (see below):* Note: in a recent prospective study of 177 courses of enoxaparin in pediatric patients (146 treatment courses and 31 prophylactic courses), considerable variation in maintenance dosage requirements was observed[16,17]

>*Relationship between anti-Factor Xa concentrations and dosage titrations:*[2]
>Goal anti-Factor Xa level 4 hours after enoxaparin dosing: prophylaxis, 0.2 to 0.4 Units/mL; treatment, 0.5 to 1 Units/mL

>>If the anti-Factor Xa level is between 0 and at most 0.35 Units/mL, then increase dose by 25% and repeat anti-Factor Xa level 4 hours after the next dose
>>If the anti-Factor Xa level is between 0.35 and 0.49 Units/mL, then increase dose by 10% and repeat anti-Factor Xa level 4 hours after the next dose
>>If the anti-Factor Xa level is between 1.1 and at most 1.5 Units/mL, then decrease dose by 20% and repeat anti-Factor Xa level before the next scheduled dose and then 4 hours after the dose is administered.
>>If the anti-Factor Xa level is between 1.6 and at most 2 Units/mL, then hold the dose for 3 hours and decrease the next dose by 30%. Repeat anti-Factor Xa level before next dose and then 4 hours after the dose is administered
>>If the anti-Factor Xa level is greater than 2 Units/mL, then hold the dose until the anti-Factor Xa level has come down to 0.5 Units/mL and decrease the dose by 40%. Repeat anti-Factor Xa level before the next dose until the level has come down to 0.5 Units/mL and then check level 4 hours after the next dose is administered

Adults: consider lower doses for patients weighing less than 45 kg
>*Treatment of acute deep vein thrombosis (DVT) and pulmonary embolism:* initiate warfarin therapy when appropriate (usually within 72 h of starting enoxaparin); continue enoxaparin for a minimum of 5 days (average, 7 days) until INR is therapeutic
>*Inpatient treatment of acute DVT with or without pulmonary embolism:* 1 mg/kg S.Q. every 12 hours or 1.5 mg/kg S.Q. once daily
>*Outpatient treatment of acute DVT without pulmonary embolism:* 1 mg/kg S.Q. every 12 hours
>*Dosage adjustment in renal impairment:*
>>S.Q., creatinine clearance (Cl_{cr}) at least 30 mL/min: no specific adjustment recommended; monitor patients closely for bleeding
>>Cl_{cr} less than 30 mL/min: DVT prophylaxis in abdominal surgery, hip replacement, knee replacement, or in medical patients during acute illness, 30 mg S.Q. once daily

DVT treatment in conjunction with warfarin (in inpatients with or without pulmonary embolism and in outpatients without pulmonary embolism): 1 mg/kg S.Q. once daily

Pharmacokinetics

Based on anti-Factor Xa, enoxaparin is 100% bioavailable after S.Q. injection with maximal effect in 3 to 5 hours and a duration of approximately 12 hours. Enoxaparin does not cross the placental barrier and does not bind to most heparin-binding proteins. Metabolism is hepatic via desulfation and depolymerization. Enoxaparin is renally excreted, 40% as active and inactive fragments and 10% as unchanged drug. The half-life for adults via S.Q. administration route is 4.5 hours for a single dose and 7 hours for repeat dosing.

Monitoring Parameters

The following should be monitored: CBC with platelets, liver function tests, stool testing for occult blood, and anti-Factor Xa activity (especially in patients with significant renal impairment, active bleeding, or abnormal coagulation parameters); and blood pressure and symptoms of bleeding; consider monitoring bone density in infants and children with long-term use.

Contraindications

Contraindications to enoxaparin use are hypersensitivity to enoxaparin, heparin, pork products, or benzyl alcohol; patients with active major bleeding; and patients with thrombocytopenia.

Precautions/Warning

There is an increased risk of epidural or spinal hematoma with concomitant neuraxial or spinal puncture and LMWHs, or concurrent use of drugs that impair hemostasis and/or postoperative use of indwelling catheters. Use enoxaparin with caution in patients with any increased risk of hemorrhage, uncontrolled hypertension, or renal impairment.

Drug/Drug Interactions

Anticoagulants, thrombolytic agents (alteplase, streptokinase, and urokinase), and platelet inhibitors (aspirin, salicylates, NSAIDs, dipyridamole, and sulfinpyrazone) may increase the risk of bleeding.

Adverse Effects

Potential adverse effects of enoxaparin use are edema, diarrhea, nausea, hematoma, normocytic hypochromic anemia, confusion, pain, dyspnea, fever, local irritation, atrial fibrillation, heart failure, eczema, skin necrosis, hemorrhage, thrombocytopenia, increased liver function tests, anaphylactoid reaction, hematoma, pneumonia, and pulmonary edema.

Poisoning Information

Therapeutic reference ranges for anti-Factor Xa levels are between 0.5 and 1 Units/mL for treatment and 0.2 to 0.4 Units/mL for prophylaxis. Treatment of severe bleeding or an overdose of enoxaparin is supportive. Protamine may be used at dosage of 1 mg of protamine for each milligram of enoxaparin administered. An additional dose of 0.5 mg protamine per 1 mg enoxaparin may be considered if the aPTT continues to be prolonged 2 to 4 hours after first dose of protamine.

Compatible Diluents/Administration

Do not administer enoxaparin I.M., only S.Q.; rotate sites between the left and right anterolateral and left and right posterolateral abdominal wall; enoxaparin dilutions of 20 mg/mL in NS have been used for smaller doses in neonates.

Heparin

Indication

Heparin is indicated for prophylaxis and treatment of thromboembolic disorders.

Mechanism of Action

Anticoagulation by heparin is mediated by the enzyme inhibitor, antithrombin III, which primarily inactivates thrombin. In addition, heparin also inactivates other proteases, including Factors IX, X, XI, XII, and plasmin, and it also prevents the conversion of fibrinogen to fibrin. Antithrombin III levels are low at birth, and preterm infants have even more significantly reduced levels. Interestingly, infants also have a decreased production of thrombin and have similar levels when compared with heparinized adults.[18]

Dosing

> **Prophylaxis for cardiac catheterization via an artery:**
> *Newborns and children:* bolus, 100 to 150 Units/kg I.V
> **Systemic heparinization:**
> *Neonates and infants:* I.V. infusion, initial loading dose, 50 to 75 Units/kg administered over 10 minutes; initial maintenance dose, 20 Units/kg/hour; adjust dose to maintain aPTT of 60 to 85 seconds (assuming this reflects an anti-Factor Xa level of 0.3–0.7); see also recommendations in Table 11-1

Table 11-1

APTT (s)	Dosage adjustment
< 50	Administer 25–50 Units/kg I.V. bolus (based on clinical judgment) and increase infusion rate by 20%
50–59	Increase infusion rate by 10%
> 90	Hold infusion for 1 h and decrease infusion rate by 10–15%

Heparin dosing adjustment (continuous infusion)

Children older than 1 year: I.V. infusion, initial loading dose, 50 to 75 Units/kg administered over 10 minutes; initial maintenance dose, 20 Units/kg/hour; adjust dose to maintain aPTT of 60 to 85 seconds; see also recommendations in Table 11-1.

Loading dose can be modified based on preexisting condition

Systemic heparin adjustment:

General guidelines: target range and dose will need to be adjusted based on clinical conditions. The adjustments given here are to be used after an initial loading dose; the maintenance dose is adjusted to maintain an aPTT of 60 to 80 seconds. Obtain blood to measure aPTT 4 hours after heparin loading dose and 4 hours after every infusion rate change

Adults:

Prophylaxis (low-dose heparin): S.Q., 5000 Units every 8 to 12 hours

Intermittent I.V.: initial, 5000 to 10,000 Units, then 5000 to 10,000 Units every 4 to 6 hours

I.V. infusion: initial loading dose, 80 Units/kg I.V.; initial maintenance dose, 18 Units/kg/hour (or 1000–1250 Units/hour), with dose adjusted according to aPTT; usual range, 10 to 30 Units/kg/hour

Pharmacokinetics

Onset of anticoagulation action when heparin is administered I.V. is immediate, and is 20 to 30 minutes when administered S.Q. However, absorption of drug when heparin is administered S.Q. or I.M. is erratic. Heparin does not cross the placenta and does not appear in breast milk. Protein binding is 95%. Heparin is metabolized via the liver and through the reticuloendothelial system. It is eliminated renally in small amounts as unchanged drug, with a half-life of 90 minutes and a range of 1 to 2 hours. Factors that can prolong the half-life include obesity, renal dysfunction, hepatic dysfunction, malignancy, infection, and the presence of pulmonary embolism.

Monitoring Parameters

Thromboelastogram, CBC, hemoglobin, hematocrit, signs of bleeding, PT, aPTT, stool occult blood tests, and liver function should be monitored.

Contraindications

Contraindications for heparin use are hypersensitivity to heparin or any component; uncontrollable active bleeding (unless secondary to disseminated intravascular coagulation); severe thrombocytopenia; and suspected or confirmed intracranial hemorrhage; shock, severe hypotension.

Precautions/Warnings
Preservative-free heparin should be used in neonates to prevent neonatal gasping syndrome.[19] Use heparin with caution in patients who may be at risk of bleeding; there is a risk of hemorrhage with I.M. injections, peptic ulcer disease, subacute bacterial endocarditis, or in patients with severe hypertension.

Drug/Drug Interactions
Thrombolytic agents (urokinase, streptokinase) and drugs that affect platelet function (e.g., aspirin, NSAIDs, dipyridamole, ticlopidine, clopidogrel, IIb/IIIa antagonists, and parenteral penicillins) may potentiate the risk of hemorrhage; I.V. nitroglycerin may decrease heparin's anticoagulant effect, antihistamines, tetracycline, quinine, nicotine, and digoxin have been reported to interfere with the anticoagulant effect of heparin.

Adverse Effects
Potential adverse effects of heparin are hemorrhage, thrombocytopenia, increased liver aminotransferase level, anaphylaxis, erythema, pain at the injection site, chest pain, fever, headache, chills, cutaneous necrosis with S.Q. injections, and osteoporosis with long-term use.

Poisoning Information
Bleeding is the primary symptom of overdose. The antidote is protamine. One milligram of protamine neutralizes 100 Units of heparin. Discontinue all heparin if evidence of progressive immune thrombocytopenia occurs.

Compatible Diluents/Administration
Because of pain, irritation, and hematoma, it is recommended that heparin not be administered I.M.; continuous I.V. infusion should be administered via a controlled infusion device; rotate the S.Q. administration site; heparin is compatible with 0.9% NaCl, dextrose solutions, and parenteral nutrition solutions.

Lepirudin

Indication
In the United States, lepirudin has been used for anticoagulation in patients with HIT and associated thromboembolic disease. Off-label use includes prophylaxis for MI.

Mechanism of Action

Lepirudin is a highly specific, direct thrombin inhibitor in which one molecule of lepirudin binds to one molecule of thrombin; lepirudin increases a PTT in a dose-dependent fashion.

Dosing

Pediatric dosing for lepirudin has not been established.

Adults:

Maximum dose: do not exceed 0.21 mg/kg/hour I.V. unless an evaluation of the coagulation abnormalities that limit the response to other agents has been completed. Dosing is weight based, however, patients weighing more than 110 kg should not receive doses greater than the recommended dose for a patient weighing 110 kg (44 mg I.V. bolus and initial maximal infusion rate of 16.5 mg/hour I.V.)

HIT: bolus dose, 0.4 mg/kg I.V. push over 15 to 20 seconds followed by continuous infusion at 0.15 mg/kg/hour; bolus and infusion doses must be reduced in renal insufficiency. *Note:* because of potential renal insufficiency in critically ill patients, some clinicians suggest that for HIT <u>without</u> thromboembolic complications, the initial infusion rate should be 0.1 mg/kg/hour I.V. (omit the initial bolus dose unless acute HIT exists)

Concomitant use with thrombolytic therapy: bolus dose, 0.2 mg/kg I.V. push over 15 to 20 seconds, followed by continuous infusion at 0.1 mg/kg/hour I.V.

Dosing adjustments during infusions: monitor first aPTT 4 hours after the start of the infusion. Subsequent determinations of aPTT should be obtained at least once daily during treatment. More frequent monitoring is recommended in renally impaired patients. Any aPTT ratio measurement out of range (1.5–2.5) should be confirmed before adjusting dose, unless a clinical need for immediate reaction exists. If the aPTT is below target range, increase infusion by 20%. If the aPTT is in excess of the target range, stop infusion for 2 hours. When the infusion is restarted, the dose should be decreased by 50%. A repeat aPTT should be obtained 4 hours after any dosing change[16]

Use in patients scheduled for conversion to oral anticoagulants: reduce lepirudin dose gradually to reach aPTT ratio just above 1.5 before starting warfarin therapy; as soon as INR reaches 2, lepirudin therapy should be discontinued[16]

Dosing adjustment in renal impairment: all patients with a Cl_{Cr} of less than 60 mL/min or a serum creatinine (SCr) of greater than 1.5 mg/dL should receive a reduction in lepirudin dosage; there is only limited information regarding the therapeutic use of lepirudin in HIT patients with significant renal impairment; the following dosage recommendations are mainly based on single-dose studies in a small number of patients with renal impairment:

Initial: bolus dose, 0.2 mg/kg I.V. push over 15 to 20 seconds, followed by adjusted infusion based on renal function; refer to the following infusion rate adjustments based on Cl_{Cr} (mL/min) and SCr (mg/dL):

Lepirudin infusion rates in patients with renal impairment:

Cl_{Cr} 45 to 60 mL/min; or SCr 1.6 to 2 mg/dL: decrease infusion rate by 50%

Cl_{Cr} 30 to 44 mL/min; or SCr 2.1 to 3 mg/dL: decrease infusion rate by 70%

Cl_{Cr} 15 to 29 mL/min; or SCr 3.1 to 6 mg/dL: decrease infusion rate by 85%

Cl_{Cr} less than 15 mL/min; or SCr greater than 6 mg/dL: stop infusion

Note: in acute renal failure or hemodialysis, infusion is to be avoided or stopped. After the bolus dose, additional bolus doses of 0.1 mg/kg I.V. may be administered every other day, but only if aPTT falls below the lower therapeutic limit[16]

Pharmacokinetics

Lepirudin is confined to extracellular fluids and is metabolized by the release of amino acids via catabolic hydrolysis of parent drug. The elimination half-life is ~10 minutes and the termimal half-life in healthy volunteers is 1.3 hours; in patients with renal impairment, the half-life is at most 2 days; 48% of lepirudin is excreted as unchanged drug in the urine.

Monitoring Parameters

The following parameters should be monitored: aPTT, with monitoring to start 4 hours after the initiation of infusion and then daily, check aPTT 4 hours after any change in dosing; CBC; liver function; renal function; and blood pressure.

Contraindications

Contraindications are hypersensitivity to hirudin products or any components of the formulation, and active major bleeding.

Precautions/Warnings

Use lepirudin with caution in patients who are at risk of bleeding, patients with severe hypertension, history of recent major surgery, history of recent major bleeding, recent cerebrovascular accident, liver dysfunction, GI ulceration, and bacterial endocarditis. Use with caution in patients with renal impairment or cirrhosis.

Drug/Drug Interactions

Thrombolytic agents (urokinase, streptokinase) and drugs that affect platelet function (e.g., aspirin, NSAIDs, dipyridamole, ticlopidine, clopidogrel, IIb/IIIa antagonists, parenteral penicillins) may potentiate the risk of hemorrhage; an increased risk of bleeding can also occur with concurrent therapy with warfarin.

Adverse Effects

Potential adverse effects are bleeding (e.g., GI, rectal), hematoma, anemia, fever, heart failure, pericardial effusion, ventricular fibrillation, eczema, maculopapular rash, abnormal liver function tests, hematuria, epistaxis, renal failure, pneumonia, sepsis, thrombocytopenia, and anaphylaxis.

Poisoning Information

There are no specific antidotes for direct thrombin inhibitors. Treatment of lepirudin overdose is symptomatic and supportive, with management directed toward the control of bleeding.

Compatible Diluents/Administration

Reconstitute a 50-mg vial of lepirudin with 1 mL of sterile water for injection or 0.9% NaCl, and shake gently. For **bolus** infusions, further dilute lepirudin to a final concentration of 5 mg/mL and administer I.V. over 15 to 20 seconds. For **continuous infusions,** further dilute lepirudin to a final concentration of 0.2 mg/mL or 0.4 mg/mL. Lepirudin is compatible with 0.9% NaCl or D5W.

Protamine

Indication

Protamine is used for the treatment of heparin overdose. Protamine is also used to neutralize heparin during surgery or dialysis procedures.

Mechanism of Action

Protamine is a weak anticoagulant that combines with strongly acidic heparin to form a stable salt complex that neutralizes the anticoagulant activity of both drugs.

In addition, it seems that protamine can inhibit the inactivation of thrombin by antithrombin III and is a competitive inhibitor of the thrombin-fibrinogen interaction.[18]

Dosing

Protamine dose is dependent on most recent dosage of heparin or LMWH. One milligram of protamine will neutralize 115 Units of porcine intestinal heparin, 90 Units of beef lung heparin, and 1 mg (100 Units) of LMWH; the maximum dose is 50 mg. Based on these dosing guidelines, Table 11-2 shows the appropriate dose of protamine to be administered according to the time that has elapsed since heparin was administered.[21]

Heparin administered by S.Q. injection: 1 to 1.5 mg protamine per 100 Units of heparin administered as 25 to 50 mg infused via slow I.V. infusion

Table 11-2

Time since last dose	Dose of protamine
<30 minutes	100% of above dosing recommendations
30–60 minutes	Administer 50–75% of dose
60–120 minutes	Administer 37.5–50% of dose
>120 minutes	Administer 25–37.5% of dose

Source: modified from Lee C, Nechyba C, Gunn VL; Drug doses. Gunn VL, Nechyba C. *The Harriet Lane Handbook.* Philadelphia; Mosby, 2002.

followed by the remaining portion of the calculated dose over 8 to 16 hours or the expected duration of absorption for the heparin

LMWH: if LMWH was administered within the last 4 hours, administer 1 mg protamine per 1 mg (100 Units) LMWH; a second dose of 0.5 mg protamine per 1 mg (100 Units) LMWH may be administered if the aPTT remains prolonged 2 to 4 hours after the first dose

Pharmacokinetics

Heparin neutralization occurs within 5 minutes after I.V. administration; elimination is unknown.

Monitoring Parameters

Coagulation studies, including aPTT and plasma thrombin time; blood pressure; and heart rate should be monitored.

Contraindications

Protamine use is contraindicated with hypersensitivity to protamine or any component.

Precautions/Warning

There is an increased risk of hypersensitivity reactions to protamine in patients who have been previously exposed to protamine or protamine-containing insulin, infertile or vasectomized men, or in patients who have hypersensitivity to fish. Heparin rebound or bleeding have been reported 8 to 18 hours after protamine administration in cardiac surgery patients. In operative settings, protamine administration has been associated with acute hypotension.

Drug/Drug Interactions

Protamine may prolong the effects of insulin.

Adverse Effects

Potential adverse effects of protamine use are bradycardia, flushing, hypotension, nausea, vomiting, dyspnea, pulmonary hypertension, circulatory collapse, capillary leak, and hypersensitivity reactions.

Poisoning Information

Signs and symptoms of protamine overdose include hypertension and bleeding. Treatment of overdose is symptomatic and supportive.

Compatible Diluents/Administration

Reconstitute the protamine vial with 5 mL of sterile water for injection (use preservative-free sterile water for injection for neonates) to yield a final concentration of 10 mg/mL. Administer the solution I.V. without further dilution over 10 minutes, but do not exceed 5 mg/min. The solution may be further diluted with either D5W or 0.9% NaCl. Rapid I.V. infusion may cause hypotension.

Tranexamic Acid

Indication

Tranexamic acid has off-label use in cardiac surgery and cardiopulmonary bypass as a prophylaxis against hemorrhage and to reduce perioperative blood loss in children and adults.

Mechanism of Action

Tranexamic acid competitively inhibits activation of plasminogen by forming a reversible complex that displaces plasminogen from fibrin, resulting in inhibition of fibrinolysis; it also inhibits the proteolytic activity of plasmin.

Dosing

A pediatric prospective, randomized, double-blinded study was conducted to compare tranexamic acid with placebo in decreasing blood loss during repeat cardiac surgery. The study enrolled 43 children (age range, 6 month–12 years) who underwent elective repeat cardiac surgery via sternotomy with cardiopulmonary bypass using a tranexamic acid dose of 100 mg/kg diluted to 20 mL with 0.9% NaCl infused over 15 minutes, after the induction of anesthesia and before incision. A continuous infusion dose of 10 mg/kg/hour was then administered after the initial dose until transport to the intensive care unit.[22]

> **Dosing adjustment in renal impairment (adult data): IV dose (or) oral dose**
> *SCr 1.36 to 2.83 mg/dL:* 10 mg/kg I.V. twice daily; 15 mg/kg orally twice daily
> *SCr greater than 2.83 to 5.66 mg/dL:* 10 mg/kg I.V. once daily; 15 mg/kg orally once daily

SCr greater than 5.66 mg/dL: 10 mg/kg I.V. every other day or 5 mg/kg I.V. once daily; 15 mg/kg orally every other day or 7.5 mg/kg orally once daily

Pharmacokinetics

Systemic bioavailability for oral tranexamic acid tablets is between 30 and 50%, with greater than 95% of drug renally excreted as unchanged drug; 3% is protein bound, and the elimination half-life is 2 to 10 hours.

Monitoring Parameters

Reduction of bleeding with a reference range of 5 to 10 µg/mL is required to decrease fibrinolysis. Ophthalmic exam. Before and after with chrone therapy.

Contraindications

Tranexamic acid is contraindicated with hypersensitivity to tranexamic acid or any component; subarachnoid hemorrhage; or active intravascular clotting process.

Precautions/Warnings

Do not administer tranexamic acid concomitantly with Factor IX complex concentrates or anti-inhibitor coagulant concentrate because of increase risk of thrombosis. Use tranexamic acid with caution in patients with disseminated intravascular coagulation, history of thromboembolic disease, and in patients with cardiovascular, renal, cerebrovascular disease, or transurethral prostatectomy.

Drug/Drug Interactions

Antifibrinolytic agents may enhance the thrombogenic effect; chlorpromazine may increase cerebral vasospasm and ischemia; coadministration of Factor IX complex or anti-inhibitor coagulant concentrates may increase risk of thrombosis.

Adverse Effects

Potential adverse effects are nausea, diarrhea, vomiting, hypotension (caused by rapid injections), and thrombosis.

Poisoning Information

Treatment of tranexamic acid overdose is symptomatic and supportive.

Compatible Diluents/Administration

Tranexamic acid may be administered by direct I.V. injection at a maximum rate of 100 mg/min (use plastic syringe only for I.V. push). Tranexamic acid is compatible with D5W and 0.9% NaCl solutions.

Warfarin

Indication
Warfarin is used as treatment and prophylaxis for atrial fibrillation, thromboembolism related to prosthetic cardiac valves, prosthetic cardiac valve thrombosis, pulmonary embolism, venous thrombosis, and thrombotic disorders.

Mechanism of Action
Warfarin inhibits the vitamin K-dependent clotting factors (II, VII, IX, and X) and the anticoagulant proteins C and S by blocking the regeneration of vitamin K (1) epoxide.

Dosing

> **Infants and children:** oral, goal is to maintain an INR between 2 and 3. Table 11-3 describes initial loading and titration doses
> **Adults:** oral/I.V, 5 to 15 mg/day for 2 to 5 days, then adjust dose according to INR or PT (usual maintenance doses, 2 to 10 mg/day)

Table 11-3

Loading dose	Dose
Day 1 (if baseline INR is 1–1.3)	0.2 mg/kg (maximum dose of 10 mg); 0.1 mg/kg if patient has liver dysfunction
Days 2–4: dose is dependent on patient's INR	
INR	Dose
1.1–1.3	Repeat initial loading dose
1.4–3	Administer 50% of the initial loading dose
3.1–3.5	Administer 25% of the initial loading dose
> 3.5	Hold drug until INR is < 3.5, then restart at 50% less than the previous dose
Maintenance dosing (Day 5 and beyond) based on INR	
INR	Dose
1.1–1.4	Increase dose by 20% of previous dose
1.5–1.9	Increase dose by 10% of previous dose
2–3	Do not change the dose
3.1–3.5	Decrease dose by 10% of previous dose
> 3.5	Hold drug and check INR daily until INR is < 3.5, then restart at 20% less than the previous dose

Pharmacokinetics

Warfarin is rapidly absorbed, with peak concentrations in 4 hours. Warfarin is highly protein bound (99%). Warfarin is metabolized in the liver through the cytochrome P450 system, with a half-life of approximately 42 hours (highly variable). Ninety-two percent of the drug is excreted renally (mainly as metabolites), with the remaining excreted through the biliary tract.

Monitoring Parameters

INR, signs and symptoms of bleeding, stool guaiac tests, hemoglobin, and hematocrit should be monitored.

Contraindications

Contraindications to warfarin use are hypersensitivity to warfarin or any component, severe renal or hepatic impairment, hemorrhagic tendencies, cerebral or dissecting aortic aneurysms, active ulceration, malignant hypertension, bacterial endocarditis, pericarditis and pericardial effusions, surgery, spinal punctures or lumbar block, and pregnancy (severe birth defects have been associated with fetal exposure).

Precautions/Warnings

Skin necrosis and gangrene or systemic cholesterol emboli may occur with warfarin use; use warfarin with caution in patients with diabetes, congestive heart failure, renal or hepatic disease, or malignancy. Use caution in patients with prolonged dietary insufficiencies such as Vitamin K deficiency.

Drug-Drug Interactions

Alcohol, aspirin, NSAIDs, sucralfate, carbamazepine, gemfibrozil, phenytoin, sulfonylureas, statins, amiodarone, anabolic steroids, fluconazole, ketoconazole, miconazole, metronidazole, cholestyramine, omeprazole, amoxicillin, chloral hydrate, chloramphenicol, phenobarbital, prednisone, propranolol, rifampin, streptokinase, sulfamethoxazole and trimethoprim, urokinase, ritonavir, nevirapine, garlic, ginkgo biloba, coenzyme Q_{10}, St. Johns wort, any herbal remedies, and food that contain vitamin K can interact with warfarin. Concurrent use of delavirdine and warfarin is not recommended. Breast milk has decreased levels of vitamin K and therefore, breast-fed infants may be more sensitive to warfarin.

Adverse Effects

Potential adverse effects to warfarin use are skin necrosis, lesions, gangrene, fever, hair loss, tracheal calcification, hemoptysis, and hemorrhage.

Poisoning Information

Vitamin K reverses the anticoagulation effects of warfarin. Free frozen plasma may be needed. Use extreme care administering vitamin K or fresh-frozen plasma in patients with prosthetic valves, because valve thrombosis can occur.

Compatible Diluents/Administration

Protect warfarin from light. Warfarin for injection should be reconstituted with sterile water for injection to a final concentration of 2 mg/mL and used within 4 hours. Administer I.V. over 1 to 2 minutes.

References

1. Monagle P, Chan A, Massicotte P, et al. Antithrombotic therapy in children: The Seventh ACCP Conference on Antithrombotic and Thrombolytic Therapy. *Chest* 2004; 126: 645S–687S.

2. Monagle P, Michelson AD, Bovill E, et al. Antithrombotic therapy in children. *Chest* 2001; 119: 344S–370S.

3. Balaguru D, Dilawar M, Ruff P, Radtke WA. Early and late results of thrombolytic therapy using tissue-type plasminogen activator to restore arterial pulse after cardiac catheterization in infants and small children. *Am J Cardiol* 2003; 91(7): 908–910.

4. Duncan BW, Hraska V, Jonas RA, Wessel DL, del Nido PJ, Laussen PC, MayerJE, Lapierre RA, Wilson JM. Mechanical circulatory support in children with cardiac disease. *J Thorac Cardiovasc Surg* 1999; 117: 529–542.

5. Wilson JM, Bower LK, Fackler, JC, Beals DA, Berhus BO, Kevy SB. Aminocaproic acid decreases the incidence of intracranial hemorrhage and other hemorrhagic complications of ECMO. *J Pediatr Surg* 1993; 28: 536–541.

6. Horwitz JR, Cofer BR, Warner BH, Cheu HW, Lally KP. A multicenter trial of 6-aminocaproic acid (Amicar) in the prevention of bleeding in infants on ECMO. *J Pediatric Surg* 1998; 33: 1610–1613.

7. Thompson, CA. Don't give aprotinin again within 12 months, FDA says. *American Society of Health System Pharmacists* December 15, 2006.

8. Lexi-comp© 1978–2007; Poison and Toxicology.

9. Hursting MJ, Dubb J, Verme-Gibboney CN. Argatroban anticoagulation in pediatric patients. A literature analysis. *J Pediatr Hematol Oncol* 2006; 28: 4–10.

10. John TE, Jallisey RK. Argatroban and lepirudin requirements in a 6-year-old patient with heparin-induced thrombocytopenia. *Pharmacother* 2005; 25: 1383–1388.

11. Israels SJ, Michelson AD. Antiplatelet therapy in children. *Thrombosis Research* 2006; 118: 75–83.

12. Macdonald S. Aspirin use to be banned under 16 year olds. *BMJ* 2002; 325: 988.

13. Finkelstein Y, Nurmohamed L, Avner M, Benson LM, Koren G. Clopidogrel use in children. *J Pediatr* 2005; 147: 657–661.

14. Soman T, Rafay MF, Hune S, Allen A, MacGregor D, deVeber G. The risks and safety of clopidogrel in pediatric arterial ischemic stroke. *Stroke* 2006; 37: 1120–1122.

15. Newburger JW, Takahashi M, Gerber MA, Gewitz MH, Tani LY, Burns JC, et al. Diagnosis, treatment, and long-term management of Kawasaki disease: A statement for health professionals from the Committee on Rheumatic Fever, Endocarditis, and Kawasaki Disease, Council on Cardiovascular Disease in the Young, American Heart Association. *Circulation* 2004; 110: 2747–2771.

16. Lexi-Comp© 1978–2007; Pediatic Lexi-Drugs.

17. Dix D, Andrew M, Marzinotto V, Charpentier K, Bridge S, Monagle P, deVeber G, Leaker M, Chan AK, Massicotte MP. The use of low-molecular-weight heparin in pediatric patients: A prospective cohort study. *J Pediatr* 2000; 136: 439–445.

18. Schmidt B, Ofosu FA, Mitchell L, Brooker LA, Andrew M. Anticoagulant effects of heparin in neonatal plasma. *Pediatr Res* 1989; 25: 405–408.

19. Gershanik J, Boecler B, Ensley H, et al. The gasping syndrome and benzyl alcohol poisoning. *N Engl J Med* 1982; 307: 1384–1388.

20. Cobel-Geard RJ, Hassouna HI. Interaction with protamine sulfate with thrombin. *Am J Hematol* 1983; 14: 227–233.

21. Lee C, Nechyba C, Gunn VL, Drug doses. Gunn VL, Nechyba C. *The Harriet Lane Handbook*. Philadelphia; Mosby, 2002.

22. Reid RW, Zimmerman AA, Laussen PC, Mayer JE, Gorlin JB, Burrows FA. The efficacy of tranexamic acid versus placebo in decreasing blood loss in pediatric patients undergoing repeat cardiac surgery. *Anesth Analg* 1997; 84: 990–996.

12. Sedative Hypnotic and Anesthetic Agents: Their Effect on the Heart

Charles I. Yang, Pravin Taneja, and Peter J. Davis

Propofol

Indications

Propofol is a nonopioid, nonbarbiturate sedative hypnotic used extensively as an induction agent for general anesthesia and as a sedative in intensive care units (ICUs). The prompt recovery without residual sedation and low incidence of nausea and vomiting make propofol an appropriate choice for use in ambulatory surgery procedures.

Mechanism of Action

Propofol has a sedative-hypnotic effect through an interaction with γ-aminobutyric acid (GABA), the principle inhibitory neurotransmitter in the central nervous system (CNS). Propofol interacts with the GABA receptor complex and decreases the rate of dissociation of GABA from its receptor, thereby enhancing inhibitory neurotransmission and depressing nervous system activity. Propofol has proconvulsant and anticonvulsant properties. The antiepileptic property of propofol presumably reflects from its GABA-mediated presynaptic and postsynaptic inhibition action.

Dosing

Induction of anesthesia:
   Healthy adults and children between 6 and 12 years of age: 1.5 to 2.5 mg/kg intravenous (I.V.)
   Younger children and infants: 2.5 to 3.5 mg/kg I.V.
Maintenance dose: 200 to 300 µg/kg/min continuous I.V. that should immediately follow the induction dose. Infusion rates should subsequently be decreased 30 to 50% (125–150 µg/kg/min) during the first half hour of maintenance

Elderly patients: elderly patients require a 25 to 50% decrease of the induction dose as a result of a smaller central distribution and decreased clearance rate.[1] The short context-sensitive half-time of propofol, even with prolonged periods of infusion, makes it the drug of choice for producing I.V. "conscious sedation" as a part of balanced or total I.V. anesthesia (TIVA)[2]

Sedation:

Continuous infusion: continuous infusion can be used for sedation in the ICU. Sedating doses of 25 to 75 μg/kg/min are 20 to 50% of those required for general anesthesia. Patients recovering from the effects of general anesthesia or deep sedation will require maintenance rates of 5 to 50 μg/kg/min (0.3–3 mg/kg/h) individualized and titrated to clinical response and the level of other hypnotics

Pharmacokinetics

Onset: rapid onset of anesthesia and loss of consciousness after an I.V. bolus dose. There is rapid equilibration of propofol between the plasma and the highly perfused brain tissue

Distribution: large volume of distribution; plasma levels initially decline rapidly as a result of both high metabolic clearance and rapid redistribution into muscle and fat

Protein binding: highly protein bound; pharmacokinetics may be affected by conditions that alter serum protein levels

Half-life (t 1/2β): 30 to 60 minutes

Metabolism: extensively metabolized in the liver by microsomal hydroxylation primarily involving cytochrome P450 and, to a lesser extent, by nonspecific uridine diphosphate (UDP)-glucuronosyl transferases to inactive water soluble sulfate and glucuronide conjugates, respectively

Clearance: clearance from the plasma exceeds hepatic blood flow, suggesting tissue uptake, as well as anhepatic metabolism (possibly in the lungs). This is important in removal of the drug from the plasma. These lesser active metabolites are renally excreted, with less than 0.3% of a dose excreted unchanged. The activity of UDP-glucuronosyl transferases is severely reduced in the neonates, so that overall propofol clearance may be decreased compared with the older infant and child

Drug-Drug Interactions

- Coadministration of propofol with intramuscular (I.M.) or I.V. premedication drugs, anesthetics, sedatives, hypnotics, and opioids may result in an enhancement of its effects on mean arterial blood pressure and cardiac output

- Propofol does not cause a clinically significant change in onset, intensity, or duration of action of depolarizing and nondepolarizing neuromuscular blocking agents
- Propofol also does not significantly interact with commonly used premedication agents or inhalational agents, analgesics and local anesthetics

Systemic and Adverse Effects

Cardiovascular

Propofol causes a dose-dependent decrease in systemic blood pressure (25–40% reduction in systolic, diastolic, and mean blood pressure), associated with a 15% decrease in cardiac output/cardiac index (CI), stroke volume, and systemic vascular resistance.[3] This is caused both by vasodilation and myocardial depression. Propofol may also decrease sympathetic nervous system activity to a greater extent than parasympathetic nervous activity, resulting in a predominance of parasympathetic activity.[1,4] Propofol has greater negative inotropic effects on the heart than other induction agents such as etomidate and thiopental. These effects may be exaggerated in hypovolemic or elderly patients, and patients with compromised left ventricular function caused by coronary artery disease. Adequate hydration before I.V. administration of propofol may minimize the blood pressure effects of this drug. Despite decreases in systemic blood pressure, heart rate often remains unchanged. An infusion of propofol results in a significant reduction in both myocardial blood flow and myocardial oxygen consumption, which suggests that the global myocardial oxygen supply/demand ratio is preserved. Bradycardia and asystole have been observed after induction of anesthesia with propofol, resulting in the recommendation that anticholinergic drugs be administered when vagal stimulation is likely to occur. The risk of bradycardia-related death during propofol anesthesia has been estimated to be 1.4 in 100,000. Clinical studies have shown that propofol causes prolongation of the QT interval and a relatively high incidence of bradycardia and junctional rhythm, even in children premedicated with atropine.[3] Baroreceptor reflex control of heart rate may be depressed by propofol and seems to be more prominent in children younger than 2 years of age.[5–7]

Central Nervous System

Spontaneous, nonpurposeful movements may occur during induction and recovery in younger children and infants. These movements are not associated with cortical epileptic activity and are caused by depression of subcortical areas of the brain. Propofol decreases cerebral metabolic rate for oxygen ($CMRO_2$), cerebral blood flow, intracranial pressure (ICP), and intraocular pressures. Cerebrovascular blood pressure autoregulation is not affected by propofol. In high doses, propofol produces electroencephalographic (EEG) burst suppression[1] and decreases the early component of somatosensory evoked potentials (SSEPs) and motor evoked potentials (MEPs). Unlike thiopental, propofol does not have a neuroprotective effect.

Respiratory

Induction with propofol causes depression of ventilation and apnea in 25 to 35% patients. A maintenance infusion of propofol further decreases the tidal volume and rate of respiration. When propofol is administered by infusion to spontaneously breathing children, it causes a significant decrease in minute ventilation and carbon dioxide retention. Pharyngeal and laryngeal reactivity are also depressed by propofol, and it can be used to facilitate tracheal intubation in children without the use of muscle relaxants. Propofol can produce some bronchodilation and relief from bronchospasm.[8] It does not inhibit hypoxic pulmonary vasoconstriction.

Hepatic and Renal

Propofol does not adversely affect hepatic or renal function. Prolonged infusions of propofol may result in excretion of green urine, reflecting the presence of phenols in the urine.

Other

Propofol has no effects on coagulation or platelet function. Unlike thiopental, propofol has no effect on adrenocortical function and is safe in patients with hereditary coproporphyria. Propofol readily crosses the placenta and is considered safe for use in pregnant women. It transiently depresses activity in the newborn and is also rapidly cleared from the neonatal circulation.[9]

Propofol should not be administered to patients with a history of allergy to muscle relaxants or eggs or to those with multiple drug allergies. When injected in a small vein, propofol causes severe pain at the site of injection, which is related to the aqueous concentration of propofol in the emulsion directly stimulating venous nociceptive receptors and also stimulating the release of kininogens.[10] The pain during injection may be decreased by previous administration of 1% lidocaine or a short-acting opioid.

Poisoning Information

Propofol is classified as a pregnancy category B drug. Propofol crosses the placenta and is excreted in human milk. It may be associated with neonatal depression and should be used during pregnancy only if the potential benefits justify the potential risk to the fetus. In vitro and in vivo animal tests do not show any potential for mutagenicity by propofol.

Standard Concentrations and Compatible Diluents

The active ingredient in propofol, 2,6 di-isopropyl phenol, is insoluble in water and is formulated in a white, oil-in-water emulsion for I.V. administration. In addition to the active compound, 1% propofol (10 mg/mL), the aqueous solution also contains 10% soybean oil (100 mg/mL), 2.25% glycerol (22.5 mg/mL), and 1.2% egg lecithin (12 mg/mL).[1,2] Because the lipid moiety supports rapid bacterial growth (*E. coli and P. aeruginosa*) at room temperature, in the United States, 0.05 mg/mL disodium EDTA with sodium hydroxide or sodium metabisulfite (0.25 mg/mL) are added to adjust the pH and thereby inhibit bacterial growth. Nevertheless, significant bacterial contamination of open containers has been associated with serious patient infection.[2] Propofol should be either administered or discarded within 6 hours after removal from sterile packaging.

Propofol is an isotonic emulsion with a pH of 7 to 8.5 and a pKa of 11. Propofol injectable emulsion is available in ready to use 20-mL, 50-mL, and 100-mL infusion vials containing 10 mg/mL propofol. Propofol undergoes oxidative degradation in the presence of oxygen, and it is, therefore, packaged under nitrogen to eliminate this degradation path.

Propofol should be stored at room temperature between 4°C and 22°C (40–72°F). It is not recommended to mix or dilute the emulsion before use, because it supports the growth of microorganisms. Propofol should not be coadministered through the same I.V. catheter with blood or plasma, because aggregates of the globular component of the emulsion can occur with blood, plasma, or serum.

Etomidate

Indications

Etomidate is a nonopioid, nonbarbiturate sedative hypnotic used extensively as an induction and maintenance agent for general anesthesia and as a sedative in ICUs, including prolonged sedation in critically ill patients. Because of its effects of hemodynamic stability and reduction of ICP, it is frequently used as an induction agent in rapid sequence intubations in adults and increasingly in children. There is limited published evidence that supports the safety and efficacy of etomidate in pediatric patients. Etomidate exists as two isomers, but only the (+) isomer is active as a hypnotic.[11] It produces unconsciousness within one arm-brain circulation time after a rapid I.V. injection.

Mechanism of Action

Etomidate (Amidate) was introduced into clinical practice in 1972, and is the ethyl ester of a carboxylated imidazole.[11] Etomidate is a sedative hypnotic and its CNS depression effect is caused by its ability to enhance the effects of

GABA$_A$ receptors, the principle inhibitory neurotransmitter in the CNS. It acts like GABA and is thought to exert its mechanism by depressing the activity of the brainstem reticular system. Etomidate has no analgesic activity.

Dosing, Uses/Indications

Induction dose: 0.2 to 0.4 mg/kg by I.V. injection

Onset of general anesthesia: is rapid after induction (5–30 s) and can be maintained with an infusion at 10 µg/kg/min I.V. along with a volatile anesthetic and an opioid

Etomidate is a strong hypnotic sedative but has no analgesic properties. It can be used as an alternative to other hypnotic drugs, such as propofol or barbiturates, for induction of anesthesia, especially in the presence of an unstable cardiovascular system. Awakening and recovery from a single I.V. dose of etomidate is more rapid than after barbiturates, and there is little or no evidence of hangover or cumulative drug effect. The duration of anesthesia after induction is linearly related to the dose used. Etomidate at 0.1 mg/kg provides approximately 100 seconds of sleep, and repeat doses provide a longer duration of sedation. Hypnosis with etomidate is achieved at plasma levels of 300 to 500 ng/mL. Sedation and analgesia with etomidate can be achieved with 5 to 8 µg/kg/min I.V. infusion. Loss of consciousness occurs after 1.5 to 2 minutes, and the infusions can be stopped 10 minutes before desired awakening.

Etomidate used in doses of 0.15 to 0.3 mg/kg I.V. has minimal effect on the duration of electrically induced seizures and, thus, may serve as an alternative to drugs that decrease the duration of seizures in patients undergoing electroconvulsive therapy (ECT).

In children, etomidate at a dose of 6.5 mg/kg can be used rectally for induction of anesthesia. Sedation occurs within 4 minutes and recovery is still rapid.

Pharmacokinetics

Onset of action: 5 to 30 seconds

Duration of effect: 5 to 15 minutes. The duration of anesthesia is directly related to the dose used.[12] The hypnotic effects usually last for 10 to 20 minutes, and are somewhat dose dependent

Volume of distribution: large (lipophilic drug) in both adults and children

Distribution half-life (t$_{1/2}$): 3 minutes

Redistribution half-life: approximately 29 minutes

Elimination half-life (t 1/2β): 2.9 to 5.3 hours[13]

Protein binding: 75% bound to albumin

Metabolism: it undergoes hydrolysis to a water soluble, inactive compound in the liver (carboxylic acid of etomidate)

Excretion: these inactive metabolites are excreted in the urine (85%) and bile (15%). Less than 3% of etomidate is excreted unchanged in urine.

Pathological conditions affecting the liver result in decreased clearance of etomidate and a prolonged and exaggerated effect[14]

Rapid recovery from the sedative effects of etomidate is a result of both large redistribution and high metabolic clearance.

Drug-Drug Interactions

- Etomidate injection is compatible with the commonly administered preanesthetic medications
- Etomidate hypnosis does not significantly alter the usual dosage requirements of depolarizing or nondepolarizing neuromuscular blocking agents
- Narcotics like fentanyl may decrease the elimination of etomidate
- Verapamil may increase the anesthetic and respiratory depressant effects of etomidate
- Long-term infusion is likely to result in inhibition of adrenal steroid synthesis with decreased levels of cortisol and aldosterone

Systemic and Adverse Effects

Etomidate has also been associated with some adverse effects when used for induction.

Gastrointestinal

Potential gastrointestinal effects of etomidate are nausea and vomiting (the most frequent, in approximately 30–40% of patients). Use of opioids along with etomidate worsens this complaint.

Cardiovascular

Cardiovascular effects of etomidate need special consideration because this drug *is highly recommended to be used during induction of anesthesia in patients with little or no cardiac reserve.* Etomidate has minimal effects on cardiovascular function. An induction dose of 0.3 mg/kg of etomidate causes less than 10% change in heart rate, mean arterial pressure (MAP), mean pulmonary artery pressure (PAP), pulmonary capillary wedge pressure (PCWP), central venous pressure (CVP), CI, stroke volume, and pulmonary and systemic vascular resistance.[15] These effects of cardiovascular stability are also observed in patients with coronary heart disease, valvular heart disease, cardiomyopathy, and in patients with cardiac disease undergoing noncardiac surgery. The hemodynamic stability seen with etomidate is probably caused by its lack of effect on both the sympathetic nervous system and on baroreceptor function.[16] Etomidate has little effect on coronary perfusion pressure, while reducing myocardial oxygen consumption.

Central Nervous System

Etomidate causes cerebral vasoconstriction and decreases the cerebral blood flow by 34% and the $CMRO_2$ by 45% without altering the MAP.[17] Thus, cerebral perfusion pressure is well maintained and the ICP is decreased. Induction with etomidate does not alter the cerebral vascular reactivity, therefore, hyperventilation can further reduce the ICP. Etomidate also decreases the intraocular pressures for 5 minutes after a single dose. Similar to barbiturates, etomidate causes a biphasic EEG response with activation at low concentrations followed by inhibition at higher concentrations. At low concentrations, etomidate may activate any seizure foci and has been shown to produce increased EEG activity in epileptogenic foci in patients with a history of seizure activity.[18] This feature has been observed to facilitate intraoperative mapping of seizure foci before surgical ablation. At higher concentrations, etomidate produces burst suppression. Thus, etomidate has both proconvulsant and anticonvulsant effects depending on its dose and concentration in specific areas of the brain. It also augments the amplitude of SSEPs, making monitoring of these responses more reliable.

Etomidate has been associated with a high incidence of involuntary myoclonic movement during induction and recovery of anesthesia. This transient myoclonic activity is caused either by blockade of inhibition or by enhancement of excitability in the thalamocortical tracts.[19] Most movements are bilateral and could involve the arms, legs, shoulders, neck, chest wall, trunk, or all four extremities, with one or more of these muscle groups predominating. These movements could also be unilateral averting movements, tonic contractions, or only eye movements. Premedication with an opioid or a benzodiazepine may decrease the incidence of these myoclonic excitatory movements.

Respiratory

Etomidate has a minimal effect on ventilation. On induction, etomidate causes a decrease in tidal volume and a compensatory increase in the frequency of breathing. This resulting hyperventilation is very brief, lasting only 3 to 5 minutes and may be accompanied by apnea. The overall effect of this results in a slight increase in $PaCO_2$ and no change in PaO_2. Etomidate decreases the ventilatory response to carbon dioxide. Etomidate also seems to directly stimulate the basal ventilation, an effect that is independent of carbon dioxide tension. Induction with etomidate occasionally causes hiccups or coughing. It does not induce any histamine release, making it safe in patients with reactive airway disease.

Hepatic and Renal

Hepatic and renal functions are not altered by etomidate. Unlike other I.V. anesthetics, there is no decrease in renal blood flow. Etomidate has been used safely in porphyria without resulting in an acute attack.

Endocrine

A single induction dose or a short-term infusion of etomidate may cause adrenocortical suppression with a significant decrease in plasma cortisol, corticosterone, and aldosterone concentrations in the first 24 hours after surgery. This adrenocortical suppression effect of etomidate is a reversible, dose-dependent inhibition of the enzyme 11-β-hydroxylase, which converts 11-deoxycortisol to cortisol, and a minor inhibitory effect on enzyme 17-α-hydroxylase. This leads to an increase in the levels of cortisol precursors and adrenocorticotropic hormone (ACTH).[20] The mechanism of inhibition involved may be via the free imidazole radical of etomidate binding cytochrome P450, leading to inhibition of ascorbic acid synthesis. Ascorbic acid is required for steroid production in humans. Vitamin C supplementation has been reported to restore cortisol levels to normal after etomidate use.

Other

Pain on Injection   Pain on injection occurs in up to 80% of patients. Pain on injection worsens when using a small vein and can be eliminated by the use of lidocaine before the use of etomidate. The carrier preservative, propylene glycol, has been found to be the causative factor for the pain during injection. Preparation without a propylene glycol formulation decreases the pain with I.V. injection.

Superficial Thrombophlebitis   Superficial thrombophlebitis occurs in up to 20% of patients. This has been observed to occur 48 to 72 hours after the injection. Accidental intra-arterial injection of etomidate has not been associated with any local or vascular disease.

Poisoning Information

Etomidate is classified as a pregnancy category C drug. It should be used during pregnancy only if the potential benefits justify the potential risk to the fetus.

Although studies in animals have not shown etomidate to cause birth defects or be teratogenic, etomidate has been shown to cause other unwanted effects in the animal fetus when administered in doses many times the usual human dose. Animal studies showed no impairment of fertility in male and female rats when etomidate was administered before pregnancy.

Compatible Diluents

Etomidate is generally compatible with most drugs and can be mixed and diluted with crystalloids such as 0.9% sodium chloride and 5% dextrose solution.

Ketamine

Indications

Ketamine was released for clinical use in the United States in 1970. Ketamine can be used as an agent for sedation, anesthesia, and procedural sedation. Ketamine is distinct among the anesthetic agents not only for its mechanism of action, but also because it produces profound analgesia. It produces a cataleptic state characterized clinically by a functional and electrophysiological dissociation between the thalamic, cortical, and limbic systems in the brain. During this hypnotic state of ketamine, the patient is noncommunicative, although wakefulness may be present. The eyes remain open with a slow, nystagmic gaze and varying degrees of involuntary limb movements. The patients are amnesic, breathe spontaneously, and have intense analgesia. This cataleptic state has been termed "dissociative anesthesia."

Mechanism of Action

Ketamine is 2-(o-chlorophenyl)-2-(methylamino) cyclohexanone hydrochloride, a congener of phencyclidine. The structure of ketamine has a "chiral" center and is available as the racemic mixture of its two enantiomers (S-R). The S($+$) isomer of ketamine produces more effective anesthesia than racemic or R($-$) ketamine. Clinically, ketamine produces general as well as local anesthesia along with analgesia. It also produces sympathomimetic effects that are mediated by interactions with various receptors of the nervous system.[21] Ketamine interacts on multiple receptors, including N-methyl-D-aspartate (NMDA) receptors, opioid receptors, monoaminergic receptors, muscarinic receptors, and voltage-sensitive Ca+ channels. The pharmacological effects of ketamine are derived from a collective interaction on these various receptors.

Ketamine is a noncompetitive antagonist of the NMDA receptor calcium channel pore. This leads to significant inhibition of the receptor activity and is associated with general anesthesia and analgesic effects. Action of ketamine with the opioid receptors contributes to its analgesic and dysphoric reactions. Ketamine acts on all opioid receptors, mu (μ), delta (δ), and kappa (κ). Its action of analgesia is two- to three-fold more stereoselective at μ and κ receptors than at δ receptors ($\mu > \kappa > \delta$).

The sympathomimetic properties of ketamine result from enhanced central and peripheral monoaminergic transmission. Ketamine also blocks dopamine uptake and elevates the synaptic dopamine levels. It also inhibits central and peripheral cholinergic transmission and contributes to the induction of anesthesia and a state of hallucinations. The local anesthetic property of ketamine is derived from its ability to block Na+ channels at high dose. However, unlike other general anesthetic agents, such as propofol and etomidate, ketamine does not interact with GABA receptors.

Dosing, Uses/Indications

Ketamine can be administered by either the I.V. or I.M. routes to provide surgical anesthesia.

I.V., I.M.:
Induction dose:
1 to 2 mg/kg I.V., with peak effect in 30 to 60 seconds
2 to 4 mg/kg I.M., with onset of action in 5 minutes and peak in 20 minutes
Maintenance of anesthesia: 15 to 45 μg/kg/min (1–3 mg/min) by continuous I.V. infusion. Excellent analgesia and sedation can be obtained with smaller I.V. doses
Orally, rectally, or via intranasal route: 7.5 to 15 mg/kg as a form of premedication and pain management

Ketamine may be used as anesthetic agent for a large number of minor surgeries and procedures in both adults and children. Common procedures undertaken with ketamine anesthesia include minor to intermediate orthopedic surgery, gynecological surgery, drainage of abscesses, debridement of burns, change of dressings and minor dental procedures, bone marrow biopsies and spinal taps in children, intubations for patients with status asthmaticus, as well as a variety of examinations under anesthesia.

A combination of ketamine and benzodiazepine, such as midazolam, is commonly used for rapid induction of anesthesia and can also be used for maintenance of anesthesia and sedation during TIVA. Analgesia begins at plasma concentrations of approximately 100 ng/mL. During anesthesia, blood ketamine concentrations of 2000 to 3000 ng/mL are used, and patients may begin to awake from a surgical procedure when concentrations have been naturally reduced to 500 to 1000 ng/mL.

Pharmacokinetics

Volume of distribution: large, ketamine readily crosses the blood-brain barrier
Peak plasma concentrations: within 1 minute I.V. and within 5 minutes I.M.
Bioavailability: 93% (I.M.), 25 to 50% (intranasal), 15 to 25% (oral)[22]
Distribution: rapidly distributed into brain and other highly perfused tissues
Protein binding: 12%
Distribution half-life ($t_{1/2}$): 11 to 16 minutes
Elimination half-life (t $1/2\beta$): 2 to 3 hours
Clearance (Cl) rate: 12 to 17 mL/kg/min (high)
Metabolism: ketamine is metabolized by the hepatic microsomal cytochrome P450 3A4 system to form norketamine, which has 20 to 30% of the activity of ketamine[23]
Elimination: norketamine has an elimination half-life (t 1/2 β) of 6 hours, and contributes significantly to the analgesic property
Excretion: norketamine is hydroxylated to hydoxynorketamine followed by conjugation with glucuronide to form inactive metabolites that are

excreted in the urine. Oral administration of ketamine produces lower peak concentrations, but increased amounts of the metabolites norketamine and dehydronorketamine. Less than 4% of the drug is excreted in the urine unchanged and ketamine use can be detected in urine for approximately 3 days. Pathological conditions affecting liver function result in decreased clearance of ketamine with prolonged and exaggerated effect

Drug-Drug Interactions

Prolonged recovery time may occur if barbiturates and/or narcotics are used concurrently with ketamine. Benzodiazepines have significant effects when administered with ketamine. Midazolam attenuates altered perception and thought processes. Lorazepam may decrease ketamine-associated emotional distress but does not decrease cognitive or behavioral effects of ketamine. Acute administration of diazepam increases the half-life of ketamine. Haloperidol may decrease impairment by ketamine in executive control functions, but does not affect psychosis, perceptual changes, negative schizophrenic-like symptoms, or euphoria.

- Opioids have an additive effect with ketamine in decreasing pain and increasing cognitive impairment
- Ketamine is clinically compatible with the commonly used general and local anesthetic agents
- Ketamine has been reported to potentiate nondepolarizing neuromuscular blockade
- Physostigmine and 4-aminopyridine can antagonize some pharmacodynamic effects of ketamine
- Ketamine's preservative may be neurotoxic, therefore epidural or subarachnoid administration is prohibited in the United States

Systemic and Adverse Effects

Cardiovascular

Ketamine is the only anesthetic that routinely produces cardiovascular stimulation and does not cause hypotension in healthy patients. These effects resemble a direct stimulation and excitation of the central sympathetic nervous system.[24] In addition, ketamine also inhibits the extraneuronal uptake of catecholamine at the sympathetic nerve terminals. Increases in plasma epinephrine and norepinephrine levels occur as early as 2 minutes after I.V. ketamine administration and return to control levels 15 minutes later. This results in an increase in systemic and pulmonary arterial blood pressures, heart rate, cardiac output, cardiac work, and myocardial oxygen requirement, associated with appropriately increased coronary artery dilation and flow. The peak increases in these variables occur 2 to 4 minutes after I.V. injection and slowly decline to normal over the next 10 to 20 minutes. In vitro ketamine produces a direct negative inotropic effect, myocardial depression, and vasodilatation, emphasizing the importance of an intact sympathetic nervous.[25] The tachycardia and hypertension effects can be blunted or prevented by previous administration of benzodiazepines, barbiturates, or β-blockers, or by delivering ketamine by continuous infusion rather than by boluses. The use of inhaled anesthetic agents concomitantly with ketamine may block its cardiovascular effects as well.[26]

Ketamine used in critically ill patients caused a significant decrease in blood pressure, contractility, and cardiac output. This reflects the depletion of their endogenous catecholamine stores and exhaustion of their sympathetic drive, leading to unmasking of ketamine's direct myocardial depressant effect.[27] Ketamine is considered useful for poor-risk geriatric patients and patients in shock because of its cardiostimulatory properties. Ketamine is also used in children undergoing painful procedures, such as dressing changes on burn wounds.

In neonates with congenital heart disease, ketamine usually causes no significant change in the shunt or arterial oxygen saturation ($SaPO_2$). Ketamine does cause an increase in PAP and pulmonary vascular resistance more than systemic vascular resistance.

Central Nervous System

Ketamine is traditionally considered a potent cerebral vasodilator that increases the ICP and cerebral blood flow by 60%. Unlike other I.V. anesthetics, which actually reduce the ICP and cerebral metabolism, ketamine is relatively contraindicated in patients with increased ICP. Previous administration of thiopental, diazepam, or midazolam, along with hyperventilation, has been shown to blunt this ketamine-induced increase in cerebral blood flow.

The behavioral effects of ketamine are distinct from those of other anesthetics. The cataleptic state induced is accompanied by nystagmus with papillary dilation, salivation, lacrimation, and spontaneous involuntary muscle movements and gaze into the distance without closing the eyes. These eye effects, along with increased intraocular pressure by ketamine, make its use controversial in open eye injury cases.

Induction with ketamine produces a hypnotic state and a dose-related anterograde amnesia, during which the patients are unresponsive to painful stimuli. The added advantage over other parenteral anesthetics is the intense analgesia produced by ketamine. Induction with ketamine is associated with a decrease in EEG amplitude and frequency, followed by intermittent high-amplitude polymorphic δ activity, although overt epileptiform seizures are not produced. At high doses, ketamine produces a burst suppression pattern.

Emergence and recovery from ketamine anesthesia has been accompanied with both pleasant and unpleasant dreams. Illusions, visual disturbances and hallucinations, "weird trips," floating sensations, alterations in mood and body image, and delirium have been reported. The psychedelic effects of dreams and hallucinations can occur up to 24 hours after the administration of ketamine. The incidence of these phenomena occurs less frequently in young children, and premedication with a benzodiazepine may decrease these effects. Emergence delirium probably occurs secondary to the ketamine-induced depression of the inferior colliculus and medial geniculate nucleus, leading to misinterpretation of auditory and visual stimuli.[28]

Respiratory

Ketamine does not produce significant depression of ventilation. Upper airway muscle tone and airway reflexes such as cough, gag, sneeze, and swallow are relatively intact and well maintained. The patients may be capable of maintaining an intact airway and swallowing during ketamine anesthesia. Ketamine is a potent bronchodilator and inhibits bronchial constriction. This effect is secondary to inhibition of extraneuronal uptake of catecholamines, by inhibition of calcium influx through calcium channels in the bronchial smooth muscle cells, and by inhibition of postsynaptic nicotinic or muscarinic receptors in the tracheobronchial tree. Thus, ketamine can be used to treat bronchospasm in the operating room and ICU, to treat asthmatic children refractory to more conventional therapy, and may be the I.V. induction drug of choice in the presence of active bronchospasm.

Under anesthesia with ketamine, salivary and tracheobronchial secretions are increased, the ventilatory response to carbon dioxide is maintained, and functional residual capacity in spontaneously breathing healthy young children is unaffected. Perhaps the most important property of ketamine is that, despite the induction of anesthesia and dissociation, the cough and gag reflexes usually are not affected.

Hepatic and Renal

Ketamine does not significantly alter hepatic and renal functions. Ketamine has been used safely in patients with myopathies and a history of malignant hyperthermia. Although ketamine increases the liver enzyme ALA synthetase, it has been safely used in patients with acute intermittent porphyria and hereditary coproporphyria.

Other

Allergy (rarely because not followed by histamine release); cardiovascular stimulation; partial airway obstruction; and minor postanesthetic complications (profuse salivation, lacrimation, sweating, involuntary purposeless movements, unpleasant dreams with restlessness, and a more prolonged recovery) have also been observed.

Poisoning Information

Drowsiness, perceptual distortions, and intoxication may be dose related in a concentration range of 50 to 200 ng/mL.

Ketamine is considered a drug with abuse potential and is currently a Schedule C controlled substance in the United States. Ketamine crosses the placenta but studies in animals have not shown ketamine to cause any birth defects. Recreationally, ketamine is used as a psychedelic and for its dissociative effects. Long-term exposure leads to high tolerance, drug craving, and flashbacks. Abrupt discontinuation in chronic users causes a physiological withdrawal syndrome.

Standard Concentrations and Compatible Diluents

The S(+) isomer of ketamine preparation in sodium chloride solution has a pH of 3.5 to 5.5 and is available in three concentrations of ketamine, 10, 50, and 100 mg/mL, with benzethonium chloride added as a preservative. Ketamine is partially water soluble at pH 7.4 (pK$_a$, 7.5), and is 5 to 10 times more lipid soluble than thiopental.

Ketamine is manufactured commercially as a powder or liquid. Ketamine hydrochloride injection is supplied as the hydrochloride in concentrations equivalent to ketamine base. Each 10-mL vial contains 50 mg/mL. The color of the solution may vary from colorless to very slightly yellowish and may darken after prolonged exposure to light. This darkening does not affect the potency of the ketamine. Ketamine is stored at controlled room temperature, 15°C to 30°C (59°F to 86°F). Barbiturates and ketamine, being chemically incompatible because of precipitate formation, should not be injected from the same syringe. Ketamine is compatible with crystalloids, such as 0.9% sodium chloride and 5% dextrose solution.

Dexmedetomidine

Indications

Dexmedetomidine is a selective, centrally acting, α2-adrenoceptor agonist with centrally mediated sympatholytic, sedative, and analgesic effects. It is being increasingly used in anesthesia and ICUs, because it not only decreases sympathetic tone and attenuates the stress responses to anesthesia and surgery, but also causes sedation and analgesia. Dexmedetomidine is also used as an adjuvant during regional anesthesia. Clonidine, which was initially introduced as an antihypertensive, is the most commonly used α2 agonist by anesthesiologists. Dexmedetomidine is the most recent agent in this group approved by the US Food and Drug Administration (in 1999) for use in humans for analgesia and sedation.

Mechanism of Action

The mechanism of action of dexmedetomidine differs from clonidine because dexmedetomidine possesses selective α2-adrenoceptor agonism, especially for the 2A subtype of this receptor, which causes dexmedetomidine to be a much more effective sedative and analgesic agent than clonidine. The α2-adrenoceptors are found primarily in the peripheral nervous systems and the CNS. They are located both prejunctionally and postjunctionally and are generally inhibitory, whereas α1-adrenoceptors are excitatory. An exception is in vascular smooth muscle, where α2-adrenoceptor stimulation causes vasoconstriction. Presynaptically, α2-receptor activation reduces norepinephrine release, and activation of postsynaptic α2-receptors hyperpolarizes neutral membranes. Activation of these receptors by norepinephrine, thus, acts as an inhibitory feedback loop, reducing further release of norepinephrine. Decreases in norepinephrine levels reduce brain noradrenergic activity and inhibit sympathetic outflow and tone, causing hypotension, bradycardia, sedation, and analgesia.[29]

The sedative action of dexmedetomidine seems to be mediated by the activation of postsynaptic α2-receptors in the locus coeruleus (LC), the brain's predominant noradrenergic nucleus, which serves as a key modulator of vigilance in the CNS.

The mechanism of antinociceptive action of α2-receptor agonists involves the stimulation of noradrenergic descending inhibitory system originating in the LC. Analgesia produced by stimulation of the LC is mediated by release of norepinephrine activating α2-receptors in the substantia gelatinosa in the spinal cord.

Additionally, α-receptors are found in platelets and many other organs, including the liver, pancreas, kidney, and eye. The responses from these organs include decreased secretion, salivation, and bowel motility; increased glomerular filtration, secretion of sodium and water, and inhibition of renin release in the kidney; decreased intraocular pressure; and decreased insulin release from the pancreas.

Dosing, Uses/Indications

Dexmedetomidine is an anesthetic agent used to reduce anxiety and tension, and promote relaxation and sedation. It can be used for premedication, especially for patients in whom preoperative stress is undesirable. Dexmedetomidine has also been found to be an effective drug for premedication before I.V. regional anesthesia,[30] because it reduces patient anxiety, sympathoadrenal responses, and opioid analgesic requirements.

In mechanically ventilated patients, dexmedetomidine has been continuously infused before extubation, during extubation, and after extubation. It is not necessary to discontinue dexmedetomidine before extubation.

The sympatholytic effect of dexmedetomidine provides improved hemodynamic stability, slows the heart rate, and helps in reducing intraoperative blood loss. It also attenuates the stress response to laryngoscopy and decreases excessive hemodynamic effects during recovery and extubation.

Loading infusion: 1 µg/kg I.V. over 10 minutes
Maintenance infusion: 0.2 to 0.7 µg/kg/h I.V. The rate of the maintenance infusion should be titrated to achieve the desired level of sedation

Dexmedetomidine has also been used for sedation in children for computed tomographic (CT) scan and magnetic resonance imaging (MRI) scan in large doses of $2\,\mu g/kg$ I.V. as a loading dose followed by infusion of $1\,\mu g/kg$.[31]

Concurrent dexmedetomidine treatment lowers the dosage requirements for sedative agents, such as midazolam or propofol, and opioids in mechanically ventilated patients.

Epidural/subarachnoid administrations of α2-adrenergic agonists produce analgesia partly by causing spinal acetylcholine and nitric oxide (NO) release, because clonidine-induced analgesia is enhanced by subarachnoid neostigmine and inhibited by N-methyl-L-arginine (NMLA), a blocker of NO synthesis. Bouaziz et al.[32] administered clonidine and dexmedetomidine in the subarachnoid space to ewes and found that both clonidine and dexmedetomidine produced dose-dependent analgesia with similar potency.

Dexmedetomidine also causes muscle flaccidity and prevents opioid-induced muscle rigidity. This muscle relaxant effect is mediated via a central action, not at the neuromuscular junction.

Overall, dexmedetomidine administration during anesthesia maintains hemodynamic stability and allows lower doses of anesthetics and opiates to be used, resulting in more rapid recovery from anesthesia and a reduced need for pain medication after procedures, thereby reducing the length of hospital stay.

Pharmacokinetics

Distribution half-life ($t_{1/2}$): rapid (6 min)
Elimination half-life (t $1/2\beta$): approximately 2 hours
Onset of action: within 5 minutes
Protein binding: 94%. The unbound fraction of dexmedetomidine is significantly decreased in subjects with hepatic impairment compared with healthy subjects
Metabolism: dexmedetomidine undergoes almost complete hydroxylation through direct glucuronidation and oxidative metabolism via the cytochrome P450 system in liver
Elimination: the major excreted metabolites are N-glucuronides and N-methyl o-glucuronide dexmedetomidine. These metabolites are inactive and excreted in the urine (approximately 95%) and in the feces (4%)

Drug-Drug Interactions

- In vitro studies in human liver microsomes demonstrated no evidence of cytochrome P450-mediated drug interactions that were of clinical relevance
- Coadministration of dexmedetomidine with anesthetics, sedatives, hypnotics, and opioids is likely to lead to an enhancement of their effects.

Thus, because of pharmacodynamic interactions, a reduction in dosage of dexmedetomidine may be required
- Dexmedetomidine does not significantly interact with neuromuscular blockers, antihypertensives, ACE inhibitors, calcium channel blockers, or inotropes
- Although dexmedetomidine is highly protein bound, it does not result in protein-binding displacement of digoxin, phenytoin, warfarin, propranolol, theophylline, lidocaine, or ketorolac[33]

Systemic and Adverse Effects

Adverse events are generally reported after continuous infusions of dexmedetomidine when used for sedation in the ICU setting. Overall, the most frequently observed adverse events included hypotension (30%), hypertension, nausea/vomiting (11%), sinus bradycardia (8%), atrial fibrillation (7%), fever, hypoxia (6%), sinus tachycardia, and anemia (3%).

Cardiovascular

Dexmedetomidine does not have any direct effects on the heart. A biphasic cardiovascular response has been described after the administration of dexmedetomidine.[34] The bolus of 1 μg/kg dexmedetomidine initially results in a transient increase of the blood pressure and a reflex fall in heart rate, especially in younger, healthy patients.[34] Stimulation of αB-2-adrenoceptors in vascular smooth muscle is responsible for the initial rise in the blood pressure. Transient hypertension has been observed, primarily during the loading dose in association with the initial peripheral vasoconstrictive effects of dexmedetomidine, and may be associated with the rate of infusion. This initial response lasts for 5 to 10 minutes and is followed by a slight decrease in blood pressure caused by the inhibition of the central sympathetic outflow. The presynaptic α2-adrenoceptors are also stimulated, decreasing norepinephrine release, resulting in a fall in blood pressure and heart rate. These effects may also be observed in the postoperative period. Because dexmedetomidine decreases sympathetic nervous system activity, hypotension and/or bradycardia may be expected to be more pronounced in patients with hypovolemia, diabetes mellitus, or chronic hypertension, or patients with fixed stroke volume. Caution should also be used in patients with preexistent severe bradycardia and conduction problems, in patients with reduced ventricular function (ejection fraction > 30%), and in patients who are hypovolemic or hypotensive. Predictable, dose-dependent decreases in heart rate and blood pressure are observed during infusions. The transient hypertension can generally be attenuated by reducing the infusion rate. The hemodynamic values return to baseline when the infusion is discontinued. If medical intervention is required for hypotension or bradycardia induced by α2 agonism, treatment may include decreasing or stopping the infusion of dexmedetomidine, I.V. fluid resuscitation, elevation of the lower extremities, and the use of atropine and pressor agents, such as ephedrine.

Rapid I.V. bolus or rapid I.V. injection of dexmedetomidine has been associated with bradycardia and cardiac arrest in healthy subjects.[33] Patients older than 65 years may have a stronger reaction to the sedative and antihypertensive effects of dexmedetomidine and need smaller doses.

Central Nervous System

Dexmedetomidine is an adrenoceptor agonist that has been used for its sedative, anxiolytic, and analgesic properties and does not produce respiratory depression because of its nonopioid mechanism of analgesia. Dexmedetomidine has a 1600-fold greater affinity for the α2-receptor compared with α1-receptors.[33] One of the highest densities of α2-adrenoceptors has been detected in the pontine LC, a key source of noradrenergic innervation of the forebrain and an important modulator of vigilance. The sedative effects of α2-adrenoceptor activation have been attributed to the inhibition of this nucleus.[35]

Dexmedetomidine has no direct effect on ICP. Stimulation of the receptors in the brain and spinal cord inhibits neuronal firing, causing hypotension, bradycardia, sedation, and analgesia. Qualitatively, dexmedetomidine induces a sedative response that exhibits properties similar to natural sleep. Patients receiving dexmedetomidine experience a clinically effective sedation, yet are still easily and uniquely arousable and alert when stimulated from sedation and quickly return to their sleep-like state,[36] an effect not observed with any other clinically available anesthetic or sedative.

Dexmedetomidine lacks amnesic properties, and an overzealous reduction in the anesthetic dose because of suppression of hemodynamic responses to surgical stimulus may lead to awareness. Coadministration of dexmedetomidine with anesthetics; sedatives and hypnotics, such as propofol, barbiturates, or benzodiazepines; opiate agonists; or other anxiolytics may enhance the effects of these drugs and lead to depression of the CNS.[37] This is also true with volatile anesthetics such as sevoflurane and isoflurane. Dexmedetomidine decreases the minimum alveolar concentration (MAC) of isoflurane by 90% and decreases the MAC of sevoflurane by 17%. Dexmedetomidine decreases opioid and barbiturate requirements. Parenteral, epidural, and intrathecal placement cause analgesia and synergistically enhance opioid analgesia, decreasing their side effect of respiratory depression.

Dexmedetomidine is observed to reduce the incidence of postoperative shivering. It reduces the vasoconstrictive threshold by 1.4°C and the shivering threshold by 2°C. Administration of dexmedetomidine causes reduction in intraocular pressure. The reduction of central sympathetic activity by α2 agonists decreases the extent of neuronal damage.

Respiratory

Dexmedetomidine has no deleterious clinical effects on respiration and produces no clinically apparent respiratory depression[36] when used in doses that are sufficient to provide adequate sedation and effective analgesia in the surgical population requiring intensive care. There are no clinically important adverse effects on respiratory rate or gas exchange. Dexmedetomidine can be continued safely in the extubated, spontaneously breathing patient. In spontaneously breathing volunteers, I.V. dexmedetomidine caused marked sedation with only mild reductions in resting ventilation at higher doses.[38]

Hepatic and Renal
The pharmacokinetics of dexmedetomidine clearance decrease with the severity of hepatic impairment. Although dexmedetomidine is dosed to effect, dosage reduction may be necessary in patients with hepatic impairment. Dexmedetomidine pharmacokinetics are not significantly different in subjects with severe renal impairment (creatinine clearance < 30 mL/min) compared with healthy subjects.[33]

Dexmedetomidine is unlikely to be removed by hemodialysis because of its high protein binding and minimal renal excretion.

Other
Infrequent, but clinically relevant systemic adverse events reported in 1% patients are diaphoresis, hypovolemia, light anesthesia, and rigors. Most of these adverse effects occur during or briefly after bolus dose of the drug. Omitting or reducing the loading dose can reduce adverse effects.

Withdrawal Symptoms
After chronic administration, dexmedetomidine could potentially lead to withdrawal symptoms similar to those reported for another α2 adrenergic agonist, clonidine: nervousness, agitation, and headaches, accompanied or followed by a rapid rise in blood pressure and elevated catecholamine concentrations in the plasma.[37]

Poisoning Information

Dexmedetomidine is classified as a pregnancy category C drug. It should be used during pregnancy only if the potential benefits justify the potential risk to the fetus.

Standard Concentrations and Compatible Diluents

Dexmedetomidine hydrochloride is the S-enantiomer of medetomidine and is chemically described as (+)-4-(S)-[1-(2, 3-dimethylphenyl) ethyl]-1H-imidazole monohydrochloride. The active ingredient is dexmedetomidine, the pharmacologically active d-isomer of medetomidine.[28] Medetomidine is a highly lipophilic agent that has demonstrated selectivity for α2-adrenoceptors.

Dexmedetomidine is available in 2-mL vials and is a clear, colorless, isotonic solution freely soluble in water with a pH of 4.5 to 7.0 and has a pKa of 7.1. Dexmedetomidine should be diluted in 0.9% sodium chloride solution before administration. Dexmedetomidine has been shown to be compatible when administered with lactated Ringers, 5% dextrose in water, 20% mannitol, thiopental sodium, etomidate, depolarizing and nondepolarizing neuromuscular blockers, glycopyrrolate bromide, atropine sulfate, midazolam, morphine, fentanyl, and a plasma substitute.

Future of Dexmedetomidine

Intrinsic anesthetic properties and effects of dexmedetomidine can be selectively reversed by administering the α2-adrenoceptor antagonist atipamezole (A-17). This drug reverses sedation and sympatholysis caused by dexmedetomidine and has a half-life of 1.5 to 2 hours. The combination of dexmedetomidine and atipamezole might be the basis for a "reversible intravenous anesthetic technique." Antagonizing the sedative and hypnotic effects of dexmedetomidine with atipamezole will allow rapid recovery from anesthesia, regardless of its duration. This technique could provide timely and independent recovery from anesthesia and sedation in the future.[39]

Remifentanil

Indications

Remifentanil is a potent opioid used for anesthesia, analgesia, and sedation.

Mechanism of Action

Remifentanil is a synthetic opioid, piperidine derivative, and a hydrochloride salt of 3-(4-methoxycarbonyl-4-[1-oxopropyl phenylamino]-1-piperidine) propanoic acid, methyl ester. It binds strongly to stereospecific μ receptors at many sites within the CNS. It has less affinity for δ and κ receptors.[40,41] It is competitively antagonized by naloxone.[42] Remifentanil has a rapid onset of action, in 1 to 3 minutes. Its main metabolite, remifentanil acid (GI90291), is 800 to 2000 times less potent.[43] Remifentanil has a rapid onset and offset.

If postoperative pain is anticipated, adequate analgesia should be initiated before the discontinuation of the remifentanil infusion.

Dosing

Neonates: 0.4 to 1 µg/kg/min I.V. continuous infusion, supplement dose, 1 µg/kg
Infants: 0.4 to 1 µg/kg/min I.V. continuous infusion, supplement dose, 1 µg/kg
Children: 0.05 to 1.3 µg/kg/min I.V. continuous infusion, supplement dose, 1 µg/kg
Adults: 0.05 to 2 µg/kg/min I.V. continuous infusion, supplement dose, 0.5 to 1 µg/kg

Dosing should be based on an ideal body weight. The use of remifentanil as the sole induction agent is limited by variable sensitivity and associated side effects. The calculated ED_{50} for loss of consciousness is 12 µg/kg. Nevertheless, even at doses of 20 µg/kg, not all patients lose consciousness. A high percentage of patients have also been reported to develop rigidity. For effective induction of loss of consciousness, a hypnotic agent should be combined with 0.5 to 5 µg/kg of remifentanil. Then, an infusion of 0.1 to 0.5 µg/kg/min should be immediately started. Clinical effect can be readily achieved through titration of the infusion dose.

In children aged 2 to 7 years old and breathing spontaneously, there is a large variation (0.053–0.3 µg/kg/min) in the dose tolerated. Reduction in respiratory rate (< 10 breaths per minute) seems to be the best predictor of apnea. A dose of 0.05 µg/kg/min will allow spontaneous respiration in greater that 90% of children, whereas a dose of 0.3 µg/kg/min will prevent spontaneous respiration in 90% of children.[44]

For conscious sedation in adults, remifentanil can be combined with midazolam. A dose of 0.06 µg/kg/min results in an average sedation level of 3 (eyes closed; arousable to verbal command) on the Ramsay Scale. Titrating to effect at increments of 0.025 µg/kg/min has been recommended.

Pharmacokinetics

A pharmacokinetic study in children aged 0 to 18 years old suggested a profile similar to that of adults:

Volume of distribution: small (100 mL/kg in adults)
Distribution phase: rapid
Half-life: mean of 3.4 to 5.7 minutes. Because of its zero-order kinetics, the time to reach steady-state concentration is very rapid
Protein binding: 70% (primarily to α1-acid glycoprotein)
Metabolism: it undergoes rapid esterase hydrolysis in blood and tissue
Elimination: extremely rapid

Systemic and Adverse Effects

Cardiovascular

Cardiovascular effects of remifentanil seem to be similar to those of other opioids, such as fentanyl and alfentanil, although bradycardia seems to be more pronounced with remifentanil. The exact mechanism responsible for the bradycardia and hypotension effects is not known. An echocardiographic study of healthy children treated with remifentanil showed that a decrease in mean blood pressure and heart rate was associated with a dose-dependent decrease in CI, whereas the stroke volume remained stable. The decrease in mean blood pressure was ameliorated by an increase in systemic vascular resistance.[45]

Respiratory

Remifentanil produces respiratory depression in a dose-dependent fashion. The respiratory depression is not expected to last more than 10 to 15 minutes because of its rapid metabolism. In children with spontaneous breathing under anesthesia, a large variation in the dose of remifentanil tolerated exists, ranging from 0.053 to 0.3 μg/kg/min with a median 0.127 μg/kg/min.[44] The incidence of muscle rigidity after I.V. delivery is similar to that with alfentanil and can make ventilation difficult. This can be alleviated by naloxone or muscle relaxants. An infusion bolus of remifentanil at 1.0 μg/kg followed by a continuous infusion of 0.5 μg/kg/min was more effective than alfentanil (20 μg/kg bolus; 2 μg/kg/min) in obtunding the response to endotracheal intubation.

Neuromuscular

Side effects of remifentanil are similar to those of other opioids. A high incidence of muscle rigidity has been reported after the initial bolus of remifentanil. The incidence seems to be similar to that observed with alfentanil. Rigidity can be readily treated or prevented with the use of neuromuscular agents.

Other

Additional potential adverse effects are nausea, vomiting, hypotension, bradycardia, hypertension, dizziness, headache, fever, pruritus, visual disturbances, respiratory depression, apnea, hypoxia, shivering, and postoperative pain.

Drug-Drug Interactions

Remifentanil is synergistic with other anesthetics and may decrease the dose required for similar anesthetic effects.

Poisoning Information

Symptoms are similar to other opioid overdose and include apnea, chest wall rigidity, seizures, hypoxemia, hypotension, and bradycardia. Treatment includes airway support, administration of I.V. fluids, administration of atropine for bradycardia, and opioid reversal with 10 µg/kg naloxone, repeated as needed.

Compatible Diluents

Remifentanil is stable with the following diluents: sterile water injection, 5% dextrose injection, 5% dextrose and 0.9% sodium chloride injection, 0.9% sodium chloride injection, 0.45% sodium chloride injection, lactated Ringer's injection, and lactated Ringer's and 5% dextrose injection.

Standard Concentrations

One milligram, 2 mg, or 5 mg injectable powder is reconstituted to desired concentrations.

Fentanyl

Indications

Fentanyl is a potent opioid used for anesthesia, analgesia, and sedation.

Mechanism of Action

Fentanyl is a synthetic opioid related to the phenylpiperidines. It has a strong affinity for µ receptors located throughout the CNS. Fentanyl is 75 to 200 times more potent than morphine and approximately 7000 times more lipophilic.[46] The relative potential to enter the CNS is approximately 133 times greater than morphine. The pharmacological activity of fentanyl metabolites is unknown, but thought to be minimal.

Dosing

Fentanyl is primarily administered I.V. However, other techniques of administration, including transdermal, transmucosal via oral and intranasal, epidural, and intrathecal applications are well documented. Dosing should be titrated to desired effect.

> **Neonates:**
> - 0.5 to 3 μg/kg/dose; continuous infusion of 0.5 to 2 μg/kg/h I.V. (analgesia)
> - 1 to 4 μg/kg/dose; continuous infusion of 0.5 to 1 μg/kg/h I.V. followed by titration (sedation with analgesia)
> - For premature neonates with a gestational age younger than 34 weeks, mean dose of 0.64 μg/kg/h I.V. is appropriate. Older neonates with a gestational age of at least 34 weeks may require a slightly higher mean dose of 0.75 μg/kg/h
>
> **Infants:** 1 to 2 μg/kg/dose; continuous infusion of 1 to 3 μg/kg/h I.V.
> **Children:** 0.5 to 2 μg/kg/dose; continuous infusion of 1 to 3 μg/kg/h I.V.
> **Adults:** 0.5 to 2 μg/kg/dose; continuous infusion of 1 to 2 μg/kg/h I.V.

During extracorporeal membrane oxygenation (ECMO), an initial I.V. dose of 5 to 10 μg/kg followed by a continuous infusion of 1 to 5 μg/kg/h I.V. can be used. Tolerance can develop rapidly, resulting in dose requirements as high as 20 μg/kg/h.

In older infants to children of 12 years of age, sedation with analgesia is achieved with fentanyl doses of 1 to 2 μg/kg/dose I.V. or I.M. The dose may be repeated at 30-minute intervals until the required effect is obtained. If continuous sedation is necessary, an infusion dose of 1 to 3 μg/kg/h can be initiated after the initial bolus. Transdermal fentanyl can be used in children at least 2 years of age and receiving at least 45 to 60 mg of oral morphine equivalents per day. An initial transdermal patch of 25 μg/h is supplemented with intermittent short acting opioids. After 72 hours, the transdermal patch can be titrated as necessary.

In children older than 12 years of age and in adults, a fentanyl dose of 0.5 to 1 μg/kg/dose I.V. can be repeated every 5 minutes to reach appropriate sedation/analgesia levels. For continuous sedation/analgesia, an infusion initiated at 1 to 2 μg/kg/h can be titrated for appropriate effects.

Pharmacokinetics

> **Absorption:** transmucosal absorption is rapid and followed by slow gastrointestinal tract absorption
>
> **Effect (analgesia) onset:** almost immediate (I.V.), 7 to 15 minutes (I.M.), 6 to 8 hours (transdermal patch), and 5 to 15 minutes (after transmucosal administration). After transdermal application, the maximum analgesic effect is achieved at 24 hours compared with 20 to 30 minutes with transmucosal administration

Duration of effect: duration of effect is dependent on the route of administration with I.M., I.V., transdermal, and transmucosal duration of activity lasting 1 to 2 hours, 0.5 to 1 hour, 24 hours, and 1 to 2 hours, respectively

Half-life: after prolonged continuous infusions, the half-life of fentanyl is reportedly age dependent, and ranges from 11 to 36 hours in children aged 0.5 to 14 years

Binding: at physiological pH, 84% is bound to erythrocytes, α_1-acid glycoprotein, and plasma albumin, whereas 8.5% of the compound is unionized in plasma

Volume of distribution: its high lipid solubility results in a high volume of distribution, including muscle and fat. In adults, the volume of distribution ranges from 3 to 6 L/kg. In neonates to 14 years of age, the volume of distribution is reportedly greater, with a range of 5 to 30 L/kg

Metabolism: fentanyl is almost exclusively metabolized in the liver to norfentanyl, hydroxyproprionyl-fentanyl, and hydroxyproprionyl-norfentanyl.[47] Metabolism occurs via N-dealkylation and hydroxylation

Elimination: less than 10% of fentanyl is excreted unchanged by kidney

Systemic and Adverse Effects

The side effect profile of fentanyl is similar to other opioids, as follows.

Cardiovascular

There is minimal effect on the cardiovascular system. In adults, fentanyl at 5 and 10 μg/kg does not result in significant changes in cardiovascular parameters. At a higher dose of 20 μg/kg, significant reduction of heart rate and mean arterial blood pressure has been reported.[48] These changes, however, were not associated with significant changes in stroke volume, cardiac output, CVP, or peripheral arterial resistance. When additional fentanyl is administered at doses up to 50 μg/kg, no further heart rate or arterial blood pressure changes are observed.[48] However, fentanyl administered in combination with diazepam or other sedatives may result in decreased cardiac output, blood pressure, and peripheral vascular resistance, even at lower doses.[48]

In infants, bolus doses of 25 μg/kg had no significant changes in heart rate, left atrial pressure, mean pulmonary arterial pressure, pulmonary vascular resistance index, or CI. Nevertheless, fentanyl as a bolus of 25 μg/kg has been reported to decrease elevated suprasystemic PAPs.[49]

Respiratory

Chest wall rigidity and respiratory depression; fentanyl produces ventilatory depression in a dose-dependent fashion. The peak ventilatory effect of fentanyl injected I.V. is within 5 to 10 minutes. It decreases the response of the respiratory centers in the brainstem to increases in CO_2. Low doses tend to decrease breathing rate while maintaining tidal volume. As the dose is increased, tidal volumes and breathing rates usually decrease. High doses may produce apnea, even in an awake patient. Combination with other CNS depressants increases respiratory depression. High doses of fentanyl can cause marked muscle rigidity, which may make ventilation difficult. This can be alleviated by naloxone or muscle relaxants.

Central Nervous System

Fentanyl can cause CNS depression, confusion, drowsiness, and sedation.

Others

Fentanyl can also cause nausea, vomiting, constipation, xerostomia, weakness, miosis, and diaphoresis.

Drug-Drug Interactions

- Fentanyl is synergistic with other anesthetics and may decrease the dose required for similar anesthetic effects
- Inhibitors of CYP3A4 may increase the level of fentanyl. These inhibitors include azole antifungals, clarithromycin, diclofenac, doxycycline, erythromycin, imatinib, isoniazid, nefazodone, nicardipine, propofol, protease inhibitors, quinidine, telithromycin, and verapamil
- With monamine oxidase inhibitors, a severe and unpredictable potentiation of opioid analgesics has been reported

Poisoning Information

Symptoms are similar to other opioid overdose and include apnea, chest wall rigidity, seizures, hypoxemia, hypotension, and bradycardia. Treatment includes airway support, administration of I.V. fluids, administration of atropine for bradycardia and opioid reversal with 10 µg/kg naloxone, repeated as needed.

Compatible Diluents

Fentanyl is stable with the following diluents: sterile water injection, 5% dextrose injection, and 0.9% sodium chloride injection.

Midazolam

Indications

Midazolam has the anxiolytic, hypnotic, anticonvulsant, muscle relaxant, and antegrade amnestic effects characteristic of benzodiazepines.

Mechanism of Action

Midazolam binds to stereospecific benzodiazepine receptor sites on the postsynaptic GABA receptor complex and, thereby, modulates GABA. These binding sites are found mainly in the CNS, with the greatest density in the cerebral cortex, hypothalamus, cerebellum, midbrain hippocampus, limbic system, reticular formation, striatum, medulla oblongata-pons, and spinal cord.[50]

Dosing

Neonates: dosage must take into account the patient's age, any underlying disease processes, and concurrent medications. Lower doses of midazolam should be used if other opioids or sedatives are used concurrently. The dose adjustment is particularly important with opioids to avoid respiratory depression and hypotension

Sedation in mechanically ventilated neonates: 0.5 µg/kg/min for neonates younger than 32 weeks. An initial dose of 1 µg/kg/min is appropriate for neonates older than 32 weeks gestational age. Severe hypotension and seizures have been reported after rapid I.V. administration, particularly with concurrent use of fentanyl[51]

Infants and children:

Sedation in mechanically ventilated older infants and children: a loading dose 0.05 to 0.2 mg/kg I.V. is administered slowly, followed by an infusion of 0.4 to 6 µg/kg/min

For procedural sedation of infants 6 months to children 5 years of age: a dose of 0.05 to 0.1 mg/kg I.V. can be titrated to effect, for a maximum dose of 6 mg

For procedural sedation of children 6 to 12 years of age: a dose of 0.025 to 0.05 mg/kg I.V. is titrated to effect, with a maximum dose of 10 mg

For procedural sedation of children older than 12 years of age: slow titration with 1 to 2 mg I.V. until the desired level of sedation is obtained. A total dose greater than 5 mg is rarely necessary. Alternatively, an I.M. dose of 0.1 to 0.15 mg/kg can be injected 30 to 60 minutes before the procedure. The maximum I.M. dose is 10 mg

For sedation, anxiolysis, and amnesia before a procedure, midazolam can be administered as a single oral dose of 0.25 to 0.5 mg/kg in infants older than 6 months and a maximum dose of 20 mg in children. In addition, an intranasal dose of 0.2 mg/kg can be administered using a 1-mL needleless syringe into the nare over 15 seconds. This can be repeated in 5 to 15 minutes

Adults: in adults, an I.M. dose of 0.07 to 0.08 mg/kg has been administered up to 1 hour before surgery for anxiety. Onset is within 15 minutes and the peak effect at 30 to 60 minutes. An I.V. dose of 0.25 mg/kg will usually suffice for anxiety. For continuous infusion, midazolam is initially bolused at 0.01 to 0.05 mg/kg then infused at a rate of 0.02 to 0.1 mg/kg/h. Individual response to midazolam can vary and, therefore, may require further titration for desired effect

Pharmacokinetics

Absorption: via oral and nasal route is rapid secondary to high lipophilicity

Bioavailability: oral bioavailability is 15 to 45%; rectal bioavailability is 40 to 50%; intranasal bioavailability is 60%

Onset of action: high lipophilicity at physiological pH results in rapid onset of activity. Onset of action, maximum effect, and duration varies by mode of administration. Onset of action is within 20 minutes when administered orally, and within 5 minutes when administered I.M., intranasally, or I.V.

Maximum effect: 15 to 30 minutes (I.M.); 5 to 7 minutes (I.V.); and 10 minutes (intranasal application)

Mean duration: 2 to 6 hours (I.M.); 20 to 30 minutes (I.V.); and 30 to 60 minutes (intranasal)

Half-life: 2.6 to 17.7 hours (preterm infants); 4 to 12 hours (neonates); 2.9 to 4.5 hours (children)

Volume of distribution: 0.4 to 4.2 L/kg (preterm infants); 1.24 to 2.02 L/kg (infants and children 6 months to 16 years old); 1 to 3.1 L/kg (adults)

Protein-binding: 97%, primarily to albumin

Metabolism: midazolam undergoes extensive metabolism by hepatic CYP450-3A4. Metabolites include 1-hydroxymidazolam (the principal metabolite), 4-hydroxymidazolam, and 1,4-dihydroxymidazolam. The 1- and 4-hydroxy metabolites have pharmacological activity, although less than that of the parent compound

Elimination: excretion occurs through urine as glucuronide-conjugated metabolites (80%) and feces (2–10%)

Systemic and Adverse Effects

Cardiovascular

In adults, midazolam administered at 0.15 mg/kg produces a significant reduction in systolic (5%) and diastolic (10%) blood pressure and increases in heart rate (18%).[52] CI and bilateral heart filling pressures are maintained, but systemic vascular resistance may decrease 15 to 33%.[53] A decrease in systemic vascular resistance, venodilation, and a transient change in portal blood flow can combine to reduce cardiac filling. Combination with opioids can exaggerate cardiovascular effects.

Respiratory

Midazolam produces centrally mediated ventilatory depression. In healthy volunteers, tidal volumes decreased but respiratory rates increased, resulting in unchanged minute ventilation. In patients with chronic obstructive pulmonary disease, midazolam produced a more profound and longer-lasting respiratory depression than it did in healthy patients.[54] Its ventilatory depression is not reversed by naloxone, but can be reversed by flumazenil. Apnea is more likely to occur after midazolam is administered to patients premedicated with opioids.

Central Nervous System

Adverse CNS effects include drowsiness, headache, seizure-like activity.

Other

Other adverse effects include nausea, vomiting, nystagmus, cough, physical and psychological dependence with prolonged use, and paradoxical reaction.

Drug-Drug Interactions

The sedative effect of midazolam is increased in the presence of other CNS depressants, particularly with narcotics. Cimetidine, erythromycin, diltiazem, verapamil, ketoconazole, and itraconazole can prolong the sedative effect of midazolam by inhibiting plasma clearance secondarily to inhibition of the CYP450-3A4 enzyme system.

Poisoning Information

Midazolam has been associated with respiratory depression and respiratory arrest. Flumazenil, in titrating doses of 0.01 mg/kg I.V., can reverse the effects of benzodiazepine.

Compatible Diluents

Midazolam formulations of 1 mg/mL and 5 mg/mL may be diluted with 0.9% sodium chloride or 5% dextrose in water. Midazolam at a concentration of

0.5 mg/mL is compatible with 0.9% sodium chloride and 5% dextrose in water for up to 24 hours and with lactated Ringer's solution for up to 4 hours.

Halothane, Isoflurane, Sevoflurane, and Desflurane

Indications

Halothane, isoflurane, sevoflurane, and desflurane are inhalation anesthetics agents used for general anesthesia.

Mechanism of Action

Halogenated general inhalational anesthetics include halothane, isoflurane, sevoflurane, and desflurane. The mechanisms of action of these agents are not fully understood. It is thought that multiple sites of activity may be involved, resulting in anesthesia. Anesthetic actions on the CNS are known to occur both in the spinal cord and the brain. The ablation of movement in response to pain is mediated primarily by the spinal cord.[55] It is still uncertain whether specific regions of the brain are targeted by the inhaled anesthetics. Nevertheless, the reticular-activating system, thalamus, pons, amygdala, and hippocampus are all thought to be involved in general anesthesia because of their importance in cognition, memory, learning, sleep, and attentiveness. The inhalation anesthetics both depress excitatory synapses and augment inhibitory synapses.[56] On the molecular level, inhaled anesthetics alter the function of protein kinase C and ion channels associated with neurotransmitter receptors, including nicotinic acetylcholine, serotonin type 3, $GABA_A$, glycine, and glutamate receptors. Inhaled anesthetics not only potentiate the action of neuromuscular blocking drugs, but also possess intrinsic muscle-relaxant properties.[57]

Dosing

The measure of inhalation anesthetic potency has traditionally been expressed in terms of the MAC. This is defined as the expired concentration of the inhaled anesthetic that prevents movement in 50% of patients in response to a surgical stimulus. The inhaled anesthetics MAC value is dependent on the age of the patient. Generally, the MAC value is higher in infants and decreases with age. Thus, infants require a higher concentration of anesthetic than older children and adults.[58] Tables 12-1 to 12-4 show MAC correlated with age for desflurane, halothane, sevoflurane, and isoflurane.

Table 12-1.   Desflurane: MAC correlated with age

Age	MAC (% expired)
0–30 d	9.16
1–6 mo	9.42
6–12 mo	9.98
1–3 yr	8.72
3–5 yr	8.62
5–12 yr	7.98
> 12 yr	6

Table 12-2.   Halothane: MAC correlated with age

Age	MAC (% expired)
1 mo	0.87
4 mo	1.2
1 yr	0.93
4 yr	0.87
15 yr	0.94
40 yr	0.77

Table 12-3.   Sevoflurane: MAC correlated with age

Age	MAC (% expired)
0–30 d	3.3
1–6 mo	3.2
6–12 mo	2.5
1–12 yr	2.5
Adults	2.6
Elderly	1.5

Table 12-4.   Isoflurane: MAC correlated with age

Age	MAC (% expired)
35 wk	1.4
0–1 mo	1.5
1–6 mo	1.8
6–12 mo	1.6
1–5 yr	1.6
Adult	1.2

Pharmacokinetics

Uptake and Distribution

The uptake and distribution of inhalation agents is more rapid in infants and children than in adults.[59] Several factors may contribute to this finding. Compared with adults, pediatric patients have a more rapid respiratory rate, increased CI, and distribution of a greater proportion of the cardiac output to vessel-rich organs. For any given anesthetic agent, the onset time and recovery time are related to the solubility of the anesthetic as well as the patient's minute ventilation and cardiac output. Frequently, nitrous oxide is used to reduce the dose of halothane, sevoflurane, desflurane, or isoflurane, which are more potent but cause more cardiovascular depression. Furthermore, the rate of induction and awakening may be related, in part, to the type of anesthetic circuit used: a nonrebreathing system produces a more rapid rise in alveolar anesthetic concentration compared with a rebreathing system.

Elimination and Metabolism

Elimination of inhalation anesthetics is by exhalation. The duration of emergence after discontinuation of the inhaled anesthetic is dependent on the blood concentration of the anesthetic. Table 12-5 shows the onset of action and degree of hepatic metabolism of the inhalation anesthetics.

Systemic and Adverse Effects

Cardiovascular

All of the halogenated inhalation anesthetics decrease arterial pressure in a dose-related manner. Generally, this occurs secondary to vasodilation, decreased cardiac output, and decreased sympathetic tone. Myocardial oxygen consumption is also decreased with inhalation anesthetics. The cardiovascular effects of these agents are summarized in Table 12.6.

Respiratory

All inhalation anesthetics depress ventilation in a dose-related manner. This depression is evidenced by their effect on $PaCO_2$, which increases in proportion

Table 12-5. Onset of action and metabolism of inhalation anesthetics

Inhalation anesthetic	Halothane	Sevoflurane	Isoflurane	Desflurane
Onset of action (min)	1.5–3	2	7–10	1–2
Metabolism	Hepatic, 20–30%	Hepatic, 3–5%	Hepatic, 0.2%	Hepatic, 0.02%

Table 12-6. Cardiovascular effects of inhalation anesthetics[a]

Effect	Halothane	Isoflurane	Sevoflurane	Desflurane
SNS	—	$+>>1$ MAC	—	$+1$ MAC
Blood pressure	$\downarrow\downarrow$	$\downarrow\downarrow$	$\downarrow$	$\downarrow\downarrow$
SVR	$\downarrow\downarrow$	$\downarrow\downarrow$	$\downarrow$	$\downarrow\downarrow$
Heart rate	NC or $\uparrow$	NC or $\uparrow$	NC or $\downarrow$ at low MAC; $\uparrow$ at >1.5 MAC	NC or $\uparrow$
Cardiac output	NC or $\downarrow$	NC	NC or $\downarrow$	NC or $\downarrow$
Myocardial contractility	$\downarrow\downarrow$	$\downarrow\downarrow$	$\downarrow\downarrow$	$\downarrow\downarrow$

[a]SNS, sympathetic nervous system; SVR, systemic vascular resistance.

to the increase in the concentration of anesthetic. The changes in $PaCO_2$ are caused by a decrease in tidal volume, but somewhat offset by an increase in the respiratory rate. Inhalation anesthetics depress the ventilatory response to hypoxemia at peripheral and central chemoreceptors. They also dilate constricted bronchial muscles. In the absence of bronchoconstriction, these agents have a minimal effect on airway resistance.

Other
Additional adverse effects include myocardial depression, apnea, nausea, vomiting, and shivering. With sevoflurane, there is a potential for renal injury from a sevoflurane degradation product, Compound A.[60] To minimize exposure to Compound A, sevoflurane exposure should not exceed 2 MAC-hours at flow rates of 1 to less than 2 L/min.

Drug-Drug Interactions

- CNS depressants add to the depression effects of the inhaled anesthetics
- With halothane, the heart is predisposed to premature ventricular extrasystoles in the presence of epinephrine[61]
- Desflurane enhances the positive inotropic effect of dobutamine
- All of the potent inhalation anesthetics increase the arrhythmogenic threshold for digitalis-like drugs
- All of the potent inhalation anesthetics increase both the intensity and duration of neuromuscular blockade induced by nondepolarizing muscle relaxants

Poisoning Information

Overdose with potent inhalation anesthetics can lead to respiratory arrest and cardiovascular collapse. Treatment for overdose is discontinuation of these agents and supportive care with ventilatory support, I.V. fluids, and inotropic medications.

Compatible Diluents

Inhalation anesthetics are not diluted.

References

1. Fulton B, Sorkin EM. Propofol: an overview of its pharmacology and a review of its clinical efficacy in intensive care sedation. *Drugs* 1995; 50:636–657.
2. Bryson HM, Fulton BR, Faulds D. Propofol: an update of its use in anesthesia and conscious sedation. *Drugs* 1995; 50:513–559.
3. Coates DP, Monk CR, Prys-Roberts C, et al. Hemodynamic effects of the infusion of the emulsions formulation of propofol during nitrous oxide anesthesia in humans. *Anesth Analg* 1987; 66:64–70.
4. Wagner BK, O'Hara DA. Pharmacokinetics and pharmacodynamics of sedatives and analgesics in the treatment of agitated critically ill patients. *Clin Pharmacokinet* 1997; 33:426–453.
5. Saarnivaara L, Hiller A, Oikkonem M. QT interval, heart rate and arterial pressures using propofol, thiopentone or methohexitone for induction of anesthesia in children. *Acta Anaesthesiology Scand* 1993; 37:419–423.
6. Deutschman CS, Harris AP, Fleisher LA. Changes in heart rate variability under propofol anesthesia: a possible explanation for propofol-induced bradycardia. *Anesth Analg* 1994; 79:373–377.
7. Aun CS, Sung RY, O'Meara ME, et al. Cardiovascular effects of I.V. induction in children; Comparison between propofol and thiopentone. *Br J Anaesth* 1993; 70:647–653.
8. James MK, Feldman PL, Schuster SV, et al. Opioid receptor activity of GI 87084B, a novel ultra-short acting analgesic, in isolated tissues. *J Pharmacol Exp Ther* 1991; 259:712–718.
9. James MK, Vuong A, Grizzle MK, et al. Hemodynamic effects of GI 87084B, an ultra-short acting mu-opioid analgesic, in anesthetized dogs. *J Pharmacol Exp Ther* 1992; 263:84–91.
10. Amin HM, Sopchak AM, Esposito BF, et al. Naloxone reversal of depressed ventilatory response to hypoxia during continuous infusion of remifentanil [Abstract] 1993; 79:A1203.
11. Glass PSA. Remifentanil: a new opioid. *J Clin Anesth* 1995; 7:558–563.

12. Ansermino JM, Brooks P, Rosen D, et al. Spontaneous ventilation with remifentanil in children. *Paediatr Anaesth* 2005; 15:115–121.

13. Chanavaz C, Tirel O, Wodey E, et al. Haemodynamic effects of remifentanil in children with and without intravenous atropine. An echocardiographic study. *Paediatr Anaesth* 2005; 94:74–79.

14. Herz A, Teschenmacher HJ. Activities and sites of antinociceptive action of morphine-like analgesics and kinetics of distribution following intravenous intracerebral and intraventricular application. *Advance Drug Research* 1971; 6:79–119.

15. Mather LE. Clinical pharmacokinetics of fentanyl and its newer derivatives. *Clinical Pharmacokinetics* 1983; 8:422–426.

16. Stanley TH, Webster LR. Anesthetic requirements and cardiovascular effects of fentanyl-oxygen and fentanyl-diazepam-oxygen anesthesia in man. *Anesth Analg* 1978; 57:411–416.

17. Hickey P, Hansen D, Wessel D. Pulmonary and systemic hemodynamic responses to fentanyl in infants. *Anesth Analg* 1985; 64:483–486.

18. Mantegazza P, Parenti M, Tammiso R, et al. Modification of the antinociceptive effects of morphine by centrally administered diazepam and midazolam. *Brit J Pharmacol* 1982; 75:569–572.

19. Burtin P, Jacqz-Aigrain E, Girar P, et al. Population pharmacokinetics of midazolam in neonates. *Clin Pharmacol Ther* 1994; 56(6 Pt 1):615–625.

20. Forster A, Gardaz JP, Suter PM, et al. IV Midazolam as an induction agent for anaesthesia: a study in volunteers. *Br J Anaesth* 1980; 52:907–911.

21. Reves JG, Samuelson PN, Lewis S. Midazolam maleate induction in patients with ischaemic heart disease: haemodynamic observations. *Can Anaesth Soc J* 1979; 26:402–409.

22. Morel D, Forster A, Bachmann M, et al. Changes in breathing pattern induced by midazolam in normal subjects (Abstract). *Anesthesiology* 1982; 57:A481.

23. Eger EI II, Bahlman SH, Munson ES. The effect of age on the rate of increase of alveolar anesthetic concentration. *Anesthesiology* 1971; 35:365–372.

24. Rampil IJ, Mason P, Singh H. Anesthetic potency (MAC) is independent of forebrain structures in the rat. *Anesthesiology* 1993; 78:707–712.

25. Violet JM, Downie DL, Nakisa RC, et al. Differential sensitivities of mammalian neuronal and muscle nicotinic acetylcholine receptors to general anesthetics. *Anesthesiology* 1997; 86:866–874.

26. Kelly RE, Lien CA, Savarese JJ, et al. Depression of neuromuscular function in a patient during desflurane anesthesia. *Anesth Analg* 1993; 76:868–871.

27. Gregory GA, Eger EI II, Munson ES, et al. The relationship between age and halothane requirements in man. *Anesthesiology* 1969; 30:488–491.

28. Johnston RR, Eger EI II, Wilson C. Comparative interaction of epinephrine with enflurane, isoflurane, and halothane in man. *Anesth Analg* 1976; 55:709–712.

29. Eger EI, II, Gong D, Koblin DD, et al. Nephrotoxicity of sevoflurane vs desflurane anesthesia in volunteers. *Anesth Analg* 1997; 84:160–168.

30. Harvey MA. Managing agitation in critically ill patients. *Am J Crit Care* 1996; 5:7–16

31. Doenicke AW, Roizen MF, Rau J, et al. Reducing pain during propofol injection: the role of the solvent. *Anesth Analg* 1996; 82:472–474.

32. Tomlin SL, Jenkins A, Leib WR, et al. Stereoselective effects of etomidate optical isomers on gamma-aminobutyric acid type-A receptors and animals. *Anesthesiology* 1998; 88:708–717.

33. Abboud TK, Zhu J, Richardson M, et al. Intravenous propofol vs thiamylal-isoflurane for caesarean section, comparative maternal and neonatal effects. *Acta Anaesthesiol Scand* 1995; 39:205–209.

34. Dundee JW, Zacharias M: Etomidate. In Dundee JW (Ed): Current topics in Anesthesia Series. 1. Intravenous Anesthetic Agents. London, Arnold, 1979, p 46.

35. Van Hamme MJ, Ghoneim MM, Ambre JJ. Pharmacokinetics of etomidate, a new intravenous anesthetic. *Anesthesiology* 1978; 49:274–277.

36. Meuldermans WEG, Heykants JJP. The plasma protein binding and distribution of etomidate in dog, rat and human blood. *Arch Int Pharmacodyn Ther* 1976; 221:150–162.

37. Gooding JM, Weng J, Smith RA, et al. Cardiovascular and pulmonary responses following etomidate induction of anesthesia in patients with demonstrated cardiac disease. *Anesth Analg* 1979; 58:40–41.

38. Ebert TJ, Muzi M, Berens R, et al. Sympathetic responses to induction of anesthesia in humans with propofol or etomidate. *Anesthesiology* 1992; 76:725–733.

39. Cold GE, Eskeen V, Eriksen H, et al. CBF and $CMRO_2$ during continuous etomidate infusion supplemented with N_2O and fentanyl in patients with supratentorial cerebral tumor: a dose dependent study. *Acta Anaesthesiol Scand* 1985; 29:490–494.

40. Ebrahim EY, DeBoer GE, Luders H, et al. Effect of etomidate on electroencephalogram of patients with epilepsy. *Anesth Analg* 1986; 65:1004–1006.

41. Ghoneim MM, Yamada T. Etomidate: a clinical and encephalographic comparison with thiopental. *Anesth Analg* 1977; 56:479–485.

42. Allolio B, Dorr H, Struttmann R, et al. Effect of a single bolus dose of etomidate upon eight major corticosteroid hormones and plasma ACTH. *Clin Endocrinol (Oxf)* 1985; 22:281–286.

43. Durrani Z, Winnie AP, Zsigmond EK, et al. Ketamine for intravenous regional anesthesia. *Anesth Analg* 1989; 68:328–332.

44. Clements JA, Nimmo WS. The pharmacokinetics and analgesic effects of ketamine in man. *Br J Anaesth* 1981; 53:27–30.

45. Geisslinger G, Hering W, Thomann P, et al. Pharmacokinetics and pharmacodynamics of ketamine enantiomers in surgical patients using a stereoselective analytical method. *Br J Anaesth* 1993: 70:666–671.

46. Lundy PM, Lockwood PA, Thompson G, et al. Differential effects of ketamine isomers on neuronal and extraneuronal catecholamine uptake mechanisms. *Anesthesiology* 1986; 64:359–363.

47. Reich DL, Silvay G. Ketamine: an update on the first twenty-five years of clinical experience. *Can J Anaesth* 1989; 36:186–197.

48. Hoffman WE, Pelligrino D, Werner C, et al. Ketamine decrease plasma catecholamines and improves outcome from complete cerebral ischemia in rats. *Anesthesiology* 1992; 76:755–762.

49. White PF, Ham J, Way WL, et al. Pharmacology of ketamine isomers in surgical patients. *Anesthesiology* 1980; 52:231–239.

50. Hayashi Y, Maze M. Alpha 2-adrenoceptor agonists and anesthesia. *Br J Anaesth* 1993; 71:108–118.

51. Morrison P, Etropolski M, Bachand R. Dexmedetomidine and sedation: a dose-ranging study. (W97-028 manuscript for publication)

52. Venn RM, Bradshaw CJ, Spencer R, et al. Preliminary UK experience of dexmedetomidine, a novel agent for postoperative sedation in the intensive care unit. *Anaesthesia* 1999; 54:1136–1142.

53. Precedex® (dexmedetomidine HCl) package insert. Lake Forest, IL: Hospira, Inc.; 2004 Apr.

54. Mason KP, Zgleszewski SE. Dexmedetomidine for pediatric sedation for computed tomography imaging studies. *Anesth Analg* 2006; 103:57–62.

55. Bouaziz H, Hewitt C, Eisenach JC. Subarachnoid neostigmine potentiation of alpha 2-adrenergic agonist analgesia. Dexmedetomidine versus Clonidine. *Reg Anesth* 1995; 20: 121–127.

56. Bloor BC, Ward DS, Belleville JP, et al. Effects of intravenous dexmedetomidine in humans. II. Hemodynamic changes. *Anesthesiology* 1992; 77:1134–1142.

57. Correa-Sales C, Rabin BC, Maze M: A hypnotic response to dexmedetomidine, an α-2 agonist, is mediated in the locus coeruleus in rats. Anesthesiology 1992; 76:948–995.

58. Khan Z, Ferguson C, Jones R: Alpha-2 and imidazoline receptor agonists: their pharmacology and therapeutic role. *Anaesthesia* 1999; 54:146–165.

59. Precedex product label, Abbott Laboratories Inc.

60. Talke PO, Caldwell JE, Richardson CA, et al. The effects of dexmedetomidine on neuromuscular blockade in human volunteers. *Anesth Analg* 1999; 88:633–639.

61. Belleville JP, Ward DS, Bloor BC, et al. Effects of intravenous dexmedetomidine in humans. I. Sedation, ventilation, and metabolic rate. *Anesthesiology* 1992, 77:1125–1133.

13. Drug Therapy for Hypercholesterolemia and Dyslipidemia

Sarah D. de Ferranti

Treatment Criteria and Guidelines

The initial and primary treatment of abnormal lipid levels (Table 13-1) in children is to change diet and activity levels. Pharmacological treatment of lipid disorders is used according to guidelines published in 1992 (Table 13-2). In adults, treatment cutpoints and goals for therapy are adjusted based on high-risk populations and in the presence of other cardiovascular (CV) risk factors; a similar approach is being taken in pediatrics (Table 13-3). New pediatric lipid guidelines are being developed and will likely reflect this type of thinking. Although atherosclerosis is known to begin in childhood, extensive outcome data are lacking in pediatrics, and parental and/or patient preferences are usually included in the decision-making process.

Nonpharmacological Lipid Lowering

Diet and Activity

Dietary counseling for abnormal lipid levels should be tailored to address the lipid profile of the child and the circumstances of the family. For elevated low-density lipoprotein (LDL), a low-fat diet beginning at age 2 years is safe and moderately successful.[1,2] The low-fat Step 1 diet calls for reducing saturated fat to at most 10% and total fat to at most 20% of total calories, while dietary cholesterol is limited to at most 300 mg/day. The Step 2 diet, which severely restricts saturated fat ($\leq$7%) and dietary cholesterol ($\leq$200 mg/day), is probably too difficult for a child to follow and is not recommended. Low-fat diets are not recommended for children younger than age 2 years because of concerns regarding adequate neuronal myelination. For high triglycerides (TG), seen more frequently with the current epidemic in childhood obesity, lowering dietary carbohydrate content and/or glycemic load is generally effective.[3] Exercise is an important part of treatment that decreases total cholesterol (TC) and increases high-density lipoprotein (HDL). We recommend 60 minutes of exercise 5 days a week.

Table 13-1. Categorization of lipid levels[a]

	TC (mg/dL)	LDL (mg/dL)	TG (mg/dL)	HDL (mg/dL)
Abnormal[b]	> 200	> 130	> 150	< 40
Borderline[c]	170–199	110–129	130–150	40–45
Acceptable	< 170	< 110	< 130	> 45
Ideal		70		> 60

[a]Cutpoints for TC and LDL are defined by the National Cholesterol Education Program (NCEP) and American Academy of Pediatrics (AAP) as published in 1992 and 1998.[1,54] The TG and HDL cutpoints are those used by the author in clinical practice and are based on normal values for children from the Lipid Research Clinics. School-aged children have lower TG and higher HDL levels than adolescents. Adolescent males have lower HDL levels after puberty, likely because of increased testosterone.
[b]Greater than 95th percentile from the Lipid Research Clinic.
[c]Greater than 75th, less than 95th percentile.

Table 13-2. AAP/NCEP recommendations for the initiation of pharmacotherapy

Indication for pharmacotherapy

Inadequate response to diet and lifestyle modification ≥ 6–12 months
Age ≥ 10 years
LDL ≥ 190 mg/dL
OR
LDL ≥ 160 mg/dL + family history of early coronary disease, OR
Two or more CV risk factors, OR
Coronary disease or equivalent (stroke, peripheral artery disease, diabetes)

Source: guidelines are extracted from reference 1 and 54. These guidelines are notable for a lack of comment on TG and HDL levels, metabolic syndrome, and other CV risk factors. New guidelines are under development.

Pharmacotherapy

Lipid-lowering medications are usually initiated if diet and exercise changes fail to improve values sufficiently (Table 13-2). A summary of treatments is shown in Table 13-4.

Bile Acid Sequestrants—Cholestyramine, Colestipol, and Colesevelam

Bile acid sequestrants are safe medications that lower TC and LDL, and CV risk. They are, however, difficult to tolerate. The longest pediatric and adult experience is with these medications. The Lipid Research Clinic Program, one of the earliest reports on pharmacological lipid lowering, showed that a 1% reduction in TC with cholestyramine use led to a 2% decrease in coronary disease events.[4] Trials in children have demonstrated decreases in TC and LDL, and reasonable increases in HDL.[5,6]

Table 13-3. Conditions associated with CV risk that modify treatment cutpoints[a]

At-risk populations	Individual risk factors
Familial hypercholesterolemia—homozygous, heterozygous	Hypertension
Diabetes mellitus—Type 1 and Type 2	Obesity
Heart transplant	Insulin resistance, fasting glucose > 100, Hb A1C > 7%
Kawasaki Disease ± coronary aneurysms	Low HDL levels
Chronic kidney disease—transplant, insufficiency	High TG levels
Chronic inflammatory disease—SLE, scleroderma	Elevated lipoprotein (a) with consistent family history
Previous chemotherapy or mediastinal radiation	Sex (male)
Congenital heart disease	First- or second-hand smoke exposure
	HIV treatment with protease inhibitors
	Marked inactivity
	Particularly severe family history

[a]Hb, hemoglobin; SLE, systemic lupus erythematosus; HIV, human immunodeficiency virus.

Indications Bile acid sequestrants are indicated for use in cases of elevated LDL AND:

1. Age younger than 10 years with severe LDL elevations consistent with genetic hyperlipidemias
2. Age older than 10 years AND prepubertal, unable to tolerate statins, parental concern regarding statins, or as additional agent

The safety and effectiveness of colestipol has not been evaluated in children.

Mechanism of Action Positively charged sequestrants bind to negatively charged bile acids in the intestines and prevent the reabsorption of cholesterol-containing bile. This increases bile production by the liver. When bile synthesis is increased, TG production is increased, which can lead to increased TG concentrations. Increased bile synthesis also increases LDL-C clearance through the liver and up-regulates LDL receptors, causing 3-hydroxy-3-methylbutaryl (HMG) coenzyme A (CoA) reductase activity to increase, so that using a bile acid binding resin with a statin is an effective combination.

Dosing See Table 13-4. Take each dose with 8 ounces of fluid before a meal.

Pharmacokinetics

Absorption: the sequestrants remain in the gut and are not systemically absorbed, thus, the side effect profile is minimal. Maximal lipid lowering effect occurs in 2 weeks

Drug-Drug Interactions Bile acid sequestrants combine well with a statin or niacin to maximally decrease LDL. However, ingestion of other medications, including

Table 13-4. Standard adult doses and dosage forms, shown in milligrams, unless otherwise noted[a]

	Initial dose per day	Maximum dose per day	Dosage forms
Cholestyramine	2–4 g[b] Children: 240 mg/kg/day (of anhydrous resin) in 3 divided doses; may need to titrate dose OR < 10 yr: initial, 2 g/day; range, 1–4 g/day	16 g	4 g/packet or scoop
Colestipol	2.5–5 g[b]	20 g	5 g/packet or scoop
Colesevelam	1.25 g[b]	4.375 g	0.625 g per tablet
Pravastatin	20	40	10, 20, 40
Atorvastatin	5–10	80	10, 20, 40, 80
Simvastatin	20	80	10, 20, 40, 80
Fluvastatin	20	80	10, 20, 40, 80
Rosuvastatin	5	40	5, 10, 20, 40
Lovastatin	20	80	10, 20, 40, 80
Ezetimibe	10	10	10
Gemfibrozil[c]	900	1200	600
Fenofibrate	48	145	48, 145 67, 134, 200 generic[d]
Niacin	500	2000	500, 750, 1000[e]
Omega-3 fatty acids	500	4000	500, 1000

[a]See text for further information on all medications.
[b]Cholestyramine, colestipol, and colesevelam should be divided into two daily doses. Each dose should be taken with 8 ounces of liquid.
[c]Gemfibrozil should be divided into two daily doses.
[d]200-mg generic fenofibrate is equivalent to 145-mg patent-protected drug.
[e]Dosages are not interchangeable—three tablets of 500 mg each is not equivalent to two tablets of 750 mg. Doses of niacin higher than 2000 mg give greater LDL decreases, but have higher risks of hepatotoxicity and are not recommended.

statins and multivitamins (MVI), should be separated from sequestrants either by 1 hour before or 4 hours after dosing to prevent a decrease in drug absorption.

Adverse Effects

Gastrointestinal: bloating, constipation can be reduced by allowing the preparation to sit for several hours before taking (it should be refrigerated), and by increasing fiber (dietary or psyllium supplements) and liquid intake

Decreased compliance: because of gritty powder or large pills. One study showed approximately 40% noncompliance in children with familial hypercholesterolemia over 18 weeks of treatment[7]

Metabolic: hypertriglyceridemia
Other: rare reports of hyperchloremic acidosis

Poisoning Information   Cholestyramine has been used as an agent to treat toxin poisonings.

Contraindications/Cautions

- TG higher than 400 mg/dL
- Inability to tolerate or understand prophylactic medications

HMG CoA Reductase Inhibitors—Pravastatin, Atorvastatin, Simvastatin, Fluvastatin, Rosuvastatin, and Lovastatin

HMG CoA reductase inhibitors, commonly referred to as statins, are used widely in adults to reduce LDL in patients with and without CV disease, and have been shown to reduce CV events by 25 to 30%. All drugs in this class seem to have similar efficacy, given the same reduction in LDL level,[8] although there may be greater improvements in HDL with particular statins at maximal doses (rosuvastatin > simvastatin > atorvastatin).[9,10] There are eight published pediatric trials of HMG CoA reductase inhibitors, ranging from 2 months to 2 years in length. Both male and female subjects are included, and the subjects are primarily those with familial hypercholesterolemia. The trials are relatively small, with the largest including 214 participants, and the agents evaluated include simvastatin,[11,12] lovastatin,[13,14] pravastatin,[15,16] and atorvastatin.[17,18] A rosuvastatin trial is presently ongoing. These trials have demonstrated good compliance (90%) and effectiveness (Table 13-5), minimal side effects, including no clinical impact on growth and development despite some increases in dehydroepiandrosterone (DHEA) and/or cortisol levels. However, there are no long-term safety data, and no trial specifically addressed whether puberty is affected, a concern because cholesterol is a precursor for sex steroid hormones.

Indication   HMG CoA reductase inhibitors are indicated for elevated LDL-C levels in patients older than 10 years of age or postpubertal. There are US Food and Drug Administration (FDA) indications for simvastatin, lovastatin, and atorvastatin for children with heterozygous familial hypercholesterolemia older than 10 years old, and for pravastatin for children older than 7 years old.

Mechanism of Action   Competitive inhibition of the key step in cholesterol synthesis in the liver leads to greater synthesis of and reduced breakdown of LDL receptors, which causes increased uptake of LDL by the liver. Additionally, levels of very low-density lipoprotein (VLDL) and intermediate-density lipoprotein (IDL) precursors of LDL are reduced, which may explain LDL reductions seen in homozygous familial hypercholesterolemic patients who generally do not have functioning LDL receptors. Statins have other effects associated with reduced CV risk, including anti-inflammatory effects lowering C-reactive protein, a risk factor for CV disease independent of cholesterol levels,[19] greater atherosclerotic plaque stability,[20] improved endothelial function,[23,24] and decreased platelet

Table 13-5. Therapeutic effects of various interventions on lipid parameters, shown in percent change

Medication	TC	LDL	HDL	TG	Comments
Bile acid binding resin	↓ 7–17	↓ 10–20	↑ 2–8	↑ 6–12	? ↑ Homocysteine
HMG CoA reductase inhibitors	↓ 13–30	↓ 17–41	↑ 3–11	↓ 2–18	
Ezetimibe		↓ 15–20	↑ 1–2	↓ 5	↓ Plant sterol absorption
Niacin		↓ 25	↑ 15–30	↓ 35–50	↓ Lipoprotein (a) 30–50%
Fibrates	↓ 13	↓ 20	↑ 15	↓ 30–50	Can see ↑ LDL
Fish oil		? ↑		↓ 25–45	
Diet—low fat	↓ 17	↓ 25	↑ 2	↓ 6	
Diet—low carbohydrate	↓ 3	↑ 4	↑ 4	↓ 48	
Diet—low glycemic load	↓ 10	↓ 9	↑ 2	↓ 35	
Aerobic activity	↓ 5–30		↑		

Source: data extracted from references 1, 12–16, and 18. Niacin and fibrate and low glycemic load data are taken from adult experience because of the lack of pediatric data (reference 3 and 21). Other dietary data are from reference 2 and 22.

aggregation.[25] There is also evidence that statins may have a role in reducing the incidence of cancer[26] and in cataract formation.[27] The response to statins is likely mediated in part by genetic polymorphisms, although genetic testing is not yet used clinically.[28]

Dosing   See Table 13-4 for HMG CoA reductase inhibitor dosing information. Atorvastatin levels are increased in those drinking more than 1 quart/day of grapefruit juice.

Pharmacokinetics

Absorption: in the upper intestines

Metabolism: in the liver, with all but pravastatin being processed by the cytochrome P450 (CYP450) system (pravastatin is sulfonated in hepatic cytosol). Simvastatin and lovastatin are more lipophilic and are converted β-hydroxy acids, whereas rosuvastatin, atorvastatin, pravastatin, and fluvastatin are more hydrophilic

Half-life: for most statins, the half-life is 1 to 4 hours, aside from rosuvastatin and atorvastatin, which have half-lives of approximately 20 hours[29]

Protein binding: statins are primarily protein bound, aside from pravastatin, which is only half protein bound

Elimination: statins are primarily excreted through the gastrointestinal (GI) track

The shorter-acting statins should be taken at night because the highest rate of cholesterol synthesis is between 12 and 2 am. LDL reductions are seen within 7 to 10 days of initiating treatment or changing doses. Statins tend to increase intestinal absorption of cholesterol, which means they combine well with cholesterol absorption inhibitors.[30]

Drug-Drug Interactions Interactions are well described with medications metabolized by the CYP450 system, including fibrates (gemfibrozil, fenofibrate), niacin, warfarin, digoxin, amiodarone, macrolides, mibefradil, antifungals, cyclosporine, nefazodone, and protease inhibitors. Most cases of rhabdomyolysis, the most serious side effect of HMG CoA reductase inhibitors, occur in the setting of possible drug-drug interactions.[29] Pravastatin may be less likely to interact with these drugs, as it is not metabolized by the CYP system. Concomitant dosing of any statin may be acceptable if the statin is administered at 25% of usual dose (maximum 20 mg for most statins, 10 mg for rosuvastatin) with careful monitoring.[29] Statins can also be combined with bile acid binding resins if administered more than 4 hours after the statin dose to prevent reduced activity of the statin. This combination produces an additional approximately 20% decrease in LDL.[31] Combination with ezetimibe gives an additional 20% LDL lowering without an increased risk of side effects.[32]

Adverse Effects

General data: despite early reports of hepatotoxicity and myopathy, statin therapy is generally safe in adults. Pediatric trials are small, but they also have not shown significant side effects, including rhabdomyolysis. In 14,236 adults randomized to atorvastatin, there were no cases of serious liver complications or rhabdomyolysis, and rates of adverse events were similar in high-dose, low-dose, and placebo arms, including liver function test (LFT) abnormalities and increases in creatine kinase (CK).[33] Chemical differences among the statins may be responsible for individual variation in tolerance; an adverse response to one statin does not predict a response to another. The author's convention, admittedly cautious, is to measure LFTs and CK at baseline, at 6 and 12 weeks after every dose change, and every 6 months when on stable dosing

Hepatic: dose-related reversible LFT elevations (> 3 times the upper limit of normal) were initially reported in 0.3 to 1.9% of adult users. However, later studies have shown rates of LFT elevations in 1.1% of those administered placebo as well. There are 30 cases of reported liver failure associated with statin use

Muscular: CK elevations greater than 10 times the upper limit of normal occur in 0.17% of adults administered statins, compared with 0.13% of patients administered placebo. Few subjects with CK elevations reported symptoms of muscle ache. The muscle ache is similar to the myalgias accompanying influenza, starting in the extremities and accompanied by weakness and fatigue. If there are changes in the urine (dark brown color) or muscle aches, the patient should stop taking the statin and have CK measured to assess whether this is indeed myopathy. Of those with true myopathy, more than 50% are receiving other drugs that increase risk, have medical problems such as hepatic or renal insufficiency, older age (particularly > 80 yr), or are small in size (relevant for pediatrics).[34] The incidence of rhabdomyolysis in hospitalized patients was 0.44 (95% confidence interval [CI], 0.20–0.84) per 10,000 patient years for atorvastatin, simvastatin, and pravastatin; for fibrates, the incidence was 2.82

(95% CI, 0.58–8.24). For individuals taking only a statin as a lipid-lowering agent, 22,727 individuals would need to be treated in a year to see 1 case of rhabdomyolysis requiring hospital admission[35]

Neurological: headache, case reports of peripheral neuropathy, sleep and mood disturbances, cognitive difficulties

Dermatological: rash, lichenoid skin eruption

Other: GI upset

Contraindications/Cautions

- Pregnancy (teratogenic)
- Liver disease, possible steatohepatitis
- See Drug-Drug Interactions

Cholesterol Absorption Inhibitor—Ezetimibe

Indication   Ezetimibe is indicated for elevated LDL with an inadequate response to statins as monotherapy; or sitosterolemia.

Mechanism of Action   Ezetimibe selectively inhibits absorption of dietary cholesterol by (by 54%[36]) and plant sterols, and prevents reabsorption of bile acids via transport protein NPC1L1 in the jejunal brush border.[33] Decreased absorption leads to decreased cholesterol in chylomicrons circulating to the liver, which up-regulates the hepatic LDL receptor and diminishes circulating LDL levels. LDL synthesis increases in response, making this drug particularly effective when combined with a statin. HDL increases and TG decreases.[37–40] Ezetimibe also inhibits the absorption of the plant sterols, campesterol and sitosterol, by approximately 40%,[36] which may make it an effective agent for sitosterolemia, a rare disorder leading to early CV disease. In a 1-week multiple-dose trial, adolescents showed similar pharmacokinetics to those seen in adults. A pediatric study is ongoing.

Dosing   Ezetimibe dosing is 10 mg/day for all ages, taken with or without food.

Pharmacokinetics

Absorption and metabolism: ezetimibe is glucuronidated in the intestinal wall and circulated enterohepatically; there is presumably minimal systemic exposure, which may explain the low side effect profile

Elimination: most is excreted in the feces

Drug-Drug Interactions   Concomitant administration with cyclosporine or gemfibrozil raises the concentrations of both drugs.

Adverse Effects

Gastrointestinal: diarrhea, nausea, taste changes, pancreatitis, cholelithiasis

Muscular: may potentiate statin-induced myopathy

Hepatic: LFT elevations, probably not greater than placebo
Hematological: thrombocytopenia
Other: angioedema, rash. No effect on fat-soluble vitamin absorption

Contraindications/Cautions   Coadministration of ezetimibe with bile acid binding resins causes inhibition of ezetimibe absorption. High doses administered to pregnant rats and rabbits caused skeletal abnormalities; administration during pregnancy is contraindicated.

Fibrates—Fenofibrate and Gemfibrozil

Indication   Fibrates are indicated with elevated TG levels unresponsive to diet, with risk of pancreatitis (TG > 600–1000 mg/dL). Increases in HDL are greater with fenofibrate than with gemfibrozil. LDL levels may increase with gemfibrozil. The greatest TG reductions are seen in those with Fredrickson Type III (dysbetalipoproteinemia); fibrates are also effective in those with chylomicronemia, along with a low-fat and alcohol-free diet. These agents may also increase fibrinolysis and inhibit coagulation.[41] Reducing TG levels reduces the risk of coronary artery disease in adults. Adults with a history of CV disease had 22% fewer future events on fibrates without significant decrease in LDL or TC levels. The effect may be related to the anticoagulative effects or the increase in HDL. The safety and efficacy of gemfibrozil has not been established in pediatric patients, and use of fibrates is confined to severe cases and older adolescents.

Mechanism of Action   Fibrates interact with hepatic peroxisome proliferator activated receptor (PPAR) α to stimulate free fatty acid oxidation and increase the production of lipoprotein lipase, which aids in TG and VLDL clearance and HDL expression.[42]

Dosing   See Table 13-4 for fibrates dosing.

Pharmacokinetics

Absorption: absorbed best when taken 30 minutes before food
Protein binding: bound to albumin
Half-life: fenofibrate has a 20-hour half-life, whereas gemfibrozil has a 1-hour half-life
Metabolism and elimination: both fenofibrate and gemfibrozil are glucuronidated and excreted in the urine

Drug-Drug Interactions   Prothrombin time is increased when fibrates are coadministered with Coumadin. There is an increased risk of myopathy if coadministered with a statin; if using both medications, decrease the statin dose and follow CK levels every 3 months until on a stable regimen. Myopathy is less common with fenofibrate than gemfibrozil. Cyclosporine levels increase approximately three-fold with coadministration.

Adverse Effects

Gastrointestinal: side effects in 5% of adults; elevated LFTs and CK levels, less commonly than with statins

Metabolic: increased LDL, particularly in those with only mildly elevated TGs (metabolic syndrome)

A small pediatric trial[43] (n = 12) showed minimal side effects in adolescents.

Contraindications/Cautions

- Concurrent statin and gemfibrozil (fenofibrate is safer) administration
- Renal insufficiency
- Pregnancy—category C, effect unknown

Niacin (Nicotinic Acid)

Indication Niacin is indicated in low HDL-C, hypertriglyceridemia, and possible use in those with elevated lipoprotein (a) with a concerning family history, but without clear hypercholesterolemia.

Mechanism of Action Pyridine-3-carboxylic acid or nicotinic acid is a B vitamin that, in large doses, decreases VLDL production and TG synthesis. It reduces TG lipolysis by lipoprotein lipase in adipose tissue and decreases free fatty acid circulation to the liver, thus, leading to less TG synthesis by the liver. There may be some inhibition on the rate-limiting enzyme of TG synthesis (diacyl-glycerol acetyltransferase 2).[44] Less TG synthesis by the liver leads to lower VLDL levels and, thus, lower LDL levels. Clearance of TG from the blood is increased by niacin because it improves the function of lipoprotein lipase. Clearance of ApoA-I is reduced, leading to increased HDL levels.[45] The ABCA 1 membrane cholesterol transporter is up-regulated by niacin.[46] Adult data show that niacin gives the greatest increase in HDL levels of the pharmacological agents.[47,48] Furthermore, niacin is the only agent that significantly decreases lipoprotein (a) (approximately 40%), although there are some "nonresponders." The effects on TG are seen within 1 week, whereas the LDL lowering occurs over 3 to 6 weeks. There is limited experience in pediatrics: one case series found 30% reductions in LDL, with common reversible side effects in 16 (76%) of 21 participants.[49] Because of the difficulty with tachyphylaxis and other side effects, niacin is rarely used.

Adult Dosing There are several niacin preparations, which are not interchangeable.

Regular preparation: initiate at 100 mg orally twice a day and increase every 7 days by 100 mg up to 1.5 to 2 g. Check LFTs, albumin, glucose, and uric acid levels, and a fasting lipid panel every 2 to 4 weeks until on a stable dose, then follow with laboratory tests every 3 to 6 months

Extended-release form: initiate at 500 mg once daily in the evening and increase no more frequently than every 4 weeks, adjusting with laboratory tests for efficacy and side effects, up to a maximum of 2 g/day

Regular (crystalline) 50 to 500 mg, available over the counter, is not recommended by most practitioners.

Sustained release (6–8 h) is available, as is extended release. The extended-release form (Niaspan) uses once-a-day dosing and is the only FDA-approved prescription form (see Table 13-4).

Pharmacokinetics

Absorption: water soluble

Onset of action: regular-preparation niacin results in rapid peak serum levels within 60 minutes

Metabolism: processed in the liver

Elimination: excreted in the urine, or excreted unchanged as nicotinic acid[50]

Drug-Drug Interactions   Niacin can be used effectively with a bile acid binding resin as long as dosing is timed appropriately. If niacin is administered with a statin, watch carefully for increased risk of myopathy and use the statin at 25% of maximal statin dose. Flushing and dizziness is seen with nicotine and alcohol use.

Adverse Effects

Tachyphylaxis: flushing, pruritus, and headache, which are mediated through prostaglandins and can be treated or prevented in some cases with antihistamines and/or aspirin; usually resolves over 1 to 2 weeks. Flushing is worse if niacin is taken with alcohol or hot beverages

Hepatic: dose-related hepatotoxicity, particularly at more than 2 g/d, and with over-the-counter preparations, including liver failure with sustained release. The extended-release form may cause less hepatotoxicity. Flu-like symptoms, and very significant decreases in LDL (>50%) may indicate liver failure. Maximal reported improvement in lipid levels are seen with doses of 4 to 6 g/day, but the risk of hepatotoxicity increases above 2 g/day

Muscular: myopathy with CK elevations and muscle cramping, and rhabdomyolysis with coadministration of a statin in a small number of reported cases

Cardiovascular: palpitations, atrial arrhythmias, hypotension

Metabolic: mild hyperglycemia, hyperuricemia

Dermatological: acanthosis nigricans (treat with topical salicylic acid preparations), dry skin

Ophthalmological: toxic amblyopia and toxic maculopathy (rare and reversible)

Other: upper GI distress (improves if niacin is taken with a meal)

Contraindications   Contraindications to niacin use include liver disease, severe gout (increases uric acid levels), peptic ulcer, active bleeding, hypersensitivity to niacin, unstable angina, diabetes (may require an increase in hypoglycemic therapy), and pregnancy (birth defects in animals).[47,51]

Omega-3 Fatty Acids

Indication   Omega-3 fatty acids are indicated as adjunctive therapy in adults with elevated TG greater than 500 mg/dL. Safety and effectiveness have not been established in children.

Mechanism of Action   Omega-3 fatty acids are found in fatty fish (tuna, salmon, and swordfish), omega-3 fatty acids seem to protect against thrombosis, arrhythmia, inflammation, and hypertension, and improve endothelial function. Studies show that they decrease the risk of recurrent CV events (GISSI).[52] Twenty children treated with DHA had favorable lipid profile changes.[53] The mechanism is not clear, but may be related to decreased TG synthesis in the liver.

Dosing

Adolescents: 1000 mg/day
Adults: 4 g/day or more

Pharmacokinetics   Response should be seen within 2 months.

Drug-Drug Interactions   There are no known drug-drug interactions.

Adverse Effects

Metabolic: increase in LDL
Dermatological: rash
Cardiovascular: angina
Other: back pain, fishy odor to breath (lessened by freezing pills and taking at bedtime)

Poisoning Information   There is some concern regarding purity and mercury content in the over-the-counter forms, which are less regulated. One purified form is available by prescription and is approved by the FDA for use with severely elevated TG levels.

Summary

Lifestyle modification is the primary treatment modality for lipid disorders, however, pharmacotherapy should be considered in children with high cholesterol and concerning risk factors. Medications to lower lipid levels are generally well tolerated and effective. However, there are gaps in our knowledge regarding long-term safety and efficacy, and each child should be considered in the context of the family's risk and attitudes toward pharmacotherapy. Improved understanding of the initiating factors of atherosclerosis and the noninvasive measurement of preclinical disease will allow us to target treatment more precisely and interpret lipid values more effectively in the context of other risk factors, which are, in reality, surrogate markers for risk.

References

1. American Academy of Pediatrics. Committee on Nutrition. Cholesterol in childhood. *Pediatrics* 1998; 101:141–147.

2. Obarzanek E, Kimm SY, Barton BA, Van Horn LL, Kwiterovich PO, Jr., Simons-Morton DG et al. Long-term safety and efficacy of a cholesterol-lowering diet in children with elevated low-density lipoprotein cholesterol: seven-year results of the Dietary Intervention Study in Children (DISC). *Pediatrics* 2001; 107:256–264.

3. Ebbeling CB, Leidig MM, Sinclair KB, Seger-Shippee LG, Feldman HA, Ludwig DS. Effects of an ad libitum low-glycemic load diet on cardiovascular disease risk factors in obese young adults. *Am J Clin Nutr* 2005; 81:976–982.

4. The Lipid Research Clinics Coronary Primary Prevention Trial results. II. The relationship of reduction in incidence of coronary heart disease to cholesterol lowering. *JAMA* 1984; 251:365–374.

5. McCrindle BW, O'Neil MB, Cullen-Dean G, Helden E. Acceptability and compliance with two forms of cholestyramine in the treatment of hypercholesterolemia in children: a randomized, crossover trial. *J Pediatr* 1997;130:266–273.

6. Tonstad S, Siversten M, Aksenes L, Ose L. Low dose colestipol in adolescents with familial hypercholesterolaemia. *Arch Dis Child* 1996;74:157–160.

7. McCrindle BW, Helden E, Cullen-Dean G, Conner WT. A randomized crossover trial of combination pharmacologic therapy in children with familial hyperlipidemia. *Pediatr Res* 2002; 51:715–721.

8. Zhou Z, Rahme E, Pilote L. Are statins created equal? Evidence from randomized trials of pravastatin, simvastatin, and atorvastatin for cardiovascular disease prevention. *Am Heart J* 2006; 151:273–281.

9. Crouse JR, III, Furberg CD. Treatment of dyslipidemia: room for improvement? *Arterioscler Thromb Vasc Biol* 2000; 20:2333–2335.

10. Jones PH, Hunninghake DB, Ferdinand KC, Stein EA, Gold A, Caplan RJ et al. Effects of rosuvastatin versus atorvastatin, simvastatin, and pravastatin on non-high-density lipoprotein cholesterol, apolipoproteins, and lipid ratios in patients with hypercholesterolemia: additional results from the STELLAR trial. *Clin Ther* 2004; 26:1388–1399.

11. Ducobu J, Brasseur D, Chaudron JM, Deslypere JP, Harvengt C, Muls E et al. Simvastatin use in children. *Lancet* 1992; 339:1488.

12. de Jongh S, Ose L, Szamosi T, Gagne C, Lambert M, Scott R et al. Efficacy and safety of statin therapy in children with familial hypercholesterolemia: a randomized, double-blind, placebo-controlled trial with simvastatin. *Circulation* 2002; 106:2231–2237.

13. Stein EA, Illingworth DR, Kwiterovich PO, Jr., Liacouras CA, Siimes MA, Jacobson MS et al. Efficacy and safety of lovastatin in adolescent males with heterozygous familial hypercholesterolemia: a randomized controlled trial. *JAMA* 1999; 281:137–144.

14. Lambert M, Lupien PJ, Gagne C, Levy E, Blaichman S, Langlois S et al. Treatment of familial hypercholesterolemia in children and adolescents: effect of

lovastatin. Canadian Lovastatin in Children Study Group. *Pediatrics* 1996; 97: 619–628.

15. Wiegman A, Hutten BA, de Groot E, Rodenburg J, Bakker HD, Buller HR et al. Efficacy and safety of statin therapy in children with familial hypercholesterolemia: a randomized controlled trial. *JAMA* 2004; 292:331–337.

16. Knipscheer HC, Boelen CC, Kastelein JJ, van Diermen DE, Groenemeijer BE, van den EA et al. Short-term efficacy and safety of pravastatin in 72 children with familial hypercholesterolemia. *Pediatr Res* 1996; 39:867–871.

17. Raal FJ, Pappu AS, Illingworth DR, Pilcher GJ, Marais AD, Firth JC et al. Inhibition of cholesterol synthesis by atorvastatin in homozygous familial hypercholesterolaemia. *Atherosclerosis* 2000; 150:421–428.

18. McCrindle BW, Ose L, Marais AD. Efficacy and safety of atorvastatin in children and adolescents with familial hypercholesterolemia or severe hyperlipidemia: a multicenter, randomized, placebo-controlled trial. *J Pediatr* 2003; 143:74–80.

19. Pearson TA, Mensah GA, Alexander RW, Anderson JL, Cannon RO, III, Criqui M et al. Markers of inflammation and cardiovascular disease: application to clinical and public health practice: A statement for healthcare professionals from the Centers for Disease Control and Prevention and the American Heart Association. *Circulation* 2003; 107:499–511.

20. Williams JK, Sukhova GK, Herrington DM, Libby P. Pravastatin has cholesterol-lowering independent effects on the artery wall of atherosclerotic monkeys. *J Am Coll Cardiol* 1998; 31:684–691.

21. Brunton LL, Lazo JS, Parker KL, eds. Goodman & Gilman's the pharmacological basis of therapeutics. 11th ed. New York: McGraw-Hill; 2006.

22. Sondike SB, Cooperman N, Jacobson MS. Effects of a low-carbohydrate diet on weight loss and cardiovascular risk factor in overweight adolescents. *J Pediatr* 2003;142: 253–258.

23. O'Driscoll G, Green D, Taylor RR. Simvastatin, an HMG-coenzyme A reductase inhibitor, improves endothelial function within 1 month. *Circulation* 1997; 95:1126–1131.

24. Laufs U, La FV, Plutzky J, Liao JK. Upregulation of endothelial nitric oxide synthase by HMG CoA reductase inhibitors. *Circulation* 1998; 97:1129–1135.

25. Aviram M, Hussein O, Rosenblat M, Schlezinger S, Hayek T, Keidar S. Interactions of platelets, macrophages, and lipoproteins in hypercholesterolemia: antiatherogenic effects of HMG-CoA reductase inhibitor therapy. *J Cardiovasc Pharmacol* 1998; 31:39–45.

26. Sleijfer S, van der GA, Planting AS, Stoter G, Verweij J. The potential of statins as part of anti-cancer treatment. *Eur J Cancer* 2005; 41:516–522.

27. Klein BE, Klein R, Lee KE, Grady LM. Statin use and incident nuclear cataract. *JAMA* 2006; 295:2752–2758.

28. Kajinami K, Okabayashi M, Sato R, Polisecki E, Schaefer EJ. Statin pharmacogenomics: what have we learned, and what remains unanswered? *Curr Opin Lipidol* 2005; 16:606–613.

29. Bellosta S, Paoletti R, Corsini A. Safety of statins: focus on clinical pharmacokinetics and drug interactions. *Circulation* 2004; 109:III50–III57.

30. Miettinen TA, Gylling H. Synthesis and absorption markers of cholesterol in serum and lipoproteins during a large dose of statin treatment. *Eur J Clin Invest* 2003; 33:976–982.

31. Comparative efficacy and safety of pravastatin and cholestyramine alone and combined in patients with hypercholesterolemia. Pravastatin Multicenter Study Group II. *Arch Intern Med* 1993; 153:1321–1329.

32. Pearson TA, Denke MA, McBride PE, Battisti WP, Brady WE, Palmisano J. A community-based, randomized trial of ezetimibe added to statin therapy to attain NCEP ATP III goals for LDL cholesterol in hypercholesterolemic patients: the ezetimibe add-on to statin for effectiveness (EASE) trial. *Mayo Clin Proc* 2005; 80:587–595.

33. Newman C, Tsai J, Szarek M, Luo D, Gibson E. Comparative safety of atorvastatin 80 mg versus 10 mg derived from analysis of 49 completed trials in 14,236 patients. *Am J Cardiol* 2006; 97:61–67.

34. Pasternak RC, Smith SC, Jr., Bairey-Merz CN, Grundy SM, Cleeman JI, Lenfant C. ACC/AHA/NHLBI Clinical Advisory on the Use and Safety of Statins. *Stroke* 2002; 33:2337–2341.

35. Graham DJ, Staffa JA, Shatin D, Andrade SE, Schech SD, La Grenade L et al. Incidence of hospitalized rhabdomyolysis in patients treated with lipid-lowering drugs. *JAMA* 2004; 292:2585–2590.

36. Sudhop T, Lutjohann D, Kodal A, Igel M, Tribble DL, Shah S et al. Inhibition of intestinal cholesterol absorption by ezetimibe in humans. *Circulation* 2002; 106:1943–1948.

37. Altmann SW, Davis HR, Jr., Zhu LJ, Yao X, Hoos LM, Tetzloff G et al. Niemann-Pick C1 Like 1 protein is critical for intestinal cholesterol absorption. *Science* 2004; 303:1201–1204.

38. Gagne C, Bays HE, Weiss SR, Mata P, Quinto K, Melino M et al. Efficacy and safety of ezetimibe added to ongoing statin therapy for treatment of patients with primary hypercholesterolemia. *Am J Cardiol* 2002; 90:1084–1091.

39. Knopp RH, Dujovne CA, Le Beaut A, Lipka LJ, Suresh R, Veltri EP. Evaluation of the efficacy, safety, and tolerability of ezetimibe in primary hypercholesterolaemia: a pooled analysis from two controlled phase III clinical studies. *Int J Clin Pract* 2003; 57:363–368.

40. Dujovne CA, Ettinger MP, McNeer JF, Lipka LJ, LeBeaut AP, Suresh R et al. Efficacy and safety of a potent new selective cholesterol absorption inhibitor, ezetimibe, in patients with primary hypercholesterolemia. *Am J Cardiol* 2002; 90:1092–1097.

41. Watts GF, Dimmitt SB. Fibrates, dyslipoproteinaemia and cardiovascular disease. *Curr Opin Lipidol* 1999; 10:561–574.

42. Staels B, Dallongeville J, Auwerx J, Schoonjans K, Leitersdorf E, Fruchart JC. Mechanism of action of fibrates on lipid and lipoprotein metabolism. *Circulation* 1998; 98:2088–2093.

43. Büyükçelik M, Anarat A, Bayazit AK, Noyan A, Ozel A, Anarat R, et al. The effects of gemfibrozil on hyperlipidemia in children with persistent nephritic syndrome. *Turk J Pediatr* 2002;44:40–44

44. Ganji SH, Tavintharan S, Zhu D, Xing Y, Kamanna VS, Kashyap ML. Niacin noncompetitively inhibits DGAT2 but not DGAT1 activity in HepG2 cells. *J Lipid Res* 2004; 45:1835–1845.

45. Jin FY, Kamanna VS, Kashyap ML. Niacin decreases removal of high-density lipoprotein apolipoprotein A-I but not cholesterol ester by Hep G2 cells. Implication for reverse cholesterol transport. *Arterioscler Thromb Vasc Biol* 1997; 17:2020–2028.

46. Carlson LA. Nicotinic acid: the broad-spectrum lipid drug. A 50th anniversary review. *J Intern Med* 2005; 258:94–114.

47. Knopp RH, Ginsberg J, Albers JJ, Hoff C, Ogilvie JT, Warnick GR et al. Contrasting effects of unmodified and time-release forms of niacin on lipoproteins in hyperlipidemic subjects: clues to mechanism of action of niacin. *Metabolism* 1985; 34:642–650.

48. Vega GL, Grundy SM. Lipoprotein responses to treatment with lovastatin, gemfibrozil, and nicotinic acid in normolipidemic patients with hypoalphalipoproteinemia. *Arch Intern Med* 1994; 154:73–82.

49. Colletti RB, Neufeld EJ, Roff NK, McAuliffe TL, Baker AL, Newburger JW. Niacin treatment of hypercholesterolemia in children. *Pediatrics* 1993; 92:78–82.

50. Iwaki M, Ogiso T, Hayashi H, Tanino T, Benet LZ. Acute dose-dependent disposition studies of nicotinic acid in rats. *Drug Metab Dispos* 1996; 24:773–779.

51. Henkin Y, Oberman A, Hurst DC, Segrest JP. Niacin revisited: clinical observations on an important but underutilized drug. *Am J Med* 1991; 91:239–246.

52. Marchioli R, Barzi F, Bomba E, Chieffo C, Di Gregorio D, Di Mascio R, et al. Early protection against sudden death by n-3 polyunsaturated fatty acids after myocardial infarction: time-course analysis of the results of the Gruppo Italiano per lo Studio della Sopravvivenza nell'Infarto Miocardico (GISSI)-Prevenzione. *Circulation* 2002;105:1897–1903.

53. Engler MM, Engler MB, Malloy M, Chiu E, Besio D, Paul S et al. Docosahexaenoic acid restores endothelial function in children with hyperlipidemia: results from the EARLY study. *Int J Clin Pharmacol Ther* 2004; 42:672–679.

54. American Academy of Pediatrics Committee on Nutrition: Statement on cholesterol. *Pediatrics* 1992; 90:469–473.

14. Medication Errors in Children

Robert L. Poole

The Institute of Medicine's report: "To Err Is Human: Building a Safer Health System" made the headlines with startling figures on the human costs of medical errors. Highlights of the report included the following findings: 44,000 to 98,000 annual deaths are a result of medical errors, and medication errors are the leading cause, followed by surgical mistakes and complications; more Americans die from medical errors each year than from breast cancer, AIDS, or car accidents; 2% of patients admitted to hospitals experience an adverse drug event that results in an increased length of stay and nearly $4,700 increase in cost per event; the total cost of medical errors in the United States is estimated to be between $8.5 billion and $17 billion annually; and Computerized Provider Order Entry (CPOE) can improve the safety of medication use.[1]

Medication errors in pediatric and neonatal inpatients continue to be reported with an increased frequency during the past two decades. A medication error is defined as an error that originates at any point in the medication use process, from prescribing and transcribing, to dispensing, administering, or monitoring. Errors may occur at any time during a patient's hospital stay and may result from the action or inaction of physicians, pharmacists, nurses, other hospital personnel, or the patient. The top 10 causes of pediatric errors for the 2-year period of the calendar year 1999 to 2000 reported by the United States Pharmacopeia (USP) were the following: 1) performance deficit, 2) procedure or protocol not followed, 3) miscommunication, 4) inaccurate or omitted transcription, 5) improper documentation, 6) drug distribution system error, 7) knowledge deficit, 8) calculation error, 9) computer entry error, and 10) lack of system safeguards.[2]

Each day, physicians, pharmacists, and nurses in children's hospitals address the special medication needs of pediatric and neonatal patients weighing between 400 g and 200 kg. The dosing of most drugs is weight-based in pediatrics, which results in the potential for a 500-fold dosing error.[3] In contrast, in adult patients, a two-fold dosing error potential is usually the maximum encountered, because pharmaceutical manufacturers provide medications in ready-to-administer unit dose packaging. Very few drugs are available from manufacturers in ready-to-administer pediatric or neonatal unit dose or dosage forms. Pediatric pharmacists are routinely required to prepare dilutions, repackage, or compound dosage forms. Examples of the most common errors are listed in Table 14-1.[4,5]

Most of the more than 10,000 drugs on the market in the United States are not labeled with a pediatric indication, nor have they been studied in pediatric or neonatal populations. These problems put pediatric and neonatal patients at increased risk for medication errors. Studies have also shown that the majority of medication errors in pediatrics occur in patients younger than 2 years of age.[6]

Table 14-1. The most common medication errors

Type of error	Examples
Prescribing (49%)	Inaccurate dose calculation; illegible hand-writing; verbal orders; abbreviations/acronyms
Transcribing (11%)	Wrong patient; inaccurate copy of drug orders
Dispensing (14%)	Calculation error; labeling error; wrong drug; wrong concentration; dilution/compounding error
Administration (the 5 "wrongs") (26%)	Wrong drug; wrong dose; wrong patient; wrong route; wrong time
Monitoring (% included above in prescribing)	Failure to monitor patient after a dose; adverse reactions; failure to respond to abnormal laboratory test results

Source: Bates DW, Cullen DJ, Laird LA, Peterson SD, et al. Incidence of adverse drug events and potential adverse drug events. Implications for prevention. ADE Prevention Study Group. JAMA 1995;274:29–34.

Pediatric and neonatal intensive care units are prime sites for medication errors. The therapeutic regimens of intensive care patients are often complex and require numerous calculations. Medications are often needed quickly, which puts added pressure on staff members in a stressful environment, which can additionally result in mistakes. Errors, adverse drug reactions (ADRs), and drug interactions are commonplace. Table 14-2 lists the medications considered high risk or high alert. These medications require special attention, because they have been associated with serious morbidity and mortality in pediatric patients.

Several excellent reports that provide strategies and guidelines for the prevention of medication errors in pediatrics have been published recently.[6–8] They provide recommendations for systems improvements, education, the use of automation, and the benefits of CPOE systems. The value of unit-based clinical pharmacists has been demonstrated to reduce both potential and actual medication errors.[9] CPOE has also been shown to reduce medication errors. The potential benefits from CPOE are numerous and include the following: reductions in duplicate laboratory testing; the ability to recommend less expensive drug therapy; increased adherence to therapy pathways; annual savings in the millions of dollars; decreased turnaround times; pharmacy time saved; nursing time saved; and a 50% reduction in prescribing errors.[9] However, hospital computer systems and software applications are usually developed for adult patient populations. The healthcare provided for adult patients represents 95% of all health care. Although pediatrics makes up the remaining 5% of healthcare, only 1% (75) of the 7000 hospitals in the United States are children's hospitals. The safety of CPOE systems designed for adults is slowly being adapted for use in pediatrics. Computer order entry errors will most likely increase as more systems are automated and CPOE is implemented.[10] The careful implementation of technology will be important to avoid developing a whole new set of errors.

Table 14-2. High risk-high alert medications

Potassium chloride
Sodium chloride (concentrated)
Insulin
Narcotic analgesics
Heparin, warfarin
Chemotherapeutic agents
Magnesium
Calcium
Dopamine, vasoactive agents
TPN (total parenteral nutrition)

Table 14-3. Environmental factors associated with medication errors

Distractions: telephones, pagers
Excessive workload; fatigue
Staffing: temporary, inexperienced, or insufficient numbers of staff
Shift changes
Patient transfers
Poor communication among providers
Verbal orders
Emergencies: Code Blue, STAT orders
Information not available
Patient names same or similar
Drugs "similar or sound alike" or spelled similarly
Space inadequate
Computer system down

Recently, CPOE software has come to the market for Total Parenteral Nutrition (TPN) ordering and compounding process and made this high-risk therapy much safer.[11]

Workplace factors also contribute to the occurrence of medication errors. Frequent interruptions, working long or double shifts, excessive noise, and inadequate lighting are but a few of the common hospital environmental factors that can contribute to medication errors. A more complete list appears in Table 14-3. Awareness and continued efforts to minimize the impact of these factors is critical to the prevention of medication errors.

Prevention of medication errors should focus on the following basic concepts: 1) enforce standards for prescribing: complete orders; generic names only; no abbreviations for drug names, list of "do not use" abbreviations; 2) standardization where possible: doses; time of administration; storage, packaging, and labeling; dosing of insulin and potassium; use of protocols and storage of potentially lethal injectable drugs; 3) unit dose system of drug distribution; 4) simplification: limit the number of infusion pump types; 5) pharmacy-based admixture of all intravenous (I.V.) medications and solutions; 6) allergy information reliably displayed; 7) eliminate double shifts and long shifts; 8) computerized drug profiles; and 9) effective adverse drug event monitoring systems.[6–8]

The Joint Commission for the Accreditation of Healthcare Organizations (JCAHO) has developed National Patient Safety Goals each year since 2003 to improve patient safety and patient care.[12] These goals, as they relate to medication safety, are listed below in Table 14-4.

JCAHO has also developed an official "Do Not Use" list for common abbreviations that have led to medication errors (see Table 14-5).[12]

The best approach to reduce medication errors is to assume that errors occur in your institution. Recognize that medication errors are usually system failures and not human errors. Errors are almost always multifactorial. Encourage the reporting of errors. Know which patient populations are at high risk. Understand which processes are error prone and focus improvement projects in these areas. Know which medications are high alert and put patients at a higher risk, and develop procedures that require extra care to ensure safety.

Additional references regarding medication errors in pediatrics and adverse drug event reporting are available in the literature.[13-15]

Table 14-4. JCAHO Patient Safety Goals for 2006

Goal 1	Improve the accuracy of patient identification
1A	Use at least two patient identifiers when providing care, treatment, or services
Goal 2	Improve the effectiveness of communication among caregivers
2A	For verbal or telephone orders or for telephonic reporting of critical test results, verify the complete order or test result by having the person receiving the information record and "read-back" the complete order or test result
2B	Standardize a list of abbreviations, acronyms, symbols, and dose designations that are not to be used throughout the organization (see Table 14-5)
Goal 3	Improve the safety of using medications
3B	Standardize and limit the number of drug concentrations used by the organization
3C	Identify and, at a minimum, annually review a list of look-alike/sound-alike drugs used by the organization, and take action to prevent errors involving the inter change of these drugs
3D	Label all medications, medication containers (for example, syringes, medicine cups, basins), or other solutions on and off the sterile field
Goal 7	Reduce the risk of health care-associated infections
7A	Comply with current Centers for Disease Control and Prevention (CDC) hand hygiene guidelines
Goal 8	Accurately and completely reconcile medications across the continuum of care
8A	There is a process for comparing the patient's current medications with those ordered for the patient while under the care of the organization
8B	A complete list of the patient's medications is communicated to the next provider of service when a patient is referred or transferred to another setting, service, practitioner, or level of care within or outside the organization. The complete list of medications is also provided to the patient on discharge from the facility
Goal 13	Encourage patients' active involvement in their own care as a patient safety strategy
13A	Define and communicate the means for patients and their families to report concerns regarding safety and encourage them to do so
Goal 15	The organization identifies safety risks inherent in it`s patient population

Table 14-5. JCAHO official "Do Not Use" list (adapted)

Do not use	Potential problem	Use instead
U (unit)	Mistaken for "0" (zero), the number "4" (four) or "cc"; potential $10 \times$ error	Write "unit"
IU (international unit)	Mistaken for I.V. (intravenous) or the number 10 (ten)	Write "international unit"
Q.D., QD, q.d., qd (daily)	Mistaken for each other	Write "daily"
Q.O.D., QOD, q.o.d, qod (every other day)	Period after the Q mistaken for "I" and the "O" mistaken for "I"; potential $4 \times$ error	Write "every other day"
Trailing zero (X.0 mg)	Decimal point is missing	Write X mg
Lack of leading zero (.X mg)	Potential $10 \times$ error	Write 0.X mg
MS	Can mean morphine sulfate or magnesium sulfate	Write "morphine sulfate"
MSO_4 and $MgSO_4$	Confused for one another	Write "magnesium sulfate"

ADRs in Children

ADRs continue to be a major cause of morbidity and mortality in the United States, with a negative economic impact, estimated to be greater than $30 billion annually.[17] It has been estimated that 2 to 6% of admissions to the hospitals in the United States are the result of an adverse reaction to a prescribed medication. Somewhere between 5 and 30% of patients admitted were reported to have experienced an ADR. A fatal reaction to a drug occurs in approximately 0.3% of hospitalized patients.[18] Toxic effects from marketed drugs rank among the top 10 causes of death in the United States. There are a number of different ADR definitions. The World Health Organization (WHO), the US Food and Drug Administration (FDA), and the American Society of Health System Pharmacists (ASHP) versions are provided in Table 14-6.

ADRs can happen when you do everything right. You administer the right drug, for the right indication, in the right dose, at the right time, and a bad outcome still occurs. Most ADRs are identified during the clinical trial phase of bringing a new drug to market, a time when all ADRs are required to be reported to both the FDA and the drug's manufacturer. Once a drug has been approved for marketing by the FDA, ADR reporting is voluntary. Voluntary reporting relies on the goodwill and good intentions of healthcare professionals, and has resulted in the gross underreporting of ADRs. Because of this, the actual incidence of ADRs is not known. Carleton et al. reported in 2001 that physicians in the United States voluntarily report an ADR to the FDA once every 336 years, whereas pharmacists report at a rate of once every 26 years.[17] These rates were based on the number of physicians and pharmacists in the United States, and the number of ADRs reported to the FDA in 1997 to 1998. Conservative estimates suggest that 5% of all hospital admissions in the United States result from ADRs. In 1994, there were 7.2 million hospital patients who had serious ADRs; 106,000 of the ADRs were fatal.

Table 14-6. ADR Definitions

Organization	Definition
1. WHO	Any injurious, unintended, and undesired response to a drug administered at doses used normally among humans for prophylaxis, diagnosis, or therapy
2. FDA	Any experience associated with the use of a drug, whether or not considered to be drug related, including any side effect, injury, toxicity, or sensitivity reaction, or significant failure of expected pharmacological action
3. ASHP	Any unexpected, unintended, undesired, or excessive response to a drug that: 1. Requires discontinuing the drug 2. Requires changing the drug therapy 3. Requires modifying the dose 4. Requires admission to a hospital 5. Prolongs hospitalization 6. Requires supportive treatment 7. Complicates diagnosis 8. Negatively affects prognosis 9. Results in temporary or permanent harm, disability or death

ADRs in children are not well understood because greater than 75% of drugs currently on the market have not been studied in children and do not have a labeled pediatric indication for use. This fact has many clinicians referring to children as "therapeutic orphans." Additionally, infants and young children cannot evaluate and express their own response to medications. Information obtained from research in adults cannot be directly applied to infants and children that may have immature organ systems or different metabolic pathways. Information regarding a drug's use in pediatrics is usually not included in the drug's package insert. Instead, statements similar to the following appear: "not approved for use in children younger than 12 years of age" or "safety and efficacy in children has not been established." Active surveillance systems for monitoring and reporting pediatric ADRs have been proposed. Prospective studies of hospitalized pediatric patients reporting the incidence of ADRs will vary depending on the severity of illness and the number of concurrent drugs being administered. Reported incidences of ADRs ranged between 4.4 and 16.8%.[18] Gill et al. prospectively studied ADRs in a pediatric intensive care unit and found a 7% incidence.[19] In another prospective study, Weiss et al. studied ADRs in a pediatric isolation ward. In their study, ADRs occurred in 21.5% of patients.[20] An active monitoring system for reporting ADRs in children via a network of family pediatricians reported an incidence of 1.5% in nonhospitalized patients.[21] Clearly, in a controlled environment such as a hospital, active reporting yields better, more complete data. Le et al. conducted a retrospective cohort study that reviewed ADRs in children that were reported over a 10-year period in a community-based, tertiary care, children's teaching hospital. A total of 1087 ADRs were reported, with an overall incidence of 1.6%.[22] This incidence was very low compared with the previously reported rates with prospective, active surveillance methods. Active surveillance systems must be put in place to address this serious issue in pediatrics, because the underreporting of ADRs in children continues to be a serious problem.

The drug classes most commonly associated with ADRs reported in pediatric patients are listed in Table 14-7. The types of pediatric ADRs that have been reported in the literature are listed in Table 14-8.

Postmarketing surveillance for pediatric ADRs cannot be overemphasized. Reporting systems must be improved and reporting needs to be mandatory instead of voluntary. All hospitals are required to have an ADR reporting system. Most include the use of the FDA's MedWatch program for ADR reporting. The FDA will notify the drug manufacturer of all reported ADRs and require the manufacturer to follow-up each reported occurrence.

Current research is in progress to identify the genetic basis of severe and fatal ADRs in children. With this knowledge, it is hoped that testing can be performed before therapy to avoid treatment tragedies. Until such time, reporting must be improved.

Table 14-7. "Top 10" drug classes associated with ADRs in pediatrics

Drug class	Frequency
1. Antibiotics	More common
2. Narcotic analgesics	
3. Anticonvulsants	
4. Sedatives/anxiolytics/hypnotics	
5. Antineoplastic agents	
6. Antifungal agents	
7. Gastrointestinal agents	
8. Corticosteroids	
9. Cardiovascular drugs	▼
10. Immunoglobulins	Less common

Table 14-8. "Top 10" types of pediatric ADRs reported

Type of ADR	Frequency
1. Rash	More common
2. Flushing	
3. Pruritus; urticaria	
4. Blood pressure changes	
5. Fever, chills, rigor	
6. Neutropenia; thrombocytopenia	
7. Arrhythmias	
8. Respiratory depression	
9. Decreased renal function	▼
10. Abnormal liver function tests	Less common

References

1. Institute of Medicine, Committee on Quality Health Care in America. To *Err is Human: Building a Safer Health System. Report of the Institute of Medicine.* Kohn LT, Corrigan JM, Donaldson MS, eds. Washington, DC: National Academy Press; 2000.

2. Crowley E, Williams R, Cousins D. Medication errors in children: a descriptive summary of medication error reports submitted to the United States Pharmacopeia. *Curr Ther Res.* 2001;26;627–640.

3. Poole RL, Benitz WE. Medication Errors in Children. *JAMA* 2001;286(8):915–916.

4. Folli HL, Poole RL, Benitz WE, et al. Medication error prevention by clinical pharmacists in two children's hospital. *Pediatrics* 1987;79:718–722.

5. Bates DW, Cullen DJ, Laird LA, Peterson SD, et al. Incidence of adverse drug events and potential adverse drug events. Implications for prevention. ADE Prevention Study Group. *JAMA* 1995;274:29–34.

6. Levine SR, Cohen MR, Poole RL, et al: Guidelines for preventing medication errors in pediatrics. *J Pediatr Pharmacol Ther* 2001;6:426–442.

7. Fernandez CV, Gillis-Ring J. Strategies for the prevention of medical error in pediatrics. *J Pediatr* 2003;143(2):155–162.

8. Anderson BJ, Ellis JF. Common errors of drug administration in infants. *Paediatr Drugs* 1999;1(2):93–107.

9. Kaushal R, Bates DW, Landrigan C, et al. Medication errors and averse drug events in pediatric inpatients. *JAMA* 2001;285:2114–2120.

10. Upperman JS, Staley P, Friend K, Neches W, et al. The impact of hospital wide computerized physician order entry on medical errors in a pediatric hospital. *J Ped Surg* 2005;40:57–59.

11. URL: www.montereymedicalsolutions.com 2006 MMS.

12. URL: www.jointcommission.org 2006 JCAHO.

13. Ricci M, Goldman AP, de Leval MR, Cohen GA, Devaney F, Carthey J: Pitfalls of adverse event reporting in paediatric cardiac intensive care. *Arch Dis Child* 2004;89:856–859.

14. Cimino MA, Kirschbaum MS, et al. Assessing medication prescribing errors in pediatric intensive care units. *Pediatr Crit Care Med* 2004;5:124–132.

15. Ross LM, Wallace J, Paton JY. Medication errors in a paediatric teaching hospital in the UK; five years operational experience. *Arch Dis Child* 2000;83:492–497.

16. Sullivan JE, Buchino JJ. Medication errors in pediatrics—the octopus evading defeat. *J Surg Oncol* 2004;88:182–188.

17. Carleton B, Lesko A, Milton J, Poole RL: Active surveillance systems for pediatric adverse drug reactions: an idea whose time has come. *Current Therapeutic Research* 2001;62(10):738–742.

18. Carlton B, Poole RL, Milton J, Travis J, Grinder D: The pediatric adverse drug reaction reporting system. *Journal of Pediatric Pharmacy Practice* 1999;4(6):284–307.

19. Gill AM, Leach HJ, et al. Adverse drug reactions in a pediatric intensive care unit. *Acta Paediatr* 1995;84:438–441.

20. Wiss J, Krebs S, et al. Survey of adverse drug reactions on a pediatric ward: a strategy for early and detailed defection. *Pediatrics* 2002;110:254–257.
21. Menniti-Ippolito F, Rachetti R, et al. Active monitoring of adverse drug reactions in children. *Lancet* 2000;355:1613–1614.
22. Le J, Nguyen T, et al. Adverse drug reactions among children over a 10-year period. *Pediatrics* 2006;118(2)555–562.

Index